HERBS *in* NATUROPATHIC MEDICINE

HERBS
in
NATUROPATHIC MEDICINE

in their own words

Edited by Sussanna Czeranko, ND, BBE
Foreword by Jeanne Paul, ND

nunm PRESS
Portland, Oregon

Front cover Illustrations clockwise, starting at far left:
Broad leaf plantain [*Plantago major*], Dwarf Elder [*Sambucus ebulus*], Nettle [*Urtica dioica*], and Shavegrass [*Equisetum arvense*].

NUNM Press
National University of Natural Medicine
049 SW Porter Street
Portland, Oregon 97201, USA
www.nunm.edu

Managing Editor: Nichole Wright
Production: Fourth Lloyd Productions, LLC.
Design: Richard Stodart

NUNM Press gratefully acknowledges the generous and prescient financial support of HEVERT USA which has made possible the creation and distribution of the *In Their Own Words* historical series.
The HEVERT COLLECTION comprises twelve historical compilations which preserve for the healing professions significant and representational works from contributors to the historical Benedict Lust journals.

Printed in the United States of America

ISBN: 978-1-945785-07-8
Library of Congress Control Number: 2016955213

We are grateful to all the women and men who have for so long safeguarded and grown the wisdom of plant medicine for Naturopaths all over the world.

Table Of Contents

Foreword

I do feel honoured and humbled to share my ideas and feelings about what it is to be a contemporary Naturopath using some of the Herbs as Kneipp and Lust used in their day. In fact, I wild-craft many of the same indigenous medicines and then teach what I call "The Traditional Medicines of the First Nations in British Columbia" to my First Nations peoples. I have dedicated my life to this work as a Naturopath and as a First Nations Herbal Medicine Teacher. Both disciplines are so intertwined that as a Naturopath I use these Medicines in much the same way as our naturopathic "Ancients". This book which tells the story of these Elders of these herbal medicines helps us to understand all that went into becoming teachers in their day. We can see in these articles that their work paralleled the paths that many of our present ND's practise and enjoy. I am one of those avid students of these incredible teachers.

I was born a Coast Salish Native from British Columbia, Canada. I grew up in the times of great turmoil for our First Nations peoples here in British Columbia and across Canada. At the turn of the century the first "white man" entered our territories and thought we were for the taking along with the lands. Naturally, the culture of these "savage" people were the first to go and then in turn to educate the children away from their families and culture. Their strategy: "take the Indian out of the child and then take the land". The joint effort of the churches and the government saw to it that this was the path for the "Indian". Residential Schools were created to take the children from their families and homes. The children would acculturate and become the children of the greater society. The churches threw in scare tactics for these very young First Nations children, warning them that they would go to hell if they did not join the Christian church.

I was one of those children.

I grew up in a residential school. Devoid of home, family and the culture of my people, I became an obedient, shy, catholic girl who feared hell. This cultural genocide was rampant throughout Canada and the USA. My education was one of loneliness, hunger, depression and obedience to a god who wanted only misery for our First Nations Peoples. Along with so many of my brothers and sisters from different bands and villages, I tried to make some sense of it all. Many of the survivors of the residential school system had to relearn the lessons of life. Sadly, many lives were destroyed.

Of course now we have moved on from this horrific part of our lives to become who we are today. But, what a loss! As part of what was taken from us, our Herbal Medicines, Mother Nature's cure for our ailments were banished. The educational system did not allow this kind of cultural learning. Many of our First Nations peoples in British Columbia hid within their families some of these "secrets of the plants as Medicine" but mostly the younger generation had little or no knowledge of these plants as Medicine.

In studying this book, I ask myself, how did these Ancestors acquire this knowledge which we use today? Native teaching says that who ever has "the inner sight" is told the use of these Medicines. The Inner Guides will give this sight to the avid student. The Teachers in this book certainly used this inner skill too, as well as their dedication to observe. They used these skills to practice and see a positive outcome of these Medicines in their work, and their legacy has helped us to understand that indeed these Medicines do work.

Early in my life before I was sent to residential school my mother would send me into the woods to pick "cequak". This was an annual ritual that we must have one canned jar of these red berries. I would ask what it was used for because it tasted very bitter. Its strange taste was not much invitation to eat a lot of it. My mother added a lot of sugar to help with the taste. I learned later it was called the Red Elderberry. She had a forgotten memory of its original use as she was born at a time when culture in its every form was forbidden to be taught, spoken or practised. She was born 1900. She had a vague notion of its specific use and would just say, "It is just good for you; it's what we do".

Now I see in this book how the Ancients, our Naturopathic founders used this Medicine a great deal. I feel connected to this Medicine even more. I become joyful and sing when I am near these plants.

I am proud to say that walking with these Green Blessings, the Elderberry and so many of the other Medicines that these incredible Teachers mention in this book gives me a greater understanding of the value these brothers and sisters gift us. I can say "it is just good for you" but also offer much to our health and well-being, along with the technical knowledge that helps us to understand the deep value of why they work and that they can cure our patients of their ailments.

I am in awe and have a deep gratitude by our constant resilience; our evolving and growing this deep relationship with these Medicines, the Herbs that are mentioned throughout this book. It is a bond that Creator has given each of us to reacquaint ourselves with their inner life and their inner talk with each person that uses them. Certainly I feel and observe this in everyone of my students who study them. They now understand they "are good for you" but now add the teachings behind why they work. My mother would approve and so would the Ancestors who also had their own inner Teachers and Guides to speak to them. Now we as modern Teachers can also learn even more from our Ancients who are in this book. Bringing this knowledge from our history into the present day is a way to continue to evolve and pass this knowledge to our patients, to our children and to the rest of the world. After all, this is the Medicine of the future of our Green Nations, our Brothers and Sisters. Emawhega!

Many thanks for the inspiration and dedication of Sussanna Czeranko, ND for putting this Book together to help us understand where our Ancients came from and where they will now take us.

Green Blessings,
Dr. Jeanne Paul, N.D.
Chilliwack, British Columbia, Canada

Preface

Herbs in Naturopathic Medicine gives us a peek into how the early Naturopaths used plants in their practice. This book includes a total of 80 articles chosen from Benedict Lust's publications [1900–1923] of which he personally authored 57. As the major contributor in this book, Benedict Lust himself, inspired always by Sebastian Kneipp, had a tremendous impact upon the emerging naturopathic profession. Lust writes concisely and often sparsely, without elaborating upon the intrinsic properties of individual herbs. In an effort to enhance the appeal of herbal medicine, Lust includes line drawings of herbal plants which are found throughout his articles. Lust's surviving works certainly contribute much to satisfy our curiosity about how herbs were used in the late 19th and early 20th centuries. In his earlier writings, Lust provided many common and recognized uses of herbs but surprisingly he also includes unique and unfamiliar applications for the herbal remedies in use in his day.

A second prolific writer on the topic of herbs, M. G. Young, headed up a new column in *Herald of Health and Naturopath* entitled, "Phytotherapy Department" from 1915 to 1917. Young articulated the subject of herbs with more details and descriptions than Lust and succeeded in elevating the subject of herbs presented in his column. Eight articles are included in this compilation written by Young. In the masthead of "Phytotherapy Department", Young is referred to as "The American Herb Doctor" and we discover that he was practicing in Seattle, Washington.

A third contributor to the subject of herbs comes to us by a precarious path and sheds much understanding on the intersections between dietetics and herbal medicine. There are five articles included by George J. Drews who in 1909 with the publication of his book, *Unfired Food and Hygienic Dietetics,* ignited a new, revolutionary concept in North America: eating raw plants as a staple food. In Drews' articles we can see that the plants that he chose for his food movement, called Apyrotrophy or unfired food, contain many of the herbal plants that we use today. Drews concocted wonderful synedes or raw salads in which he incorporated plants such as dock, plantain, dandelion, mallow and other plants. All of these plants are generally thought of as tinctures or powders or capsules delivered in a prescription. Drews was well ahead of his time. In any case, as we become more familiar with this literature, we may conclude that we are just recycling trends from the past.

Among Lust, Young and Drews, two reprints from Sebastian Kneipp's writings are included. Benedict Lust borrowed heavily from his mentor, beloved Kneipp. In his early years as a publisher, Lust re-printed sections of Kneipp's books and included this material as content for his aspiring magazine. He often borrowed Kneipp's graphics to be included in his own magazines. From these four authors, we find the core of herbal lore and these writings taken from the Lust journals comprise a valuable foundation to Naturopathy's heritage. However, there are ten other contributions which are equally important to view and consider. I have included one article from each of these people in this compilation: Ludwig Staden, living in Brooklyn, New York and an early adapter to Naturopathy; Alfred Baumgarten, a German medical doctor who worked alongside Sebastian Kneipp at Wöerishofen; Karl Kahut; William Waugh; P. Heinrichs; Otto Carqué, a man who shared Drews passion for dietetics; Wallace Fritz, a Neuropath; and lastly, Louisa Lust, the life partner of Benedict and the quiet force behind the stage propelling Naturopathy always forward with love and tenacity.

In mid-1917 Young discontinued his column. In the following year, Lust launched a new column called "Selected Herbs", with the subcaption: "A Review of the Most Useful Herbs as a Curative Factor for Numerous Ailments". Lust presented small etchings of many of the herbs that he arranged in alphabetical order. Each herb was accompanied with indications for use and directions on their preparation. Occasionally, Lust included formulas for certain conditions and directions on how to administer the herbal remedy. In this new column, Lust continued to highlight those herbs of the Kneipp *Apotheca* and introduced new ones. The masthead that Lust used in his original articles is reproduced in this compilation and I have taken the liberty to assign new titles for each of the articles found in the "Selected Herbs" series using the names of the herbs that Lust presents. Lust followed, for the most part, an alphabetical format which is occasionally abandoned. Some of the titles are short consisting of two or a few herbs in his articles in 1918 and by 1920 he is presenting ten or more herbs in each monthly issue of *Herald of Health and Naturopath.*

The illustrations used in *Herbs in Naturopathic Medicine* are the same ones that Benedict Lust used in his original articles. Examining his journals and the books that Kneipp published, it is easy to see that Lust borrowed from Kneipp. However, Lust did not borrow all of Kneipp's images for this publication. Some of the images found in this compilation were obtained directly from Kneipp's book, *My Water Cure* (1896, Jos. Kœsel Publisher, Bavaria). NUNM has an exquisite collection of Rare Books on botanical medicine, from which I included a few images. I would like to express my gratitude to dear Simone and Mike Chilton for their generous donation to NUNM's Rare Book Collection, a first edition of John Gerard's *The herbal, or Generall historie of plantes* (Gerard, 1633). I gingerly and carefully scanned three images from this precious book to include in this book. A few images were borrowed from another book with superb images by J. H. Bailey who wrote a 6 book encyclopedia on plants in America entitled, *Cyclopeia of American Horticulture,* in 1906. (Bailey, 1906)

In past volumes of the *Hevert Collection*, I have provided lengthy introductions as a way to summarize each article found in the book. I realized when beginning the "Introduction" to *Herbs in Naturopathic Medicine* that this approach did not serve well the work contained in this unique compilation of historical documents. Rather than scratch the surface of each of the articles contained in this compilation, and potentially omit valuable clinical pearls, I decided alternatively to leave for you, the reader, a summary of each article listing herbs and their uses. For this reason, I have presented in a summary format a list of herbs found in each article and have listed these chronologically. We are introduced to 78 herbs by the end of the articles found in 1900. There are references to 168 herbs in this book and 7 Kneipp formulas that Benedict referred to often. With expressed gratitude, Benedict Lust endeavoured to keep Kneipp's life's work alive. Please use the comprehensive indexes at the back of the book for navigation. You will find a General Index which lists the herbs used for specific conditions. Herbs that are underlined indicate those that Kneipp, Lust and others considered highly effective. In addition, there is an Herb Index for convenient page location. The indexes are compiled alphabetically.

Our dear Dr. Jeanne Paul is a model for all of us to live our lives with purpose and gratitude. She has been practicing for over a quarter of a century. In her work she has long been providing true healing for the First Nations people in Canada. Her love of plants is a gift that she shares with her patients and her people. She does not dilute the sacred presence of these living plants by ascribing botanical names and reducing their essence to constituents as a way of making sense of the enormous and complex universe of plant life. Rather, Jeanne recognizes each plant as a blessed teacher embodying gifts to share with those who attend to such learning. Living each day and praying with the plant medicines that she cherishes are her ways of learning in the ancient, enduring ways. Plants speak to her and she listens with her spirit and her senses to learn more about the teachings that they offer us all. Jeanne's gratitude is deep and enduring. How often we hear this blessed healer and teacher iterate, *"I absolutely love what I do. I am so blessed."* So too blessed are the people that walk a path which crosses or joins hers as she journeys to bring healing knowledge to so many people.

She reminds me by her example to embrace with gratitude the teachers in my own life who have guided me in my learning to love the plants that surround me, including Dr. Gordon Smith, the late Dr. Bill Mitchell, and David Winston. To each of these champions who have taught me more than they will ever know, my heart swims with deep respect and honour for their contributions to herbal medicine. Thank you for your guidance and love of our kindred, sacred herbal plants.

The journey to manifest *Herbs in Naturopathic Medicine* was the work of a community. I am grateful to everyone who helped breathe life into this book across the many months of its creation. Hundreds of typed pages were patiently transcribed by many, superlative students at NUNM. In fact, there are cumulatively over 1,200 articles typed from the Benedict Lust journals in preparation for the books in the Hevert Collection. I want to acknowledge every NUNM student who typed those articles or scanned images while navigating his or her intense course loads and juggling personal lives. I am especially indebted to the enduring dedication of **Angela Carlson** who embraced the mission of transcribing most of the articles found in this book. Her love of herbal medicine shines forth and will endure as she follows her passion for healing plants. To the many students who also rose to the task of committing to the completion of the book, I am very grateful to you. **Thank you Aaron Potts, Adam Dombrowski, Cadence Wong, Cody Strodtman, Delia Sewell, Kate Leavens, Laura Weldon, Lauren Geyman, Meagan Hammel, Natasha McDougal, Rebecca Jennings, Stephanie Monesson, Susan Manongi, Tristian Rowe,** and all those whom I am inadvertently missing here. I especially extend kudos to **Aaron Potts** and **Adam Dombrowski** for your patience and fastidious care in scanning the many images found in this herbal book.

And, as this book project moves into the second half of our work and production plan, my appreciation for the invaluable organizational help that I had received from **Dr. Karis Tressel** during the early stages of figuring out what lay ahead and working so closely with me to organize the almost six thousand pages of invaluable core material is a daily reminder that book making is an undertaking of an entire community. I am deeply grateful for her profound love of the traditions and history of Naturopathy and for her inspiring, loving tenacity with this project.

I so much enjoyed working with each and every student who sacrificed scarce, precious study and leisure time for the hard work of meticulous research and transcription. As you launch yourselves into the Naturopathic profession, never forget how special and important your work has been. You have chosen a path of sacred work. You will be loved and cherished by your patients because you listen and truly care. Remember to trust Nature's power of healing, the *Vis medicatrix naturae*! Pay careful attention to your patients and they will feel enlivened and grateful to have found their way to you.

I am very thankful for the encouraging support of the Hevert Corporation here in America and in Germany. Thank you and my most gracious accolades to Mathias and Marcus Hevert for your generous contributions allowing this book series to become a reality. Much gratitude, as well, to the unwavering, behind-the-scenes support of the Board of NUNM, Dr. Sandra Snyder, Susan Hunter, and Jerry Bores who understood from the beginning the importance of this project.

The elegance and beauty that Fourth Lloyd Productions, Nancy and Richard Stodart, my designers and mentors, bring to this book are brilliantly magnificent. The journey to arrive at book eight has taken us across many crossroads and conversations. I am deeply indebted to your unwavering commitment to excellence. Thank you both for the exquisite care that you conveyed in bringing to life the world of herbs!

There are not enough words to express my love and gratitude for the support and editorial guidance that I receive at all hours of the day from my beloved husband, David Schleich. I am deeply blessed to have you by my side as this amazing journey hurls me back inside a previous century. You lighten me on days when my spirit traverses the hurdles when navigating the world of editorial minutia. Thank you for your precious spirit.

Lastly, I am so indebted to the men and women who occupy almost every minute of my day. They lived a hundred years ago and have left a legacy of wisdom and passion that fills me with confidence and gratitude for their contributions to a literature that I can read and implement in my own practice and, along with my wonderful collaborators, with you. So, remember to include a walk into Nature and reflect upon all that is good in your life. Give gratitude to those around you and to those who came before you. As you read these articles left behind by our dear elders, dare to practice their wise and salubrious ways. You have before you *in their own words* the secrets to health.

Blessings,
Sussanna Czeranko, ND, BBE
June, 2016

Every mother knows how to prepare tea. For one cup she takes as much of the dried herbs as she can hold with three fingers. Boiling water is poured over the herbs. They are boiled for a few minutes and a remedy is ready which will always produce the effect looked for, when the right kind of herb is used. One herb cannot do everything.

Benedict Lust, 1900, 11

Kneipp has experimented for years, has examined, dried, cut up, boiled and tasted most every little herb within his reach and has found many good healing qualities in them.

Benedict Lust, 1900, 116

Nearly all my teas, extracts, oils and powders are prepared from medical herbs which are to be had for a trifle, and which our dear Lord has planted in our own garden, in the fields, many of them around our houses, many on remote, unfrequented spots, so that we can gather them free of cost.

Mgr. Sebastian Kneipp, 1902, 384

Well-known and very popular applications recommended in Kneipp's works are hay flower compresses, hay flower shirts, as well as the addition of hay flowers to baths and steam baths.

Benedict Lust, 1906, 40

If we examine the non-poisonous plants, we find out that each one has a certain relationship to some organ of the body and that it excites and increases the metabolism in this organ as well as its special function by supplying the cells of the corresponding organs with its proper food.

Benedict Lust, 1908, 167

There are no definite rules for the selection of remedies in any given case, but art and experience teach us how to give the right treatment. It is to be mentioned that essential mistakes cannot be made, for the simple reason that we deal not with different, strongly acting or even poisonous plants and that in a mixture of numerous plants but a small quantity of each produces some effect.

Benedict Lust, 1908, 169

Fever is only an act of Nature, and Nature is never in error; she never makes mistakes, and this fever is simply her effort. Then, why should the doctor give the death dealing drug to stop this intelligent effort of Nature?

M. G. Young, 1916, 400

Many simple herbs in their natural state or made into teas afford relief for the severest ailments. Only those which are non-poisonous and produce natural physiological action are recommended in Naturopathy.

Benedict Lust, 1918, 253

Introduction And Herbs Overview

After spending eight months as a patient at Wöerishofen recovering from tuberculosis by following Father Kneipp's guidance, Benedict Lust returned to America not only as a confirmed hydrotherapy enthusiast, but also as a future health care professional with a passion for herbs. The combination of fervor for the work of Sebastian Kneipp and a conscientious premonition of doing good work, Lust conceived a plan to promote hydrotherapy and herbal medicine in his newly adopted country. Benedict opened his first business on September 15, 1896, the *Kneipp Health Store*. It would become New York City's first health food store at 111 East 59th St and a center for imported Kneipp herbs and products. (Boyd, 1997, 44) By the following year, Lust had become very successful in promoting his products and had accumulated a substantial inventory. One evening, though, a fire started in the adjoining furrier shop and spread through the walls causing extensive smoke damage in Lust's own building. Lust describes the scene:

> Brewing and smoldering for hours, smoke had found its way through the walls to my place next door. It wrought havoc with my stock of herbs long before the fire itself was discovered. And when the alarm was sounded and the firemen responded, the damage done by smoke was multiplied by the water employed to bring the blaze under control and put out. (Boyd, 1997, 82)

Lust continues, "I prided myself on having had the good forethought to have arranged for insurance coverage." (Boyd, 1997, 82) This fire destroyed Lust's offices and his entire herbal stock computed at $1,100.00 which was a small fortune at the time. A few weeks later, Lust was sent a check for a meager $75 which was not near the compensation expected. Lust describes the decision that he made at this time, "From that day to this I have invested no more money in fire insurance ... I would be my own fire insurance company, my own protection. ... I conceived the idea of laying away in a separate "protection fund" each year the amounts I would have had to pay in premiums for insurance to cover stock and quarters." (Boyd, 1997, 84)

This insurance fund, though, eventually was earmarked for the school fund. Both Louisa and Benedict envisioned that the money saved would be best served to build a permanent home for Naturopathy in a naturopathic university. Lust recounts, "Our school fund of $897,000, just short a million, disappeared with a snap of a finger." (Boyd, 1997, 94) The Great Depression of 1929 brought many to their knees including the man who began the first health food store in New York City. Benedict and Louisa had amassed the equivalent in today's money of about $13 million dollars over a number of years. If only history had taken a different twist, the money saved by the Lusts was more than enough to build a powerful naturopathic institution. This would never be.

The story of Benedict Lust's love of herbs did not end with the Depression. His publications live on and today we can read how the early Naturopaths used herbs in their clinical practice over a century ago. They used simple, common every day herbs. The herbal *Materia Medica* in use by Lust is all the more intriguing because of the specific uses indicated for each herb. For example, in his first article, Lust lists chamomile, chickweed, coltsfoot and elder flowers for four different presentations of colds. He names various herbs indicating concise indications for their use and provides insights into herbal practice 116 years ago. Other herbs discussed in Lust's first article include: dwarf elder, juniper, aloe, fennel, nettles, eyebright, fenugreek, plantain, St. John's wort, yarrow. Although these herbs are quite familiar, their applications are not. For example, regarding St. John's wort, Lust says, "All sorts of complaints of the head arising from watery matter or phlegm in the head or from the gases rising to the head are relieved by this herb. To mothers who have trouble with their little bed-wetters, St. John's wort is a real blessing. Common yarrow will do the same." (Lust, 1900, 12) Indeed, we can learn by studying these remarkable articles from Lust's publications many new uses and indications for our familiar common herbs.

In fact, the herbs used by Lust were essentially the same ones used by his mentor, Father Sebastian Kneipp. Kneipp's *Apotheca* lists 60 medicaments in his 4th Edition of *My Water Cure*. (Kneipp, 1896, 128-193) Not all of these medicaments are actual herbs, but rather include such items as almond oil, alum, different colours of bone powder, bran, chalk, cod liver oil, honey, incense, salad oil, sauerkraut, and laxative formulas. Kneipp compiled a list consisting of 51 herbs, each with a beautiful and intricate image depicting its unique characteristics. Images from both Lust's publications and also from Kneipp's book, *My Water Cure* (Kneipp, 1896) were used in the artwork for this book.

The chief distinction between Lust's herbal apothecary and one found in a current Naturopath's clinic is that Lust never included any toxic herbs in his. Sebastian Kneipp adamantly denounced the use of any herbs that had any poisonous properties. Using the same herbs as Kneipp and adding a few of his own, Lust established an herbal enterprise in New York City selling Kneipp herbs and formulas which he imported from Germany. Lust basically adopted Kneipp's *Apotheca* and eventually sold over 170 different herbal products by 1922. Plants would be sold in the form of powders, flowers, leaves, roots, barks, tea formulas, salves, honey, oils and pills. (Lust, 1922, 463) Lust's magazines helped develop and sustain a viable herbal business in North America for German immigrant customers accustomed to herbal medicines promoted by Kneipp.

Kneipp personally tasted and tested every herb that he prescribed. Lust placed complete confidence in Kneipp's herbal expertise, writing, "Kneipp has experimented for years, has examined, dried, cut up, boiled and tasted most every little herb within his reach and has found many good healing qualities in them." (Lust, 1900, 116) I was surprised that the herbal apothecary promoted by Lust was so extensive and occasionally exotic herbs from foreign lands also found a place among the common herbs of his inventory. Lust had in stock a full array of Kneipp herbs which he advertised extensively in his magazines. His writings popularized the herbs and his magazines accomplished the purpose of informing people about herbs and their uses.

Today, the science of pharmacognosy directs many scientific inquiries into herbal uses. The constituents of herbs weren't discussed by Lust, and Young only mentions very briefly properties that individual herbs exerted upon the human body. We could surmise that the scientific discipline and inquiry were diluted skills in the early naturopathic herbalist. Or perhaps, Lust torn between his love of herbs and hydrotherapy and naturopathic education chose to present the herbal information in the same language as it was presented to him. In any case, the articles in this book present essentially a Kneipp *Apotheca*. When looking at the writings of Kneipp, there is much similarity in the presentations of Lust and Kneipp. It was common practice in the early 20th century to copy segments from published works and republish these as original text. Invariably, Lust does credit Kneipp for his writings. He definitely imitated his mentor's presentation of herbal information, but only used a few of Kneipp's images, producing many of his own. Both men wrote concisely on the herbs that they chose. We have here valuable works available to us that could have been lost. Consequently, we have an opportunity to learn how pioneering Naturopaths used and classified the same herbs that we use today.

HERBS OVERVIEW

HERBS AND THEIR HEALING POWER • *1900, I (1), 11-12.*

Chamomile: cure a cold; remove a fever produced by a cold, flu, cramps, indigestion
Chickweed: chest catarrh from a cold
Coltsfoot: asthma, coughs, consumption tendencies
  Leaves on chest: remove fevers and weaknesses
  Leaves on wounds: anti-inflammatory, draws out morbid matter; foot pain [compress]
Elder leaves: tea as blood purifier, spring cleanse
Elder flowers: colds, diaphoresis
Elder berries: blood purifier
Elder root: diuretic (most powerful)
Juniper berries: eat 6-12 berries for heartburn; kidney stones; removing flatulence from liver disease
Peppermint / Watermint: strengthen stomach; aid digestion; headache (forehead); halitosis
  Made with vinegar: stops blood vomiting
Bilberries: stops diarrhea
Anise: superior to fennel for flatulence
Aloe: tea for eye wash; old wounds washed with aloe water; ulcers
  With honey: cleanses stomach
  Mixed with herbs has a evacuating effect and not a purging effect
  Formula: a pinch of aloe, elder flowers, 1 tsp fenugreek, 1 tsp fennel
Blackthorn flowers: harmless purgative
Nettle leaves: loosens phlegm in chest; cleanses stomach, invigorates kidneys
  Roots: stronger than leaves, phlegm, dropsy [edema] 1st stage
Eyebright: strengthens eyesight
Fenugreek: fever; gargle for sore throats
  Poultice: softens tumors; wounds
Plaintain: excellent dressing for wounds
Shavegrass *(Equisetum)*: old and putrid wounds; ulcers; kidney stones; bleeding; vomiting blood; epistaxis
St John's wort: phlegm (head); bed wetting
Yarrow: bed wetting
Succory/Chicory: removes phlegm from stomach, liver, gall bladder, spleen, kidneys
Violet: swollen throat

Strawberry And Purgative Remedies • *1900 (2) 29-30.*

Strawberry leaf tea: mix with woodruff and thyme
 Berries: convalescence; relieves inner heat; kidney stones; liver complaints; skin eruptions
Kneipp Stomach Formula: fennel, juniper berries, fenugreek and aloe
Kneipp Kidney and Bladder Formula: fennel, juniper berries, dwarf elder root, fenugreek and aloe
 Sx: burning urination, dropsy

Ribwort • Plantago Lanceolata • *1900, (3), 44.*

Leaf sap: wounds; impure blood
 Tea: phlegm obstructions

Primrose And Violets • *1900 (5), 81-82*

Primrose / Cowslips: articular diseases
Violet leaves: cough due to change in weather; whooping cough; headaches, sore throats, tumors [compress]; gout [boiled in vinegar]
 Roots [must be crushed before boiling]: coughs

The Kneipp Apotheca • *1900 (7), 116-118*

Cleanse bowels: agave, black alder bark, blackthorn blossoms, buckthorn bark, marigold flowers and Kneipp's Stomach Cure (Wühlhuber No. 1) or Kneipp's Laxative Tea
Digestion: buck bean leaves, calamus root, centaury, rosemary, succory [chicory], wormwood, and Kneipp's Stomach Cure
Stomach, liver and kidneys: agave, common nettle, dwarf elder, juniper berries, St. John's wort and watermint and Wühlhuber
Diarrhea: dried bilberries, elder berry tea, periwinkle
Stomach, bowels, kidney inflammation: yarrow
Impure blood: borage, blackberry leaves, common watercress, dandelion, common elder leaves and Kneipp's Depurative Tea
Bladder and kidney: bearberry leaves [stones, catarrh]; burdock root [diuretic] and Kneipp's Diuretic Tea [catarrh]
Lung catarrh: chickweed, coltsfoot and elecampane
Consumption: Iceland moss, lungwort and ribwort [plantain]
Whooping cough: violet leaves and black current leaves
Diabetes: bilberry leaves
Rheumatism and gout: birch leaves, commock, scurvy grass and veronica
Strengthening: oak bark
Colic and cramps: chamomile, Kneipp's Cramp tea, fennel
Throat: Kneipp Cough Tea
Fenugreek: fever, sore throats [gargle]
Perspiration: elder flowers, linden flowers

Ulcers, boils: fenugreek powder poultice, flaxseed and shavegrass
Epilepsy: galium
Dropsy: hen's feet, iris
Cancer, ulcerous sores, wounds: calendula, arnica
Blood circulation: mistletoe
Gout: mouse ear tea
Sore throat: mullein, sage leaves, basil, hyssop
Rheumatic pain: primrose
Blood to the head and hysteric cramps: rue
Inflammation, wounds: sanicle
Blood vomiting: shavegrass [*equisetum*]
Increase urination: shavegrass
Abdominal cramps and menstrual colic: silverweed

How Nature Cures • *1900 (7), 126*

Hay flower bath: inflammatory rheumatism

My Medicinal Herbs • *1900 (8), 143-144*

Father Kneipp lists herbs with their harvesting time.

Care Of The Teeth • *1901, (9), 224.*

Sage: tooth paste, powder mixed with linden wood charcoal powder
Juniper berries: chew berries

How To Heal Wounds Quickly By Natural Means • *1901 (11), 300.*

Shavegrass decoction: clean wounds
Arnica decoction or diluted tincture: vulnerary
Plantain (ribwort): vulnerary
Whey: vulnerary
Coltsfoot: vulnerary
Kneipp Pitch Plaster: remove small splinters and foreign material
Hay flower compress: larger splinters, glass, metal; blood poisoning

Kneipp's Popular Healing Remedies And Their Application • *1902 (8), 348-349.*

Honey water: purify and strengthen weak eyes
Eyebright: strengthens eyes
Lachrymose: aloe water
Fennel: strengthens eyes
Ulcers: alum, agave, lime charcoal powder, sage and shavegrass
  Formula: alum water and agave water
Cancerous sores and bone caries: calamus root powder; coltsfoot; Kneipp's pomade of marigold [Calendula]

Gout formula: ground juniper berries, dwarf elder, parsley and nettle root

Reduce uric acid formula: ground juniper berries, shavegrass, knotgrass and wormwood

Kneipp's Apotheca • *1902 (2), 384-386.*

Stomach herbs: althea, licorice, senna, hops

Falling Out Of The Hair • *1903 (10), 301.*

Kneipp's Hair Water and Oil: promotes hair growth

Knotgrass • *1904 (6), 137.*

Knotgrass tea: kidney and bladder stones; colic; poor digestion; food poisoning; liver diseases; stomach and intestine ulcers; external skin ulcers; gall bladder obstruction

Wine: diarrhea, dysentery

Ablution: old wounds

Birch Leaf Tea • *1905 (1), 7.*

Birch leaf tea: kidney diseases, dropsy [edema]

Allopathic Thinking And Naturopathic Thinking • *1905 (2), 36.*

Digitalis: slows heart rate

Kneipp's Medicinal Herbs • *1905 (4), 108-109.*

Old fashion and common names of some of Kneipp's herbs found in his Apotheca.

Father Kneipp's Curative Herbs II; Angelica • *1905 (6), 164-165.*

Angelica root tea: cleanses stomach; abdominal cramps; dissolves flatulence; lung congestion; phlegm; headaches caused by indigestion; poor circulation

Powder: indigestion

Kneipp's Medical Herbs • Arnica Montana • *1906 (1), 9-10.*

Arnica montana tincture: bruises, contusions; deep lacerations; stomach troubles and abscesses

Water and vinegar: abdominal compress for colic

The Effect Of Hay Flowers • Heublumen • *1906 (1), 40-41.*

Hay flowers scalded: first stage of blood poisoning; frozen limbs; abdomen diseases

Compress/shirt: rheumatism; gout; scrofulous symptoms; inflammation; infection

MEDICINAL VIRTUES OF THE OAK TREE • *1907 (3), 67.*

Quereus Sessiflora, Quereus Pedunculata:
- Oak acorn coffee: exhaustion
- Oak leaf tea: exhaustion
- Oak bark (young, fresh) tea: abdomen, rectum; goitre; swollen throats
- Bark tea compress: goitre, sore throats

TIMELY TALKS • *1907 (4), 101-102.*

Hepatica
Lungwort flowers: chest catarrh
Silverweed flowers: tetanus
Arbutus
Violet flowers: whooping cough; headaches; fever; asthma; consumption
Dandelion
Shepherd's purse
Bloodroot
Twin leaf
Marshmallow
Chickweed flowers: chest catarrh
Mouse ear flowers and leaves: liver and spleen diseases; dropsy; gall stones
Nettle leaves: lungs and kidneys
- Root powder: dropsy

Basil flowers: chest catarrh

MEDICINAL VIRTUES OF THE COMMON ELDER • *1907 (7), 199.*

Elderberry
- Leaves: blood purifier
- Flowers: blood purifier; diaphoretic; colds
- Roots: dropsy
- Berries: kidneys, lungs

MEDICINAL VIRTUES OF THE MINT PLANT • *1907 (8), 231.*

Mint tea: aids digestion; purifies blood; protracted illness; palpitations; nausea, vomiting
- Compress: headache with eye pain
- Mint tea with milk: abdominal pain
- Mint and grape juice: halitosis
- Mint decoction with vinegar: stops blood vomiting

MEDICAL VIRTUES OF FENNEL • *1907 (9), 263-264.*

Fennel boiled with milk: colic spasms
- Compress made with vinegar: colic
- Powder: flatulence; eyewash
- Vapour bath: use fennel, anise and caraway for eye vapour bath

Bogbean (Water Trefoil)•Menyanthus Trifoliate • *1907 (10), 295.*

Bogbean: bitter; strengthens digestion; blood cleansing; anemia; liver complaints; kidney

Medical Virtues Of Shavegrass • *1907 (5), 135.*

Shavegrass: cleansing solution for old injuries, putrid wounds, gangrenous ulcers
Tea: purifies stomach; relieves pain from kidney stones; best tea for blood vomiting; epitaxis; hemorrhages; menorrhagia
Vapour: healing for lungs, throat and nose; relieves colds and catarrh; skin complexion

Herbs For Stomach Troubles • *1908 (2), 40-41.*

Wormwood tea, tincture, powder: bitter that stimulates digestion
Salve: eyes
Gentian root: bitter, digestion
Formula: gentian, wormwood, shavegrass tea improves digestion, chronic stomach catarrh
Powder: involuntary loss of semen
Shavegrass: kidneys, bladder; hemostatic; purgative not for chronic constipation [contraindicated for diarrhea]
Powder: snuff for nose bleeds
Rosemary: dissolves congestion [edema] caused by slow circulation
Dwarf elder root: diuretic [stronger than rosemary or shavegrass]
Formula: dwarf elder, rosemary and shavegrass: dropsy
Buckbean tea: excessively bitter, added to other bitter herbs; stomach
Tincture: stomach
Peppermint: cramps; fainting spells; stomach complaints
Ribwort or plantain: lung ailments

The Science Of Herbotherapy • *1908 (6), 167-173.*

Metabolism: *Artemisia Absinthium* (plant), *Cochlearia officinalis, Erythraea centaruium persoon, Matricaria chamomilla, Fragaria vesca* (leaves), *Juglans regia* (leaves), *Achillea millefolium* (flowers and leaves), *Quercus robur* (bark), *Rubus fructicosus* (leaves), *Viola tricolor (plant)*
Lymphatics and liver: *Guaiacum officinale* (wood), *Smilax medica shlechtendahl* (sarsaparilla root), *Vaccinium myrtillus* (fruit and leaves), *Capsella bursa pastoris* (plant), *Equisetum arvense* (plant), *Urtica dioica* (plant), *Menyanthes trifoliate, Arctostaphylos uva ursi* (leaves), *Tussilago farfara* (leaves), *Salix peutaudra* (bark and leaves), *Filipendula ulmaria* (flowers), *Arnica montana* (roots and flowers)
Nervous system: *Archangelica officinalis hoffman* (root), *Arnica montana* (root and flower), *Capsella bursa pastoris, Mentha piperita* (leaves), *Melissa officinalis* (leaves), *Valeriana officinalis, Humulus*

lupulus (strobiles), *Thymus serpyllum* (plant), *Chenopodium ambrosioides* (plant)

Skin: *Tilia parviflora* and *grandiflora* (flowers), *Sambucus nigra* (flowers), *Juglans regia* (walnut shell), *Guaiacum officinale* (wood), *Viola tricolor* (plant), *Ononis spinosa* (root), *Salvia pratensis* (leaves)

Kidneys: *Juniperus communis* (fruit), *Levisticum officinale* (root), *Ononis spinosa* (root), *Quercus robur* (bark), *Petroselinum sativum* (seed and root), *Arctostaphylos uva ursi* (leaves), *Betula alba* (leaves)

Digestion: *Artemisia absinthium* (plant), *Acorus calamus* (rhizome), *Cnicus benedictus*, *Erythraea centaurium* (plant), *Mentha piperita* (plant), *Matricaria chamomilla* (flowers), *Marsdenia cundurango* (bark), *Foeniculum vulgare* (seed), *Gentian lutea, purpurea* (root), *Origanum vulgare* (plant), *Melilotus officinalis* (plant), *Achillea millefolium* (flowers and leaves)

Lung: *Althaea officinalis* (root), *Arnica montana* (flowers and root), *Pimpinella anisum* (seed), *Chondrus crispus*, *Tussilago farfara* (leaves), *Inula helenium* (root), *Verbascum thapsus* (leaves), *Cetraria islandica*, *Glycyrrhiza glabra* (root), *Symphytum officinale* (root), *Pulmonaria officinalis* (plant), *Plantago major* and *media* (leaves), *Polygala amara* (plant, flowers and root)

Walnut leaves: rickets

Enema herbs include the following four categories:

- Aids secretions and high in acids: *Rumex acetosa*, *Oxalis acetosella*, *Valeriana officinalis*, *Saponaria officinalis*, *Achillea millefolium*, *Vitis vinifera*, *Cochlearia officinalis*, *Taraxacum officinale*
- Tonics rich in tannic acids: *Quercus robur* (bark), *Juglans regia (leaves), Salvia officinalis (leaves)*, *Ruta graveolens*
- Anti-spasmodic and sedatives: *Valeriana officinalis*, *Tilia europaea* (flowers), *Verbascum thaspus*, *Matricaria chamomilla*
- Antiseptics: *Quercus robur* (bark), *Mentha piperita*, *Melissa officinalis*, *Eucalyptus globulus*, *Thymus vulgaris*, *Origanum vulgare*

Aromatic Powders • *1909 (1), 33.*

Irritating cough formula: plantain (ribwort), nettle, violet, sage

Stomach troubles: wormwood, mint, gentian

Hemorrhages: shavegrass, shepherd's purse and mistletoe

Kneipp's Herbs And Their Uses • *1909 (8), 482-486.*

Wormwood: eye wash for eye diseases

Silverweed: abdominal spasmodic cramps

Poultice: abdominal cramps

St. John's wort: excellent liver remedy; head complaints from phlegm; bedwetting in children [yarrow]

Formula: St. John's wort and aloe powder used for liver and expel morbid matter in urine

Succory or Chicory: removes stomach phlegm and cramps; aids digestion; reduces excessive bile; aids detoxification in liver, spleen and kidneys
Poultice: leaves and flowers used for stomach cramps and inflammation
Tonic Laxative I: fennel, juniper berries, fenugreek, aloe powder
Removes morbid matter in urine, relieves chest phlegm
Tonic Laxative II: fennel, juniper berries, dwarf elder roots, fenugreek, aloe powder
Cleanses kidney and bladder; first stage of edema [dropsy]
Valerian root: head complaints; spasms [rue]; flatulence
Wild Angelica root: removes disagreeable food from the body; bowel and stomach toxins; flatulence; heart burn; thick phlegm in lungs
Wormwood: best stomachic; liver complaints; indigestion; nausea
Incense: wormwood burned on charcoal clears foul air

Rosemay Wine ◈ *1910 (5), 291.*

Rosemary: edema, asthma, emphysema, kidney complaints

Drugs And Drugs ◈ *1910, (8), 469-471.*

Hyoscyamus: induces sleep; calming; prevents sleep and arouses delirium
Jaborandi: induces and suppresses perspiration; increases and decreases milk production
Gelsemium: soothing; causes convulsions
Opium: sedate; convulsions

Naturopath Advocate Offers Elder Blossoms As Blood Purifier ◈ *1911 (7), 443.*

Elder flower: eaten raw to purify blood
Blood purifiers: dandelion (whole plant), burdock root, bull thistle root, blackthorn blossom, poison oak

St. James's Oil ◈ *1912 (2), 114-115.*

St. James's oil: increase activity of the skin, reduces susceptibility to cold, fever, induces sleep, chronic diseases such as consumption, dyspepsia, diabetes, anemia; sprains and bruises

Curled Leaf Mallow Or Hygeia Plant ◈ *1913, (1), 56.*

Curled leaf mallow: tonifies blood

Curled Dock ◈ *1913 (4), 266.*

Curled dock (*Rumex*) leaves: spring tonic used like spinach in salads; rich in organic salts; tonifying for kidneys, blood, and glands

DANDELIONS • *1913 (4), 267.*

Dandelion leaves: used in salad for stomach tonic; stimulates digestive secretions; convalescence

AUTUMN'S PEACE • AUTUMN'S BLISS • *1913 (10), 645-646.*

Elecampane roots: chest, stomach ailments; asthma; expectorant
Angelica roots: promotes perspiration and urination; strengthens heart, stomach and liver
Anise seeds: colic, infantile cramps; chronic catarrh (stomach and intestines); flatulence
Wormwood: strengthens stomach; bowels
Barberry: contains malic acid; made into a vinegar for drinks
Marjoram: grippe [flu], chill
Oak acorns, roasted: coffee substitute; diarrhea
Elder berry syrup: fevers
Burdock root oil: for hair growth; heals abscesses and ulcers
Tea: increases urine and perspiration; herpes and skin eruptions
Iceland moss: dry cough
Juniper berries: strengthens digestion; increases urine; heals dropsy; protects effects of damp weather; fumigant in sick rooms

LICORICE • *1914 (12), 830-831.*

Licorice root: organic salts makes it a tonic food; tonic for glands, nerves and blood; lung disease; coughs; colds; sweetener that does not cause fermentation in digestive tract

HONEY • *1915 (2), 120-121.*

Honey: mild laxative; restores vital force in exhausted muscles; throat complaints; weak digestion in children; restores bowel function; chest cold (steam inhalation with honey and chamomile); whooping cough (honey with horehound); tapeworms; indigestion; frostbite; sore eyes; erysipelas

PLANTAIN • *1915 (9), 580-581.*

Plantain: poultice for fresh and chronic wounds; tea tonifies blood; nervousness, bladder and leucorrhea

YARROW • *1915 (12), 775-776.*

Yarrow: liver and kidney tonic; diaphoretic; diuretic; astringent [if boiled]; colds; rheumatism; parasites; wash for old sores; dandruff; scurvy; hair loss; cramps; colic; bowel pains; blood in urine; bloody discharge from bowels; toothache (roots chewed)

Garlic Juice And Medicine • *1916 (1), 11.*

Garlic juice diluted in distilled water: heals infected wounds

Sage • *1916 (1), 50.*

Sage: tonic, carminative, astringent, diuretic, sudorific, nervine, vermifuge; stomach inflammation; wash for catarrhal ulcers and sore eyes; night sweats [cold tea]; diarrhea, dysentery; fever; hair loss

Sassafras • Laurus Sassafras • *1916 (4), 261.*

Sassafras root bark: aromatic stimulant, alterative, diaphoretic, diuretic, nervine; colds; menses; skin diseases; spring tonic [duration: 1 week]; syphilis, scrofula, rheumatism; capillary circulation
Powdered bark: bruises; edema
Mixed with ground mullein: swollen face; chronic abscesses; all swellings and edema
Oil: nervine stimulant and relaxant; dysmenorrhea
Liniment: rheumatism, deep congestion and inflammation (pelvis and abdomen); sprains; bruises
Young branches have pith: mucilaginous; irritated stomach and bowel; eye inflammation

Comparative Therapeutics • *1916 (5), 314-316.*

Quinine (cinchona): astringent; bitter, promotes digestion; a long list of physiological effects listed by author

Cascara Sagrada • *1916 (5), 335-336.*

Cascara fresh bark: purgative causing gripping
Bark cured for 3 years: liver and stomach tonic when combined with other herbs
Herbal laxative formula: cascara, Oregon grape root, licorice root, dandelion root, burdock root and lady slipper root

Impure Blood • *1916 (6), 398-402.*

Bitters for liver: dandelion root, culver's root, yellow parilla
Stimulants: cayenne pepper, prickly ash bark, ginger
Laxatives: mandrake root, cascara bark, licorice root, senna leaves
Mucous membrane cleansers: blue flag root, sassafras bark, stillingia, tag alder bark, sarsaparilla

Dandelion • *1916 (7), 461-462.*

Dandelion: diuretic; diaphoretic; aperient; anti-spasmoidic and expectorant; tonic and alterative;
Dropsy: parsley and dandelion tea

Induce perspiration for colds with biliousness: pleurisy root, boneset (*Eupatorium perfoliatum*) and dandelion
Constipation: blue flag root, culver's root [*Veronicastrum virgincum*], dandelion root
Tuberculosis, asthma, bronchitis, catarrh; dyspepsia

MAYWEED ▪ *1917 (7), 461-462.*

Mayweed: tonic; emetic; antispasmodic; emmenagogue; diaphoretic; headaches; fever convalescence; neuralgia; sciatica; rheumatic pain; insect repellant

ELDER ▪ *1917 (3), 169-170.*

Elder flowers: diaphoretic; gentle stimulant
Cold infusion: diuretic; alterative and cooling; children's liver diseases and erysipelas
Erysipelatous diseases: maiden hair, beech drops and elder flowers
Elder berry juice: aperient; alterative; one ounce will purge; deobstruent; dropsy; scarlet fever; chronic fever diseases
Elder flowers and berry juice: scrofula, cutaneous diseases, syphilis, rheumatism
Elder leaf buds: purgative
Elder inner bark: cathartic; large doses cause vomiting; ointment used for burns and skin diseases
Elder root juice: hydrogogue cathartic and diuretic; dropsy; epilepsy

HERBS ▪ *1918 (3), 253.*

Agave, aloe: laxative, diuretic, anti-syphilitic; liver congestion; jaundice
Morello cherry: coughs; sore throat

ALOE • ANGELICA ▪ *1918 (4), 379*

Aloe juice powdered: purgative, used in formulas
Stomach and bowel formula: aloe; elder blossoms, fenugreek, fennel seeds
Aloe tea: to bathe inflamed eyes
Angelica: colic; digestive troubles; flatulence

ANISE SEED • ARNICA ▪ *1918 (5), 479.*

Anise: eradicates intestinal bacteria; colic; eye wash
Intestine formula: anise, caraway and fennel seeds
Arnica flowers: violent stomach and abdominal pains (boiled in vinegar)
Tincture: topically for painful joints and rheumatism; cleansing wounds; compresses on swellings

Ash • Asarum • Balm Mint • Rhubarb • Barberries ◆ *1918 (6), 577*

Ash leaves: gout, rheumatism
Asarum: mixed with plantain to remove mucous from respiratory tract; tuberculosis
Balm mint [lemon balm]: abdominal troubles from nervous complaints; chlorosis [anemia], hysteria; stomach cramps; flatulence; dyspepsia; nervous headache, nausea and vomiting, earache
Rhubarb: mild purgative; blood purifier; stomach and intestines
Barberries: liver and spleen

Green Beanpods • Mistle • Betony • Bearberry ◆ *1918 (7), 674.*

Green beanpods: edema, kidney diseases, sciatica, gout and rheumatism
Mistletoe: stops hemorrhages; improves blood circulation
Formula: mistletoe and shavegrass [*equisetum*]
Betony: emetic and purgative
Bearberry: diuretic; kidney and bladder diseases
Birch leaves: exceptional blood purifier, rheumatic pains, kidney and bladder complaints

Lavender • Birch • Black Alder • Black Current • Buckthorn ◆ *1918 (8), 740.*

Lavender flower decoction: flatulence; headache; faintness; congestion; rheumatism
Birch leaves: blood purifier; kidney and bladder diseases; rheumatic pains; skin eruptions; gout; edema (dropsy)
Black alder bark tea: purgative
Black currant leaf tea: whooping cough, chest catarrh
Blackthorn blossoms tea: mild purgative
Fruit juice: cough remedy

Blessed Thistle • Blueberries • Briar Hips • Basil ◆ *1918 (9), 790.*

Blessed thistle: nervous prostration, melancholia, hysteria
Blueberries: diarrhea
Leaves: anti-diabetic remedy
Briar hip tea: diuretic; kidney and bladder diseases; bladder stones
Basil tea: chest catarrh; eliminates phlegm

Blackthorn • Bramble • Burnet • Borage ◆ *1918 (10), 842.*

Blackthorn: gentlest purgative, strengthens digestion
Bramble leaf tea: blood purifier
Burnet root dried or tincture: sudorific, diuretic; throat catarrh, rheumatism, gout, kidney inflammation, bladder stones
Borage: blood purifier and nerve tonic; hysteria and nervous heart palpations

BUCKBEAN • BUCKTHORN • BROOM ◈ *1918 (11), 896.*

Buckbean tea and tincture: blood purifier, restores appetite
  Formula: wormwood, centaury, sage, buckbean
Buckthorn bark and berries: purgative
Broom: bladder stones; kidney; herpes; blood purifier

BURDOCK • CHAMOMILE • CARLINE THISTLE ◈ *1918 (12), 940.*

Burdock roots: promotes hair growth
  Hair formula: burdock root and blind nettle leaves
Chamomile: severe colds, fevers and acute diseases; stomach cramps; stomach tonic
Carline thistle roots: bladder catarrh; kidney inflammation; weak stomach

CARAWAY • CHERRY • CENTAURY • COMMOCK ◈ *1919 (1), 35.*

Caraway decoction: stomach disorders and cramps; flatulence
  Oil: flatulence in infants [topically]
Cherry stalks [stems] tea: tonic; promotes digestion; alleviates cough; sedative and antispasmodic in whooping cough; nausea
Centaury tea: bitter; dissolves all hard effete matter in bowels; constipation; pains in stomach, bowels, chest, liver or spleen
Commock: rheumatism; gout; edema (dropsy); bladder stones; gland induration; diuretic; laxative

CHICORY • COLTSFOOT • CHICKWEED ◈ *1919 (2), 92.*

Chicory: dyspepsia; over production of gall bile; purifies liver, kidneys, and spleen
Coltsfoot: tea: expectorant; stops coughs
Chickweed tea: chest catarrh

DANDELION • DWARF ELDER • ELDER ◈ *1919 (3), 144.*

Dandelion root: blood purifier
Dwarf Elder root tea: diuretic; dropsy; abdominal disturbances
Elder dried berries tea: colic and diarrhea
  Flowers tea: blood purifier
  Leaf tea: blood purifier
  Root tea: preventive for edema (dropsy)

CLOVES • ELECAMPANE • EYEBRIGHT • EUCALYPTUS • FERN ◈ *1919 (5), 248.*

Clove oil: flatulence
Elecampane: removes phlegm; relieves chest catarrh; diaphoretic
Eyebright tea: indigestion
  Eye wash: tea is used in compress

Eucalyptus tea: bitter tea for indigestion and dyspepsia; intermittent fever
Fern root: chew root to purge tapeworms

FENUGREEK • GALIUM • FENNEL ❋ *1919 (6), 298.*

Fenugreek tea: cooling; gargle for sore throats
Poultice: draws for swelling and ulcers
Galium: epilepsy; dropsy; cutaneous eruptions
Fennel seed tea: colic and flatulence; eye wash

GROUND IVY • HEARTSEASE • HAY FLOWERS • HEATHER • ICELAND MOSS • JUNIPER ❋ *1919 (10), 513.*

Ground ivy tea: expectorant; stomach phlegm
Heartsease (violet) tea: gently purgative (children)
Hay flowers vapor baths and compresses: diseases of reproductive organs
Heather: cough remedy; nasal and throat catarrh
Iceland moss: tuberculosis; general debility
Juniper berry tea: weak stomach; halitosis; flatulence; liver and kidney diseases; bladder stones
Chewing on berries: weak stomach; halitosis; flatulence

DAISY • HEN'S FEET • HYSSOP • IRIS • KNOTGRASS • LICORICE • LINDEN FLOWER • LUNGWORT • LIVERWORT • VERONICA • MARJORAM ❋ *1920 (5), 249-251.*

Daisy tea: muscle stiffness resulting from draughts
Hen's feet tea: jaundice; hypochondria, hysteria; hemorrhoids; enema; skin eruptions
Hyssop tea: chronic catarrh of respiratory and digestive organs; asthma; rheumatism; antispasmodic; vermifuge; eye wash
Iris: edema (dropsy); powerful diuretic
Knotgrass tea: dissolves bladder stones
Licorice: excellent expectorant
Linden flower tea: diaphoretic for fever patients; chronic cough; removes mucus from lungs; bronchial catarrh; mucus in kidneys
Vapor bath: diaphoretic
Lungwort tea: combined with plantain for lung catarrh
Liverwort tea: gastric hemorrhage; vomiting blood; diseases of sexual organs
Male speedwell (Veronica) tea: excellent blood purifier; scurvy
Marjoram tea: irregular menses; tonic and stimulant (stomach)

Mallow • Calendula • Althea • Yarrow • Milkwort • Mouse Ear• Mustard • Mullein • Nettle • Oak • *1920 (6), 297-299.*

Mallow flower tea: removes mucous obstructions from chest; throat and larynx complaints
Gargle formula: mallow flowers and alum for sore throats
Vapor bath: mallow flower vapor bath for earaches
Marigold (Calendula) flower tea: boils, ulcers; stomach abscesses; stops recurring vomiting
Marshmallow tea: hoarseness; cough
Milfoil (Yarrow) flower and leaves: mixed with St. John's wort for irregular menses and abdominal pains
Milkwort tea: galactagogue
Mouse ear decoction: liver and spleen diseases; edema (dropsy); bladder stones
Gargle: sore throat
Mullein flowers: sore throat; lung catarrh; shortness of breath
Mustard seeds: weak stomach
Plaster / poultice: rheumatism; pain
Nettle tea: clears mucus from lung; edema; hair tonic
Oak bark tea: goiter; swollen throat; tonic for over exertion

Nettle • Oats • Onion • Peony • Peppermint • Pepperwort • Periwinkle • Pine • Pimpernel • Primrose • Pumpkin Seeds • Ribwort, Rosemary • Rue • *1920 (7), 353-355.*

Nettle flower decoction: blood purifier; skin diseases; eczema
Oat straw decoction: used for packs and compresses; chest diseases
Oatmeal: convalescence
Onion juice: stimulating; expectorant; powerful diuretic
Peony flower: epilepsy; cramps; gout; asthma; antispasmodic; sedative
Peppermint and Watermint: improves digestion; heart palpitation; nausea; abdominal pain
Pepperwort tea: colic; griping pain; vomiting; dissolvent remedy; stomach tonic
Periwinkle tea: excellent for diarrhea; intestinal and lung obstructions from mucus; hemorrhages
Gargle: scurvy
Pine: excellent cough remedy
Pine honey: children's cough; bronchitis; catarrh of chest
Pine baths: convalescence; weakness
Pimpernel tea: dyspepsia, liver complaint; jaundice; powerful diuretic and sudorific
Primrose tea: rheumatism; chronic headache
Pumpkin seeds: tapeworms
Ribwort (Plantain) tea: loosens mucus in inner organs

Lung formula: plantain and lungwort used as infallible cough remedy
Rosemary tea: bitter; excellent stomach remedy; liver; expels morbid matter; preventative for incipient edema
Rue tea: headaches; nausea; fainting; difficult breathing; abdominal cramps

St. John's Wort• Sage • Sallow • Sandalwood • Sanicle • Sarsaparilla • Sassafras • Scurvy Grass • Sea Onion • Shavegrass • Silverweed • Shepherd's Purse ⁕ *1920 (8), 406-408.*

St. John's wort tea: constipation; mucus obstructions in chest; bed wetting
Sage tea: liver and kidney diseases; mucus in throat and stomach
Gargle: sage and alum
Sallow tea: catarrh, whooping cough; acute and chronic rheumatism; dyspepsia; promotes hair growth; disinfectant
Sandalwood tea: add to mistletoe to stop hemorrhages
Sanicle tea: violent attacks of catarrh of the chest
Decoction: clean wounds
Sarsaparilla root decoction: blood purifier; excellent for rheumatism and syphilis
Sassafras: diaphoretic stimulant: asthma; lung catarrh
Scurvy grass tea: rheumatism; edema/dropsy; scurvy; sexual diseases
Sea onion; expectorant; diuretic; purgative
Shavegrass (*Equisetum*) tea: cleans stomach; alleviates pain from bladder stones; painful urination; hemorrhage; vomiting blood; nose bleeds
Compress with decoction: suppurating wounds
Silverweed: tetanus; excellent for cramps in stomach, heart and abdomen
Shepherd's purse tea: best specific to stop hemorrhages of all kinds

Soapwort • Sorrel• Strawberry • Sweet Flag • Thyme • Tormentil Valerian • Vervaine • Violet • Wallwort • Walnut • Wormseed ⁕ *1920 (10), 450-452.*

Soapwort tea: catarrh
Root tea: gout, syphilis, skin eruptions, hard tumours
Sorrel tea: mouth ulcers
Wine: abdominal pain; diuretic
Strawberry leaf decoction: convalescents; blood purifier; liver complaint; eczema
Sweet flag tea: flatulence; scrofula
Thyme decoction: stomach cramps; diarrhea
Tormentil root tincture: chronic diarrhea, gonorrhea, leucorrhea
Decoction: used internal as a injection [enema or douche]
Mouthwash: using decoction and diluted tincture for tender gums and throat inflammation

Valerian root tea: head congestion; giddiness; fainting; nervous stomach; insomnia; hysteria; abdominal cramps; heart palpitations

Violet leaf tea: severe cough; whooping cough; dissolves mucus in tuberculosis; severe headache
Gargle: swollen throat; shortness of breath
Root: dissolves mucus in severe cough

Vervaine root tea: whooping cough; kidney and liver complaints; jaundice; edema/dropsy

Wallwort [Comfrey] root decoction: blood in sputum; intestinal troubles
External: wound wash

Walnut leaf decoction: removes phlegm in digestive tract; skin eruptions; gout; scrofula; syphilis; mercury poisoning
Topically: scrofulous, syphilitic inflammation, cancer, eye wash

Wormseed: mild cardiac stimulant; promotes secretions in skin and kidneys; anthelmintic; round worms

WATERMINT • WOODRUFF • WATERCRESS • WORMWOOD • KNEIPP'S FORMULAS * *1920 (10), 509-511.*

Watermint tea: excellent for stomach and bowel diseases
Decoction: with vinegar stops blood vomiting

Woodruff tea: mixed with strawberry leaf tea is blood purifier; excellent spring tonic

Watercress tea: blood purifier

Wood ashes (linden tree): strengthen digestive organs; regulate bowels; convalescents with weak stomachs

Wormwood tea: excellent stomach remedy; incipient edema and jaundice; parasites
Formula: wormwood with St. John's wort and centaury

Kneipp's Aromatic Nourishing tea: convalescents; weak patients

Kneipp's Bone Powder: nourishes blood, bones and nerves
White Powder: nervousness; headache; anemia and vertigo
Gray Powder: lung, kidney and bladder diseases
Black Powder: scrofulous and rachitic children

Kneipp's Cough Tea: catarrh of respiratory organs

Cramp Drops and Cramp Tea: cramps; anti-hysteric remedy

Kneipp's Depurative Tea: rids morbid matter; acts on bowels; skin eruptions; itching; cancers

Kneipp's Diuretic Tea: Diuretic hydrogogue; dropsy; Bright's disease; bladder stones

Kneipp's Liver Regulator # 1, Wühlhuber # 1: strong purgative

Kneipp's Liver Regulator # 2, Wühlhuber # 2: less purgative than No. 1; dropsy; urinary tract diseases

HERBS COMBINED WITH NATURE CURE • *1923 (8), 370-371.*

Sage: removes impurities; stomach and intestine
Hemorrhages: tormentil, thistle, shavegrass
Ribwort [plantain]: loosens mucus in throat and lungs
Rosemary: edema; kidney and liver troubles
Fenugreek: diphtheria; sore throat and nose; fever
Juniper and wormwood: stimulates kidney and bladder
Dandelion blossoms: chronic constipation
Raspberry leaves: diarrhea [enema]

1900

Herbs And Their Healing Power

Benedict Lust

Strawberry And Purgative Remedies

Benedict Lust

RIBWORT, PLANTAGO LANCEOLATA

Benedict Lust

Cowslips And Violets

Benedict Lust

The Kneipp Apotheca

Benedict Lust

How Nature Cures

Ludwig Staden

My Medicinal Herbs

Sebastian Kneipp

PRICE LIST OF THE GENUINE **PFARRER SEB. KNEIPP REMEDIES**

Oberhäusser & Landauer, of Würzburg, Germany, are the only firm in the Universe authorized to manufacture and prepare the Rev. Father Kneipp's Natural and Herbal Remedies according to his own instructions and supervision.—Purchasers of Father Kneipp's World-renowned Herbal Medicines are requested to bear in mind that, in order to defy imitations all wrappers, directions for use and labels bear their registered Trade Mark as shown here.

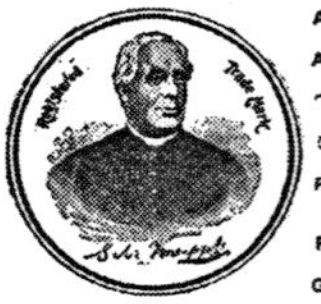

ARNICA SALVE, for sores, wounds and Eczema, ... $0 35
AUGENTROST (EYEBRIGHT), for sore, weak and inflamed eyes 50
CHOLERA DROPS, for Diarrhoe, Cholera and Bowel Complaints... 1.00
DEPURATIVE TEA for purifying the blood, also acts as tonic, ... 35
FIR CONE EXTRACT (honey), for catarrh, cough, sore & inflamed throat, etc., ... 50
FRANGULA EXTRACT, a mild purgative, may also be given to children 55
GOUT EMBROCATION, for gout and rheumatism, ... 1.00
ANTI-DIABETIC PILLS, made of Bilberry Leaves, ... 50
ANTI-DIARRHOEA PILLS, for diarrhoea and intestinal disorders 50
KNEIPP PILLS, for purifying the blood and for constipation.... 50
COUGH TEA, for coughs, colds, influenza, ... 35
COUGH DROPS, for cough and sore throat, ... 20
PECTORAL SYRUP, for affections of the respiratory organs, ... 50
WHOPING COUGH CURE, ... 50
CRAMP DROPS and **CRAMP TEA**, ... each, 40
DIURETIC TEA, for dropsy and urinary troubles, ... 35
CALENDULA SALVE (Pomade of Marigold), a healing salve for all wounds and sores, ... 35
SPIRIT OF BALM (Karmelitergeist) for stomach and bowel troubles, ... 50
MAGENTROST (Stomach Elixir), for indigestion and dyspepsia, 50
" " medium size bottle, 75c, large bottle, 1.50

EXCRETIVE OIL (Malefizöl), for toothache and headache, ... 50
WHITE BONE POWDER, for nervousness, nervous headache, anaemia and vertigo, ... 50
GREY BONE POWDER, for lung, kidney and bladder diseases, 50
BLACK BONE POWDER, for scrofulous and rachitic children, .. 50
NERVE TONIC, for nervousness, nervous headache and sleeplessness; with Dr. Baumgarten's Essay on Insomnia, ... 1.00
TRAVELLING AND HOUSE APOTHEKAS, ...$1, $2, $3, $6 and $15.00
WORM WOOD EYE SALVE, for weak eyes, cataracts, etc., ... 50
KNEIPP'S TRAVELLING DROPS, ... 75
KNEIPP'S FAMILY HEALTH TEA, replaces Chinese Tea, ... 35
" " .... large box, 65
WOERISHOFEN DIETETIC TEA, for anaemic and weak people, 35
WUEHLHUBER I (Liver Regulator No. I), a purgative for cleaning the system of all morbid matter, ... 40
WUEHLHUBER I PILLS act same as above, ... 50
WUEHLHUBER II (Liver Regulator No. 2), a gentle purgative, acting especially upon the bladder and kidneys, ... 40
WUEHLHUBER II PILLS, action same as above, ... 50
EXTRACT OF NETTLE ROOT, Kneipp's world-famous Hair Tonic, for preserving and strenghtening the hair, best dandruff cure, ... 1.00
OIL OF NETTLE ROOT, for gentlemen, ... 50
OIL OF BURDOCK ROOT, for ladies, ... 50
Either of these Oils is to be used with the Hair Tonic to keep the hair soft and to further their growth.
KNEIPP'S MOUTH AND TOOTH WASH, ... 75
KNEIPP'S HERBAL TOOTH POWDER, ... 40
KNEIPP SOAPS, made from Shave Grass, Hay Flower, Tormentil, Foenum Graecum, Curative (Heilseife) .... each, 25

We keep a full line of Father Kneipp's Articles, Herbs, Malt Coffee, Linen Underwear, Sandals and other Hygienic Supplies.

CATALOGUE AND GUIDE TO HEALTH FREE.
GOODS SENT POSTPAID ON RECEIPT OF PRICE.
AGENTS WANTED. o6m

Remember: the Trade Mark and Name of Oberhäusser & Landauer must be on every package.

SOLE GENERAL AGENTS FOR THE UNITED STATES OF AMERICA:

KNEIPP HEALTH STORE CO., 111 East 59th Street, New York.

On September 15, 1896, Benedict Lust opened up his first business, an original health food and Kniepp product store on 111 East 59th Street in New York City. This ad appeared in *The Kneipp Water Cure Monthly*, indicating some of the products available.

HERBS AND THEIR HEALING POWER

by Benedict Lust

The Kneipp Water Cure Monthly, I (1), 11-12. (1900)

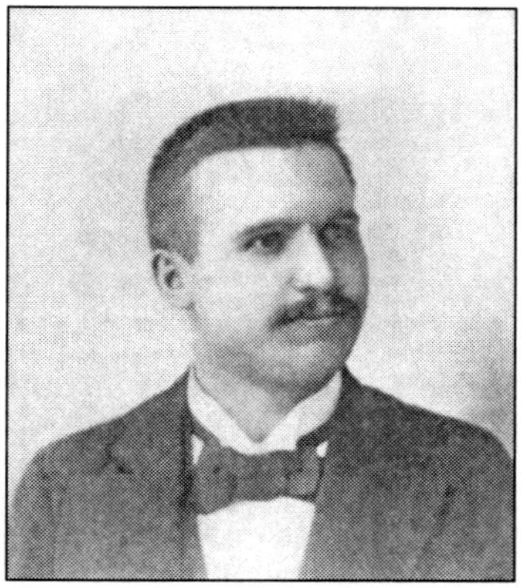

Benedict Lust

The use of herbs as a means to cure sickness is very old. Wherever we find so-called savages, human beings living according to the laws of Nature in a natural way without the slightest knowledge of drugs, we find the knowledge and the use of herbs as a factor to cure disease. Our forefathers knew the value of quite a number of herbs, but today very little was thought of them until the natural systems of healing again gave honor where honor is due.

The variety of these herbs is just as large as the different effects they have upon the human organism are great. As a first help in all diseases, herbs should be in every household; and once there, they will be valued very highly. A tea is made of these herbs and will always produce good results. Every mother knows how to prepare tea. For one cup she takes as much of the dried herbs as she can hold with three fingers. Boiling water is poured over the herbs. They are boiled for a few minutes and a remedy is ready which will always produce the effect looked for, when the right kind of herb is used. One herb cannot do everything. One herb cannot cure every ailment, but the Creator in his wisdom has given one or more herbs for every sort of sickness and has given us numberless little herbs to bring comfort to man in days of mitigation and healing his body convulsed with pain.

Everybody is liable to contract a cold. There are a number of herbs which will cure a cold. Chamomile tea will do so and remove the fever produced by the cold. But at the same time it will cure gripe, cramps and strong indigestion. If a catarrh of the chest is a consequence of the cold, chickweed is used with good results. If the chest and lungs are affected, coltsfoot will purify these organs. Asthma and coughs are easily removed by this remedy, especially if an inclination to consumption exists. If you put two leaves of coltsfoot on the chest, they will attract the heath, stop feebleness and remove fevers. Their effect upon open wounds is especially good; they remove the heat, the redness and draw out injurious matter. The leaves of coltsfoot will heal inflamed feet and stop the pain if laid on the sores.

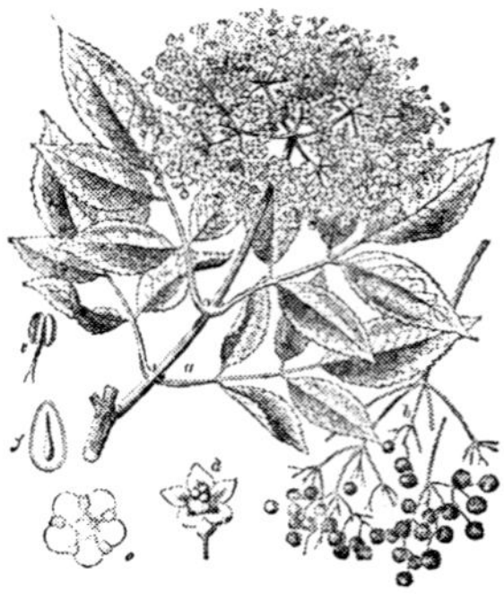

Elder (*Sambucus nigra*)

The common elder and the dwarf elder are plants of great healing power. Every part of the elder tree is a good efficacious remedy. The leaves, blossoms, berries, bark and roots are used. In springtime, vigorous nature strives to throw off matter that has gathered in the body during the winter. Whoever wishes to purify juices and blood by a spring course of medicine, whoever wishes to get rid of injurious matter in the easiest and most natural way, let him take tea of the elder tree leaves. One cup of this tea taken daily one hour before breakfast during springtime will cleanse the whole system. The leaves of the elder tree are one of the simplest and one of the best blood purifying remedies, a remedy which will also purify the blood at any other time of the year. The flowers of the elder tree should be in every household. If you want to break a cold by perspiration, take the dried elder flowers and make a cup of tea. This tea taken before going to bed will dissolve the film [mucus] and produce the looked for perspiration. Tea of the dried flowers of the elder tree will prove a remedy of excellent service. Those suffering from dropsy [edema] will find the root of the elder tree an excellent remedy. Tea prepared of the elder root will drive out the water [edema] more powerfully than any other remedy.

The berries of the elder tree are highly esteemed as a blood purifying remedy and strength giver. Tea of the dried root of the dwarf elder expels the water, purifies the kidneys and is therefore a valuable remedy in the cases of dropsy. This tea may also be used against other complaints in the abdomen arising from bad juices. All these impurities are removed by the urine.

A very valuable remedy for the home is the juniper berry. It is used for fumigation and destroys all disease germs. The juniper berry has a great effect upon the interior of the human organism. The berries, so to speak, fumigate the mouth and the stomach and ward off contagion. For a weak stomach, juniper berries are a blessing. Those who suffer from heartburn will find immediate relief after eating about from 6 to 12 berries. For stone and gravel, for complaints of the kidney and liver, for removing foul gases, foul, watery and slimy matter, there is no better remedy than the juniper berry.

Good remedies for some stomach complaints also are peppermint and watermint. They strengthen the stomach and aid digestion. Mint will relieve headaches, when bound across the forehead. A cup of mint tea taken every morning and evening will aid digestion and give a fresh and healthy appearance. Mint tea takes away a bad breath.

Prepared with vinegar, mint stops blood vomiting. During our hot summer months nobody should be without dried bilberries. They are the best *pills* to stop diarrhoea. Anise seed and fennel seed may be recommended very highly. They operate on gases and winds. The effect of the anise seed is superior to that of the fennel seed.

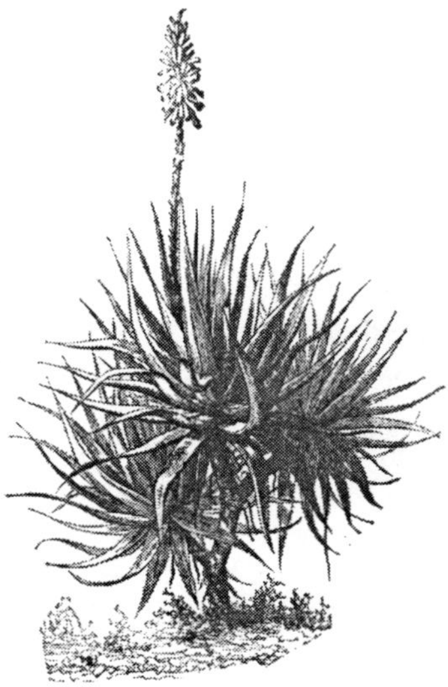

Bitter Aloe (*Agave americana*)

The powder of the Barbados aloe plant will cure quite a number of ailments. A little aloe powder boiled with a teaspoonful of honey thoroughly cleanses the stomach. Mixed with other herbs aloe has a very beneficial effect, not a very purging but a more evacuating effect. One mixture which cannot be recommended too highly consists of one pinch of aloe, sufficient elder flowers, a small teaspoonful *Foenum graecum* (Fenugreek) and one teaspoonful of fennel. Of this mixture two cups of tea are prepared and taken within two days.

Tea made with aloe powder may be used with good results in cases of sore eyes as an eyewash. Old wounds and putrefied flesh are also healed with this water. For this purpose put on the wound a piece of linen dipped into the aloe water.

Ulcers covered with aloe powder will soon heal. The powder absorbs the morbid matter; wounds quickly close if aloe powder is used.

Blackthorn blossoms are another harmless purgative.

Of the greatest medical value are nettles. Tea of dried nettles loosens the phlegm in the chest and lungs, cleanses the stomach and invigorates the kidneys. The roots of the nettle are even superior to the leaves in effect. Tea of nettle root is a good remedy for dropsy in its first stages. Nettle leaves chopped up and boiled like spinach are very wholesome for people who have had bad blood. People who suffer from rheumatism and cannot find any relief should try fresh nettle. If they strike the suffering part with this herb, relief will follow and after it the longed for healing.

Eyebright has got its name from its own merits. When other remedies failed eyebright cleared and strengthened the eyesight.

For interior use tea of fenugreek is a cooling remedy in cases of fever. In cases of throat complaints, the tea is a good gargle. For exterior use, it softens and dissolves tumor. In cases of wounds, poultices made of fenugreek heal and prevent the formation of putrid flesh as well as blood-poisoning.

The sap of ribwort [*Plantago lanceolata*] or its leaves softened and moistened by pressure are an excellent dressing for wounds and will heal rapidly.

Shavegrass [*Equisetum arvense*] affords manifold and excellent effects. On old injuries, putrid wounds and ulcers shavegrass operates in an extraordinary manner. We may say it washes away, dissolves, burns out all that is injurious. A cupful of the tea is taken from time to time. It will remove all difficulties in discharging the urine and ease the pain in cases of gravel and stone disease. It is the only herb which has this effect. It also is a good tea for cases of bleeding and blood-vomiting. Those who suffer from violent bleedings of the nose will find relief by drawing this tea through the nostrils.

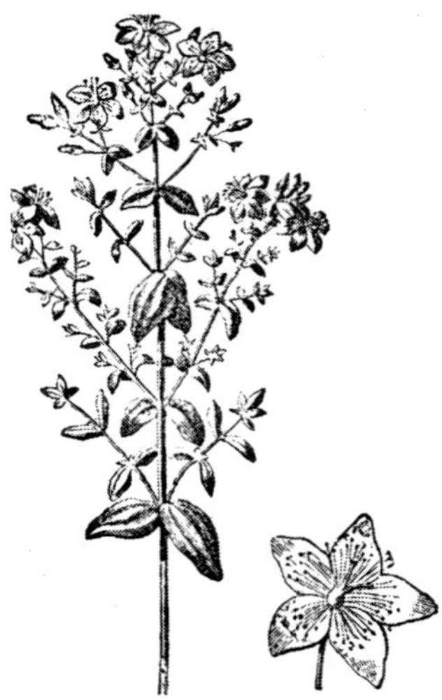

St. John's wort
(*Hypericum perforatum*]

The good effects of St. John's wort are well-known. All sorts of complaints of the head arising from watery matter or phlegm in the head or from the gases rising to the head are relieved by this herb. To mothers who have trouble with their little bed-wetters, St. John's wort is a real blessing. Common yarrow will do the same.

One who wants to remove phlegm from the stomach, superfluous gall, purify the liver, milt [spleen] and kidneys, will do so by drinking daily two cups of the tea made of the succory or chicory herb.

Great heat in the head is removed by tea of violets, while for a swollen throat this tea is a tested gargle.

Space does not permit us to mention all the herbs nor all the healing qualities of the herbs; we have called to the attention of our readers. In field and forest, in the depth of the valley and on the top of the mountain, in God's wide, wide garden we find many an herb, a valuable remedy for ailments of all descriptions. The book of Nature contains all wisdom men need to know. It is for men to read it and to profit by the knowledge it affords. This knowledge will give the power to heal through Nature's simple remedies.

One herb cannot cure every ailment, but the Creator in his wisdom has given one or more herbs for every sort of sickness and has given us numberless little herbs to bring comfort to man in days of mitigation and healing his body convulsed with pain.

Whoever wishes to purify juices and blood by a spring course of medicine, whoever wishes to get rid of injurious matter in the easiest and most natural way, let him take tea of the elder tree leaves.

The leaves of the elder tree are one of the simplest and one of the best blood purifying remedies, a remedy which will also purify the blood at any other time of the year.

Tea prepared of the elder root will drive out the water more powerfully than any other remedy.

For a weak stomach juniper berries are a blessing. Those who suffer from heartburn will find immediate relief after eating about from 6 to 12 berries.

Prepared with vinegar, mint stops blood vomiting.

During our hot summer months nobody should be without dried bilberries. They are the best pills to stop diarrhoea.

Old wounds and putrefied flesh are also healed with Aloe water. For this purpose put on the wound a piece of linen dipped into the aloe water.

Tea of dried nettles loosens the phlegm in the chest and lungs, cleanses the stomach and invigorates the kidneys. The roots of the nettle are even superior to the leaves in effect. Tea of nettle root is a good remedy for dropsy in its first stages.

For interior use tea of fenugreek is a cooling remedy in cases of fever.

To mothers who have trouble with their little bed-wetters, St. John's wort is a real blessing. Common yarrow will do the same.

Strawberry And Purgative Remedies*

by Benedict Lust

The Kneipp Water Cure Monthly, I (2), 29-30. (1900)

The Strawberry Plant

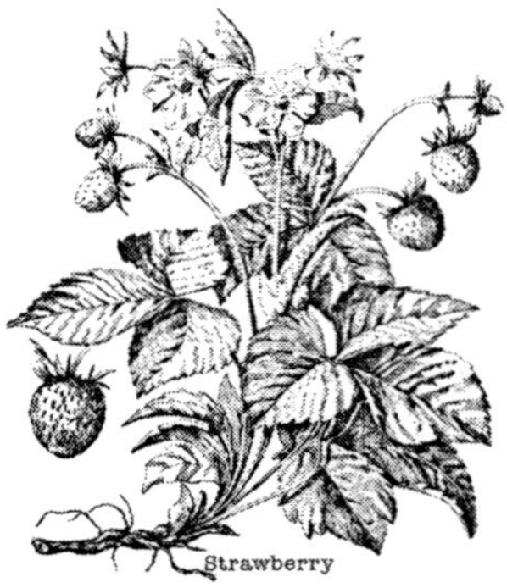

Strawberry (*Fragaria vesca*)

Strawberries! What joy for young and old! Of course, dear reader, you too only think of the delicious dishes prepared of this aromatic fruit, but there is more in this little plant than you imagine. Not only the fruit of this little plant but also the leaves have good offerings for the human being. Tea of strawberry leaves is exceedingly good and cheap nourishment. How is this tea prepared? Take as many dried strawberry leaves as you can pick up with three or four fingers, put about half a pint of boiling water on them and cover the pot [tightly]. Allow to draw for fifteen minutes, pour the tea off and your strawberry tea is ready. Mixed with hot milk and a little sugar it is a very wholesome beverage.

If a little woodroof [woodruff or *Galium odoratum*] and thyme is added, the tea will gain in taste and value.

The strawberries themselves are great strength-givers. The convalescent who feels great weakness and enervation after serious diseases should get plenty of them with other nourishment. A good wholesome and strength-giving dish is served in the southern part of Germany. This dish we recommend to the convalescent as well as to the healthy person. Mix one pint of pure milk with a quarter of a pint of strawberries and the crumbs of a slice of rye-bread or if it can be procured with the crumbs of Kneipp's 'health-bread' and a dish is ready which will soon show its exceedingly beneficial effects. In winter, preserved strawberries may be used with the same good results.

In summer, strawberries render great service to invalids in cases of great internal heat. There is not a more splendid refresher for the poor sufferer parched with thirst. Those afflicted with gravel and stone diseases may eat as many strawberries as they like and will benefit by it greatly. As much as a pint daily at different times will prove a very good thing for

*The original title of this article was "Herbs and their healing power" which was a series of articles written by Benedict Lust based on the Kneipp herbs in 1900. —*Ed.*

those suffering from liver complaints, while half a pint in the morning and half a pint in the afternoon will do a lot of good to such affected with an eruption arising from morbid blood.

If mankind only would care to know what treasures for suffering humanity are hidden in forest and field! The Creator in his wisdom has given everything plentiful what is to bring good cheer to man. This plant and its fruit is in great abundance on earth; is this fact not a sign, that God wanted to call man's attention to its usefulness? Would that our understanding and gratitude corresponded at all times to the loving bounty of our Creator!

Purgative Remedies

It was an old custom to be bled at an exact given time. At another time one had to take the yearly or half-yearly purgative. Even in our days there are people who will not give up the idea, that from time to time the stomach needs a thorough cleansing.

What makes people think so? People of a regular and healthy mind will not get such ideas. If we take in consideration how people live, it becomes a fact not very astonishing. People ought to eat in order to live and to be able to work and work in order to be able to eat and to live. But today this is changed. There are millions who do not eat only in order to live and be able to work, and there are millions who do not work only in order to eat and to live. There are those who eat for enjoyment; there are others who only work in order to get the same enjoyment. Eating has become too much of an enjoyment.

It is no longer a duty which men perform in order to live. The stomach is overloaded to a fearful degree. The stomach is only built to digest such quantities as are necessary to keep alive. Liver and kidneys etc., etc., are only able to perform a certain amount of work. The same men who know it for a positive fact that it is ridiculous to ask a boiler and engine of one horse power to perform to the work of six horses, expect their own stomachs do more than one man's stomach, liver and kidneys can stand.

If the dreadfully tormented and sinfully overstrained stomach could give a sound, it would be a cry for mercy. But as it is, it must *take in* all and be ruined. But stomach, liver and kidneys get their satisfaction from the malefactors. These headaches and kidney troubles become unbearable and purgative doses follow each other, only to make matters worse. Do not eat and drink more than is absolutely necessary to live and all these troubles and ailments will disappear.

But those who have weakened their stomachs need help and Nature provides their help. Field and forest are full of useful herbs which will heal the disorders of the stomach, cleanse liver and kidneys and make men well and healthy, providing they do not continue to sin against Nature's laws.

Kneipp says in his book, *My Water Cure* in regard to healing these disorders:

I think I have found the remedies and their mixture. Both kinds of tea shall not be a secret; on the contrary I wish that very many may use them and prepare them for the relief of others.

The first recipe is this:

KNEIPP STOMACH FORMULA

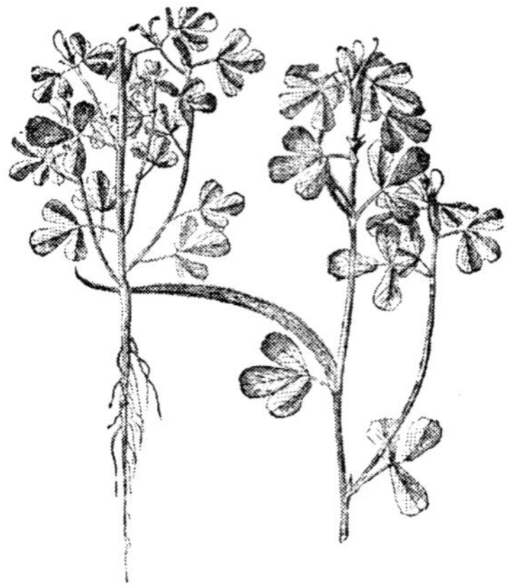

Fenugreek
(*Trigonella foecum graecum*)

Take two tablespoonful of pounded fennel, two tablespoons of crushed juniper berries, one tablespoonful of *Foenum graceum* and one tablespoonful of aloe powder. Mix them all well together, put the mixture in a box and keep it in a dry place. The remedy operates after twelve to thirty hours. The tea is taken generally at night before bed; a small cupful is a dose. One teaspoonful of the mixture is sufficient for a cupful. It is boiled for a quarter of an hour, then poured off and drunk either cold or warm with or without sugar.

Kneipp recommends to strong people to drink a cup of the tea on two succeeding days; to weak people to divide the cupful for two or three days so that they take four or six tablespoonful like medicine every evening. There will be no uncomfortable feelings, but the beneficial effect will be felt at once.

Those who only imagine ailments will feel the effect but experience no results. Where there is no sickness there can be no cure. The tea seeks impurities in stomach, liver and kidneys, but where there are none it cannot remove them. The tea does not disturb the organs, only the impurities in them. It does not weaken the organs and does not produce that tired feeling which will always follow the use of purgative doses medicine prescribes. In the same manner as upon the evacuation of the bowels, this tea operates also on the urine. Even great obstructions of phlegm on the chest are removed by it.

One small cupful taken in three portions during the day will be sufficient in cases of tedious diarrhoea, difficult to stop. The tea in such cases will remove the impurities causing the diarrhoea and quiet the organs.

Kneipp has left another recipe for the mixture of another tea, the effect of which is not so much purging as the first one but works more upon the kidneys and bladder.

Kneipp Kidney And Bladder Formula

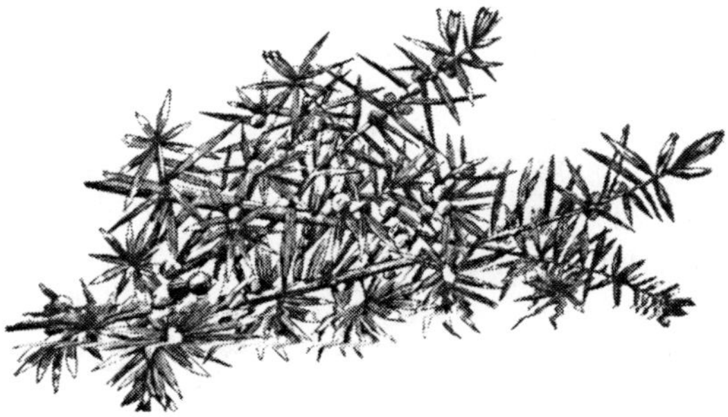

Juniper (*Juniperus communis*)

Two tablespoonful of pounded fennel, three tablespoonful of crushed juniper berries, three tablespoonful of powder from dwarf elder roots, one tablespoonful of *Foenum graceum* and one tablespoonful of aloe powder are mixed well together.

This tea will drive out morbid matter through the urine. It will be very beneficial to those who feel uneasiness in the abdomen (in the vicinity of the bladder) and experience difficulties in making urine or a burning in the bladder or kidneys. In cases of dropsy in its first stages, no remedy will produce better and more lasting results.

This tea is prepared in the same way as the first one. Its rules for application are also the same. Strong people may take one cupful at night before retiring; weak people should divide this dose in three parts and take it on three succeeding nights.

In summer strawberries render great service to invalids in cases of great internal heat.

Do not eat and drink more than is absolutely necessary to live and all these troubles and ailments will disappear.

Field and forest are full of useful herbs which will heal the disorders of the stomach, cleanse liver and kidneys and make men well and healthy, providing they do not continue to sin against Nature's laws.

Ribwort, Plantago Lanceolata

by Benedict Lust

The Kneipp Water Cure Monthly, I (3), 44. (1900)

Our readers have learned in our February issue the value of the strawberry plant. In this issue, we will dwell upon the good the little ribwort affords to mankind.

Take a farmer making hay. He may cut one of his fingers while performing his work. He is far from his home, a drugstore, etc., etc. The blood flows freely. But that does not bother him much. He knows, no, he is sure that right near him Nature allows a little insignificant plant to grow which will not only stop the bleeding immediately, but at the same time will heal the wound. He will pick a few of the leaves of the ribwort plant and squeeze a few drops of sap out of them. This sap, he will put direct on the wound or allow it to drop on a piece of cloth which he will tie around it.

Should the leaves refuse to give up their medical sap and only become soft and moist, one may wrap the moist leaves themselves around the wound. The effect will be the same and in most cases will be the best dressing for the wound; for wounds dressed in this way will heal very rapidly. There will be no putridness or proud flesh; ribwort does not allow such things.

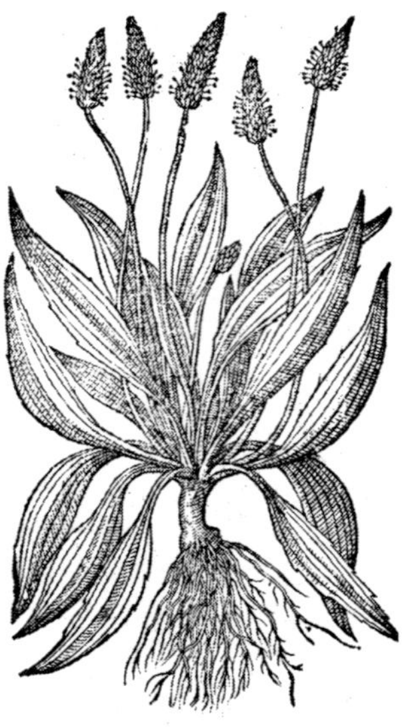

Ribwort or Plantain (*Plantago lanceolata*). This illustration was found in John Gerard's *The herbal, or generall historie of plantes* (1633).

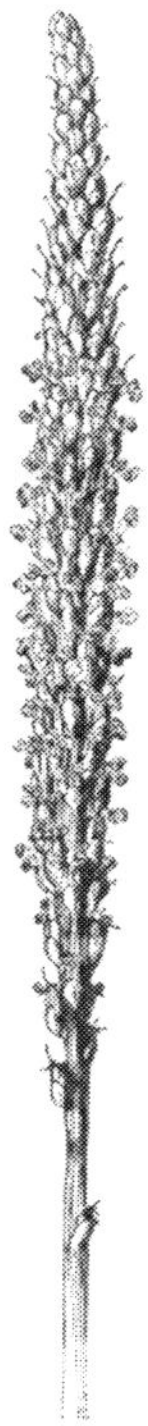

Ribwort Spike

Used internally ribwort offers great advantages. The sap pressed out of these leaves and drank is a wonderful remedy and will make impossible all the numberless interior complaints which are a consequence of impure blood and impure juices.

Against obstructions by phlegm in the interior organs a tea made of the dried leaves of ribwort will work very successfully and remove these obstructions in short order.

He knows, no, he is sure that right near him Nature allows a little insignificant plant to grow which will not only stop the bleeding immediately, but at the same time will heal the wound.

The sap pressed out of these leaves and drank is a wonderful remedy and will make impossible all the numberless interior complaints which are a consequence of impure blood and impure juices.

COWSLIPS AND VIOLETS*

by Benedict Lust

The Kneipp Water Cure Monthly, I (5), 81-82. (1900)

COWSLIPS (PRIMROSE)

One of the best remedies for articular diseases is tea of cowslips. This tea should be drank for a considerable time to effect a cure, but the violent pains will soon give way and gradually disappear altogether.

Only the dark yellow cowslips are valuable as a remedy. Their perfume already indicates of what great healing power these flowers are. If our readers will chew two or three of these little funnels they will soon feel what medical qualities they hide.

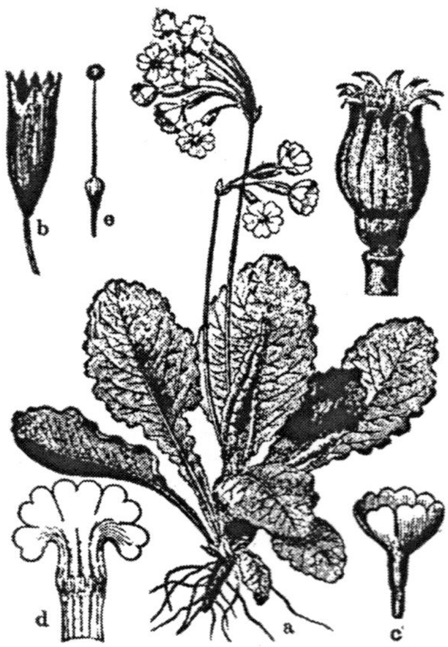

Cowslip (*Primula officinalis*)
a. Complete plant, b. calyx, c. and d. corolla, e. pistil, f. fruit.

VIOLETS

Springtime is here and with the beginning of spring violets are in blossom.

When children get bad coughs in consequence of frequent changes in the weather, boil a handful of green or dried violet leaves in half a pint of water and give the children two or three spoonful of such tea every two or three hours. One may use the roots of the plant too, but they

---

*This article belongs to a series entitled, "Herbs and their healing power". —*Ed.*

must be crushed before boiling. For whooping cough there is no better cure than a cup of this tea three times a day.

Tea of violet leaves is also a good and effective remedy for headaches and great heat in the head. A piece of linen is moistened with violet leaf tea and bound across the forehead, or to get results quicker one may wash the back of the head with a strong decoction of violet leaves.

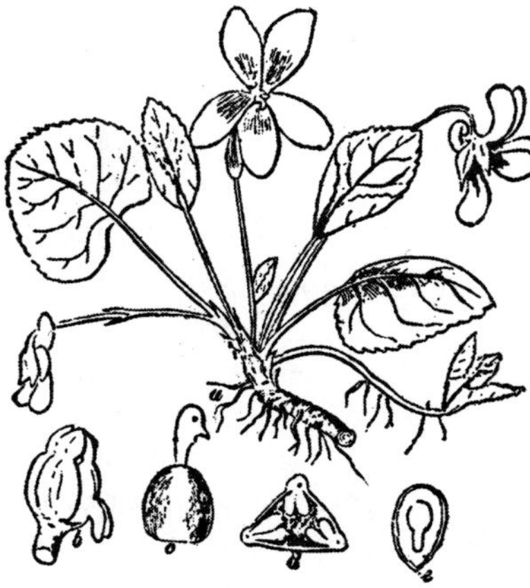

Violet (*Viola odorata*)

This tea also serves well as a gargle for swollen throats and at the same time a throat bandage dipped in the decoction may be applied.

In all cases where difficulty in breathing is produced by a gathering of gases or morbid matters in the stomach and bowels violet tea should be taken for some time about two or three cups daily.

Crushed violet leaves bound as a compress on inflamed tumors have a cooling effect, while when boiled in vinegar, they will heal gout.

No Kneipp apotheca should be without dried violet leaves.

One of the best remedies for articular diseases is tea of cowslips.

Only the dark yellow cowslips are valuable as a remedy. Their perfume already indicates of what great healing power these flowers are.

For whooping cough there is no better cure than a cup of this [violets] tea three times a day.

This [violet] tea also serves well as a gargle for swollen throats and at the same time a throat bandage dipped in the decoction may be applied.

Crushed violet leaves bound as a compress on inflamed tumors have a cooling effect, while when boiled in vinegar, they will heal gout.

THE KNEIPP APOTHECA

by Benedict Lust

The Kneipp Water Cure Monthly, I (7), 116-118. (1900)

ITS USEFULNESS IN EVERY HOUSEHOLD

No household should be without a Kneipp Apotheca, for it is a good deal easier to prevent a disease than cure one. How often does it happen that a member of the family complains about a certain feeling of uneasiness, restlessness, a little headache or dizziness, etc? How often is a mother of a family confronted by cases of diarrhoea or constipation! How often does not one little accident or other happen to the little ones! In all such cases, the Kneipp Apotheca will come in very handy and save a good deal of money which otherwise doctor and druggist would get.

Kneipp has experimented for years, has examined, dried, cut up, boiled and tasted most every little herb within his reach and has found many good healing qualities in them.

All the articles contained in his Apotheca have a threefold aim. They dissolve and evacuate any morbid matters which ought not to be in the system and strengthen the organism.

Every house apotheca should consist of four divisions:

- The teas
- The extracts
- The powders
- The oils

Some clean pieces of linen for bandages as well as some cotton wool may also be kept on hand. Its usefulness we will explain later on.

We consider first the teas.

THE TEAS

Every mother knows how to prepare tea. For one cup she takes as much of the dried herbs as she can hold with three fingers, pours boiling water into the pan upon the leaves of the blossoms, let it boil for some minutes to get a good decoction and the tea is ready to be taken.

Which herbs should be in the house apotheca? There are many. It is not the object of this article to consider the herbs themselves but only their healing power, therefore we will give the names of the herbs only and mention for what ailment they will afford relief.

There is no other part of the body which ought to be looked after with more care than the bowels. There originate quite a number of diseases which in their first states are easily cured while if not seen to from the beginning may do a lot of harm to the whole system.

To Cleanse The Bowels

To cleanse and remove the bowels there are no better remedies than agave, black alder bark, blackthorn blossoms, buckthorn bark, marigold flowers and Kneipp's Stomach Cure (Wühlhuber No. 1) or Kneipp's Laxative Tea. Either of these remedies will do its work well. Of course children should get a weaker dose than adults.

The utmost attention should be given to the kind of food partaken of by the family. The evil consequences of the taking of unwholesome food are numerous and such foods especially hurtful to little children. Quite a number of disorders of the digestive organs in general and especially of the stomach will be experienced in such cases. To overcome the effects of such unwholesome foods, we recommend the following herbs: tea of angelica is an excellent remedy in such cases which will also remove that uncomfortable cold feeling in the stomach and bowels. Often the food ought not to be blamed, but more so the stomach itself which does not possess gastric juices of the necessary regular strength to overcome this weakness of the stomach.

To Aid Digestion

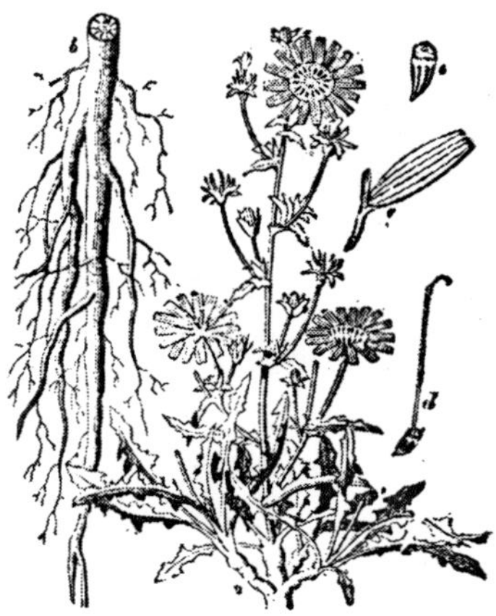

Succory or chicory
(*Cichorium intybus*)
a. Complete plant, b. root, c. flower, d. pistil, e. fruit.

We recommend tea of buckbean leaves, tea of the calamus root, tea of centaury, tea of rosemary, tea of succory [chicory], tea of wormwood, and Kneipp's Stomach Cure which is a composition of several herbs.

Often the stomach is full of phlegm which causes all sorts of ailments. In such cases, it will be easily understood, liver and kidneys are soon affected.

Stomach, Liver And Kidneys

The following herbs will cleanse the stomach, liver and kidneys. Before all other teas, Kneipp's Wühlhuber No. 1 and 2 must be mentioned here. The word Wühlhuber is one of those powerful expressions which the good people in Bavaria indulge in. It is, too, one of those words which are very hard to translate; it means something like raking or Rummaging Jack for this Wühlhuber tea will rake in and remove while rummage through the system every bit of mucous matter or phlegm which may have settled in the stomach, kidneys, or liver.

No machinist or engineer would allow the principal parts of the machinery in his control to become dirty nor would he allow dirt to accumulate in any part of the machinery. He knows too well that either the machine would not work properly or, if too much dirt would have got into it, it would not work at all. What else is the human body but a fine machine and this machine, the human organism, must be kept very clean too in order to work well. Man is the engineer, but we are sorry to say that there are too many men who allow their machinery to become clogged by dirt. Of course, they have to suffer for their neglect and often very long at that, for they do not know the simple remedies which Nature has in store for the purpose of cleansing the human body. There are quite a number of herbs which possess the power of cleansing to a great extent. A tea is made of them, a cupful of this tea taken before going to bed we recommend either one or the other of the follow teas for the purpose. There are agave, common nettle, dwarf elder, juniper berries, St. John's wort and watermint.

The most effective of all is the Wühlhuber

The stomach, the kidneys and the liver are the seat of a whole lot of ailments. We have learned about some herbs which cure constipation and make the bowels move, but it often happens that the bowels move too freely and too often. There are herbs for this ailment too.

Diarrhea

Diarrhea will be stopped in a very natural way by dried bilberries which the patient may chew, tea of elder berries will also prove a valuable remedy for violent diarrhoea and for diarrhoea in general, tea of periwinkle can be recommended.

Inflammation Of The Stomach, Bowels Or Kidneys

Often disorders of the stomach are caused by inflammation of the stomach, bowels or kidneys, etc. In such cases, it is not only necessary to cleanse those organs inflamed but the inflammations must be healed too. For such inflammation in the bowels and stomach, tea of yarrow is an excellent remedy.

When stomach, kidneys or liver, parts of the great blood manufacturing machinery, have been full of morbid or mucous matter for some time, it is not astonishing that the blood made is not as pure as it ought to be. In consequence of the impure blood, the skin becomes covered by all sorts of eruptions. The science of natural healing knows quite a number of herbs which will cleanse the blood and secrete all morbid or mucous matter in short order.

Impure Blood

Some herbs which Kneipp recommended for impure blood are very effective. Among these are borage, blackberry leaves, common water-cress, dandelion, and common elder leaves. The best and surest cure in all cases of impure blood may be expected from the use of Kneipp's Depurative Tea. This tea will remove all eruptions, itch, lupus and cancerous affections when used for a longer period of time. As it took some time to fill the blood with impurities of all kinds, patients expect that it takes time to remove these secretions of the urine.

Disorders Of Bladder Or Kidneys

[Disorders of bladder or kidneys] will find relief by using tea of the following herbs regularly for some time. For all such troubles in general, or catarrh of the bladder, dilatation of the bladder, for gravel and stone tea of bearberry leaves will prove a good remedy, tea of briar hips has an excellent effect upon all cases of gravel, while tea of broom herb will cleanse the bladder and free it of gravel and stones. Burdock root promotes the secretion of urine while Kneipp's Diuretic Tea will be found a very good remedy in all cases of catarrh or urinary disorders.

Lungs

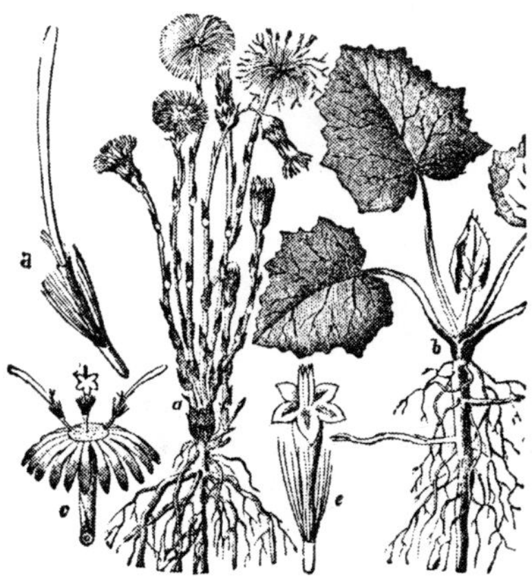

Coltsfoot (*Tussilago farfara*)

a. Flowering plant, b. plant with leaves, c. calyx and receptacle, d. female floret as in the ray, e. hermaphrodite floret. as in the disk.

Quite a number of people suffer from all sorts of troubles and ailments of the lungs or chest. From a slight cold to the first cases of consumption, all kinds of disorders of the lungs have been treated successfully by herbs in combination with some simple water application. For catarrh in the chest, tea of chickweed will always be used with good results; chest and lungs are cleansed of all impurities, phlegm, etc., by tea of coltsfoot or by tea of elecampane. Tea of group ivy has healed many cases of consumption in its first stages, while tea of Iceland moss is used with very good results for chest and lung troubles, consumption and general disability produced by disorders of the lungs. Tea of lungwort and ribwort mixed in equal parts will remove all slimy obstructions in the lungs and chest and will cure consumption in its first stages.

Those who suffer from bleedings of the lungs will get relief by taking tea of shepherd's purse hourly.

WHOOPING COUGH

While treating the subject of lung troubles, we may mention right here one which nearly every child has to suffer from former [sooner] or later. We mean the whooping cough. For this cough, there is no better remedy than tea of violets, or tea of black current leaves.

DIABETES

Diabetes has been treated with excellent results by tea of bilberry leaves.

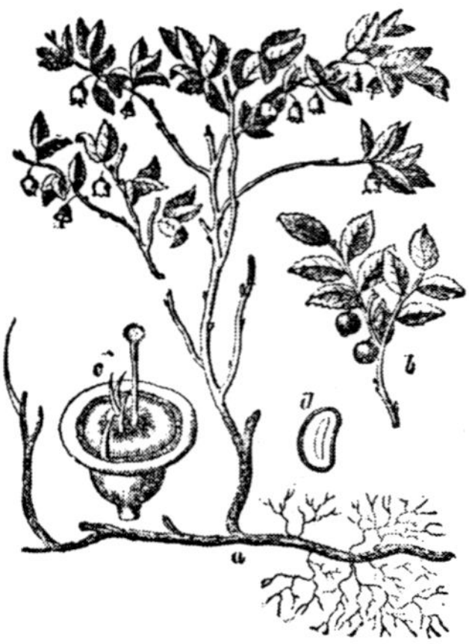

Bilberry (*Vaccinium myrtillus*)

a. Flowering plant, b. branch bearing fruit, c. receptacle with stamen, the corolla being removed, d. cross-section of the seed.

RHEUMATISM AND GOUT

Rheumatism and gout attack many and many who suffer constantly but are never healed from their ailments for their remedies don't remove the cause of the disorders. This will be done by tea made of several herbs. The tea of the leaves of the birch tree is a wonderful remedy for rheumatism and gout; the same can be said of tea of commock [*Ononis spinose*], tea of scurvy grass and tea of veronica.

A STRENGTH GIVER

A strength giver for all interior organs is tea of oak bark. This tea possesses great healing and strengthening qualities.

FOR COLIC AND CRAMPS

For colic and cramps, one may use the following teas with very beneficial results: tea of chamomile, Kneipp's Cramp Tea and fennel tea for children cannot be recommended too highly.

For Affections Of The Throat

Kneipp has an excellent combination of herbs which renders a very beneficial tea and which he called Cough Tea. This tea will cure all affections of the throat, lungs and respiratory organs in general as colds, coughs, **Bronchitis**, influenza, hoarseness, sore throat, **Croup,** etc.

Fenugreek Seeds

There are herbs which have several healing qualities as for instance the pulverized seed of fenugreek. It is used as a tea for fever with very good results in all cases and for sore throats prepared in the same way as a gargle. The gargle has to be taken hourly until relieved.

Perspiration

Perspiration often removes quite a lot of impurities and in this way prevents disease. Tea of elder flowers will purify as well as dissolve all obstructions in the system and secrete them by means of the organs of perspiration. The same will be affected by tea of linden flowers.

Weak And Sore Eyes

Weak and sore eyes are strengthened and healed when daily bathed in a decoction of eyebright for some time.

Ulcers And Boils

For ulcers and boils there is not a better remedy than a poultice of fenugreek powder. Flaxseed too has been used with good results.

Epilepsy

Epilepsy will be cured by tea of galium, while in cases of **Dropsy** tea of hen's feet [*Caucalis platycarpos*], or iris has been used very successfully.

Cancer, Ulcerous Sores And All Kinds Of Wounds

Cancer, ulcerous sores and all kinds of wounds are healed when washed hourly with a decoction of marigold flowers or arnica. After the process of healing has set in the salves made of these herbs may be used instead.

Blood Circulation

The circulation of the blood is regulated and obstructions removed by tea of mistletoe.

Gout

Tea of mouse ear [*Hieracium pilosella*], a little herb of powerful effect in all cases of gout taken regular before going to bed for some time every evening will cure even the worst cases.

Throat Complaints

All sorts of throat complaints are often to be treated. They range from a simple catarrh in the throat to the worst obstructions of phlegm in the throat and chest. All such disorders are removed by either tea of mullein, tea of sage leaves, tea of basil or tea of hyssop.

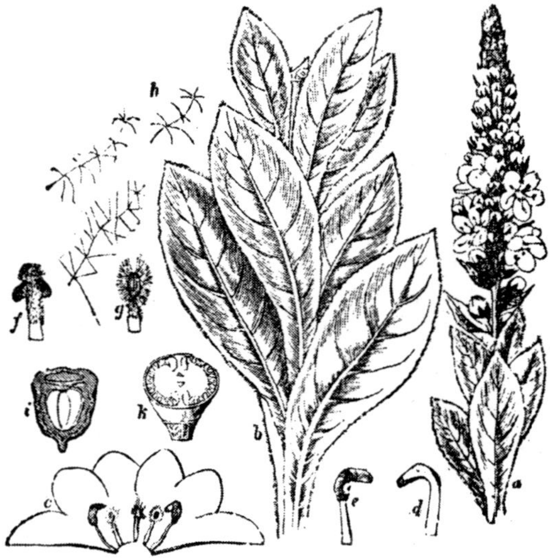

Mullein (*Verbascum schraderimeyer*)

a. and b. Parts of the stem, c. extended flower, d. stamen with declinate filament, e. side view of stamen, f. stamen with regular, erect filament, g. the same seen from the side, h. hairs of the villous filament, i. section of the seed.

Rheumatic Pain

Violent pains of a rheumatic nature in the joints are cured by tea of primrose but to produce a lasting effect it is necessary to use this tea for a considerable length of time.

Rush Of Blood To The Head

Rush of blood to the head as well as painful menses and hysteric cramps will be cured by tea of rue.

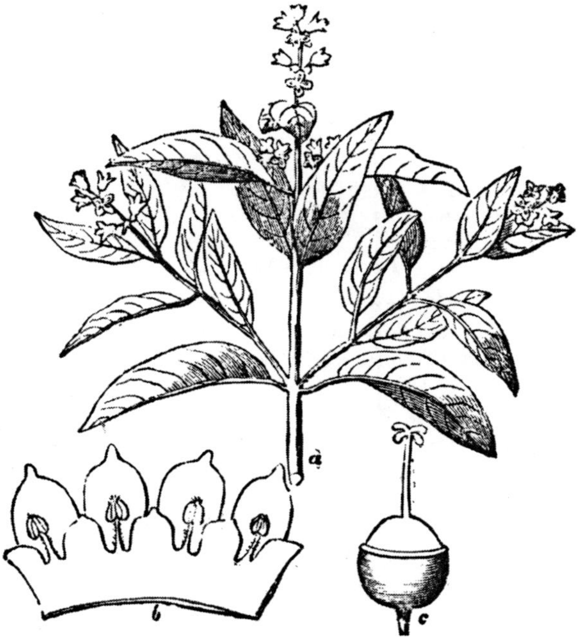

Sandal (*Pterocarpus santalinus*)
a. Branch, b. corolla, extended, c. pistil.

Wounds And Inflammation

Wounds and inflammation are best treated with a decoction of sanicle [*Sanicula europaea*]. A piece of linen is soaked wet this decoction and applied the wound or inflammation. It will be of great healing effect.

Blood-Vomiting

Blood-vomiting is stopped by tea of shavegrass, a little herb of manifold medical qualities. It will render excellent service in all cases of ulcers and putrid wounds and will overcome all difficulties which patients may experience in discharging their urine.

Menstrual Pain And Colic

Cramps in the abdomen or menstrual colic are cured by tea of silverweed. There is not one sickness for which there is not an herb which will cure it. As we have often repeated Nature is perfect everywhere, all what man only needs to do is to study Nature's simple laws, obey them and then very little sickness will trouble mankind.

All the articles contained in [Kneipp's] Apotheca have a threefold aim. They dissolve and evacuate any morbid matters which ought not to be in the system and strengthen the organism.

There is no other part of the body which ought to be looked after with more care than the bowels.

*To cleanse and remove the bowels there are no better remedies than agave, black alder bark, blackthorn blossoms, buckthorn bark, marigold flowers and Kneipp's Stomach Cure (*Wühlhuber No. 1*) or Kneipp's Laxative Tea.*

Diarrhea will be stopped in a very natural way by dried bilberries which the patient may chew, tea of elder berries will also prove a valuable remedy for violent diarrhoea and for diarrhoea in general, tea of periwinkle can be recommended.

For such inflammation in the bowels and stomach tea of yarrow is an excellent remedy.

Some herbs which Kneipp recommended for impure blood are very effective. Among these are borage, blackberry leaves, common watercress, dandelion, and common elder leaves.

For catarrh in the chest tea of chickweed will always be used with good results; chest and lungs are cleansed of all impurities, phlegm, etc., by tea of coltsfoot or by tea of elecampane.

Tea of lungwort and ribwort mixed in equal parts will remove all slimy obstructions in the lungs and chest and will cure consumption in its first stages.

We mean the whooping cough. For this cough there is no better remedy than tea of violets, or tea of black current leaves.

The tea of the leaves of the birch tree is a wonderful remedy for rheumatism and gout; the same can be said of tea of commock [Ononis spinose], tea of scurvy grass and tea of veronica.

Tea of mouse ear [Hieracium pilosella], a little herb of powerful effect in all cases of gout taken regular before going to bed for some time every evening will cure even the worst cases.

Rush of blood to the head as well as painful menses and hysteric cramps will be cured by tea of rue.

How Nature Cures

by Ludwig Staden

The Kneipp Water Cure Monthly, I (7), 126. (1900)

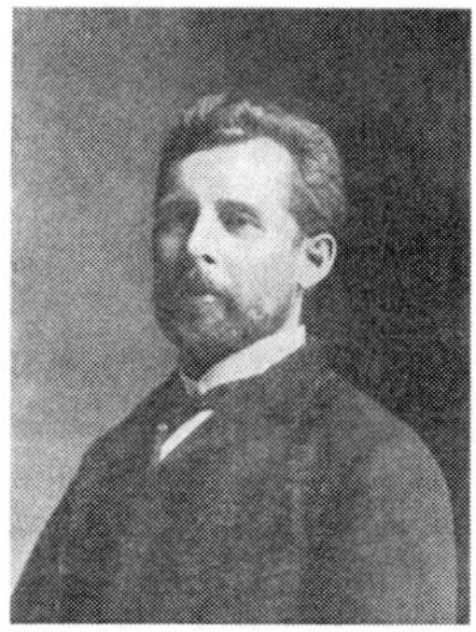

Ludwig Staden

With just a little knowledge, how easy it is to "Press the Button" of Mother Nature and "Let her do the rest".

Her ways are so simple and harmonious that people are confounded by her very simplicity. Besides, her remedies do not cost enough money to make sufficient impression upon the minds of the ignorant (?) intellectualists.

To give an example, and contrast the methods of Mother Nature with those of pure intellectualism, I will give the details of a case which recently came under my notice.

Some weeks ago, Mr. B. of Westport, Connecticut requested me to attend his four years old child who was suffering intensively, and whose case evidently puzzled the physicians.

On May 6th, upon my arrival at the home of Mr. B., I found the little boy, lying upon his left side, both legs drawn up, (he could not straighten them out,) the knee of one leg and his thigh considerably swollen.

The gentlest touch upon the arms and hands caused him intense pain and the little fellow cried pitiably night and day, his suffering was so extreme. He slept very little and had more or less fever. The entire body, even the eye lids were covered with red and yellow spots and little ulcers of a scrophulous nature. This was no doubt in my mind that the child was suffering from inflammatory rheumatism. In seven weeks, three doctors attended the child, two from Westport, and one from Norwalk, and not one of them told or seemed to know what ailed the child. After repeated questioning by the mother, one of the physicians told her it was a nervous trouble.

It was not the lack of medicine that the child's anguish continued, for the mother showed me about 2 dozen bottles of various medicines which the doctors had prescribed. Indeed, the more the child was dosed, the worse he became, until in despair they sent for a disciple of the Natural Method of Healing.

Immediately upon my arrival, after diagnosing the case I sent the father to the barn for a few handfuls of hay blossoms, and with this we made an infusion, giving the child a lukewarm bath. It was with great difficulty that we removed the little shirt and night gown of the child, his agony was so intense at the slightest touch. However, the moment we got him into the bath, his cries ceased, and after a few moments he began to talk and ask questions about the bath. After the bath, he was put in a wet pack of the same infusion and to the astonishment of the parents and the delight of all, the child fell into a calm quiet sleep. He slept about an hour; (the first quiet sleep he had had in a long time). Immediately he awoke, we removed him from the burning hot pack, put him into the bath again, (the water having become considerably cooler) about 80° F/27° C.

By this time the child was as lively as a young duck; indeed after the bath, he would not return to bed, but insisted upon sitting on his father's lap and having his dinner. His appetite was good, eating spinach, potatoes, strawberries, a piece of bread and butter and a piece of light cake. The parents were nearly dumb-founded at the quick and radical change in the child's condition, and all look of care and anxiety vanished from their faces as the child regained his natural condition.

As I left in the evening, the little fellow shook hands with me (the hands I could not touch in the morning, without causing intense agony). He looked bright and looked up at me, as much to say, "You need not come again for you have showed me my true Mama (Mother Nature)."

Neither was it necessary for me to pay another visit. I left directions to the parents for the continued treatment of abdominal bandages, and injections. I insisted upon a vegetable diet, with fruit and milk but no medicine whatsoever.

A week later, the child played on the street as usual.

The gentlest touch upon the arms and hands caused him intense pain and the little fellow cried pitiably night and day, his suffering was so extreme.

Immediately upon my arrival, after diagnosing the case I sent the father to the barn for a few handfuls of hay blossoms, and with this we made an infusion, giving the child a lukewarm bath.

My Medicinal Herbs

by Sebastian Kneipp

The Kneipp Water Cure Monthly, I (8), 143-144. (1900)

It is certainly not a very hard task to keep everything in readiness and so avoid the usual heedless confusion.

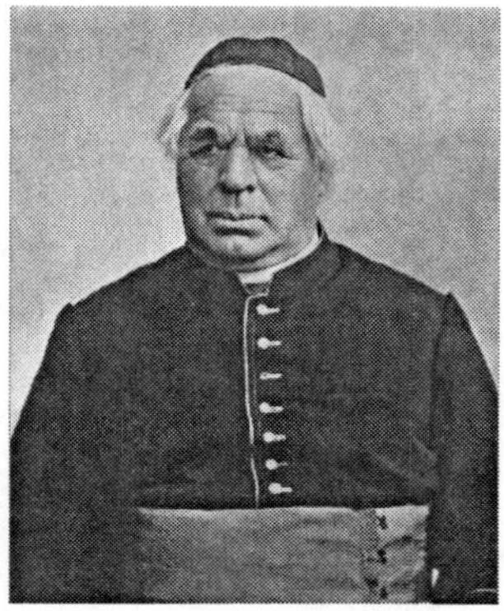

Father Sebastian Kneipp (1821-1897)

Most of my medicinal herbs are easy to recognize and many people will doubtless have taken the trouble to furnish for themselves a sort of chemist's shop containing the herbs they have personally collected.

Many herbs can be reared as decorative [indoor] plants or they may be planted and grown in little gardens. For the rest, it is not difficult if one has a room at one's command in the garden to plant and tend many medicinal herbs. There are some, however, which will not prosper and thrive in a garden because the conditions of the ground are not favorable to all plants alike.

The dear God has so well cared for that every plant should have its appointed place where it can best grow. I will enlarge on this and indicate also where the herbs I recommend may be found and when they blossom and should be plucked.

Absinthe or wormwood is generally cultivated in gardens but it grows also in uncultivated places. Flowering season: July and August.

Aloe (*Agave americana*) grows wild in Mexico and Italy; with us it thrives in hot houses where after many years it blossoms. Its flowering season is June.

Aloe vulgaris may easily be grown as a room plant; its flowering time in Southern Europe is the month of June. This plant also grows wild in Southern Europe.

Angelica grows in damp meadows, on the edge of brooks and streams, ditches and moats, also in wet places in woodlands. It flowers from July to September.

Silverweed grows freely in the neighborhood of manure heaps. Flowering time: from May to July.

Arnica grows in meadows which are near woods; on mountains, damp places and especially in marshy meadows. The flowering time is June and July. The arnica blossoms are very easy to recognize. Nearly every part of the plant is usable. The leaves make a good tea for liver diseases, and from the roots one prepares the well-known tincture of arnica.

Dwarf elder root is usually found in damp rocky glens, in marshy woods, among ruins and in fields. Flowering time: July and August.

Eyebright is to be found in meadows, wooded glades, pastures, fields and moors. It blossoms from July to October.

Valerian grows in thin woods, on the edge of thickets, generally in rather damp places though it will grow in dry soil and on sparsely covered slopes. It flowers in June and July.

Bogbean, called also **marsh-trefoil**, is mostly found in marshes, on swampy, wet meadows and in meadow ditches. Flowering time: April and May.

Fenugreek is to be found everywhere; one sees cornfields over run with it. The seed is made into powder and called ***Foenum graecum***. The seed is excellent for dissolving swellings and gatherings. It flowers in June and July.

Water cresses are cultivated in many places but grow best near fountains and brooks. One may eat this plant also as a salad.

Blackthorn blossom is known to everyone. It flowers in April and May.

Gentian grows mostly in mountainous districts, on the Alps and Lower Alps, and specially thrives on calcareous soil. Time of flowering: July and August.

Strawberries (wild) grow in wooded glens and groves but are also cultivated in gardens. They flower from April to June and the blossoms may be collected in April or May.

Fennel is mostly cultivated, but it also grows wild on rocks and stony slopes. It flowers from July to September.

Broom grows on very dry, fruitful soil in woods, or on the borders of the same. It is a bristly weed and somewhat larger than the heath herb. The plant is used to make tea for gravel and stone diseases.

Ground ivy grows in somewhat damp grass plots, in woods, bushes and on damp fields and gardens. It blooms in April and May and in some places until the autumn.

Briar hips or sweet briar is to be found in districts on the borders of woods and hedges. The flowering time is June. The fruit may be taken in October.

Bilberries grow best in a sandy soil, in leafy as well as in pine and fir woods, on heaths and on moors. Blossoming time is May and June.

Shepherd's purse is a weed which grows everywhere, even on houses. It blooms nearly the whole year through.

Black elder is found all over Germany; it grows wild but is planted also in gardens, and country people grow large quantities of it near their houses. Time of blossoming: June and July. The blossoms make a sudorific tea (sweating).

Coltsfoot grows best in damp places, on roadside mounds, on stony plains and on loam soils. It blossoms from February to April. It is an excellent curative herb.

St. John's wort thrives on dry heaths, grassy plains and thin woods. It blooms in July and August. It differs from other St. John's herbs in its round stem and the two lines running up from the same.

Chamomile is pretty generally known and it grows readily on sandy soil and on all kinds of cultivated land. It blooms from May to July.

Lime tree blossoms are plucked in the months of June and July. The lime tree is peculiar to mountainous districts but may also be found planted elsewhere too.

Lungwort grows in shady leafy woods on all sorts of soil. It blossoms in March, April, and May.

Mallow flowers are plucked in July. In Germany the mallow is a cultivated garden plant.

Mistletoe is a parasitical plant and grows on old trees. Time of flowering: March and April. Mistletoe mixed with santala makes an astringent tea.

Peppermint is mostly cultivated in gardens. In Baden it grows wild and blooms from July to October. Its leaves are used for tea.

Pimpernel or beaver root is a cultivated plant and found both in gardens and in fields. It blooms in July and August and it acts very like fennel.

Bark of oak or Quercus is obtained from the young oak trees or boughs; it is used as an astringent.

Rue is a native of Southern Europe, cultivated by us in gardens and naturalized in sunny places. Blossoms in June and July.

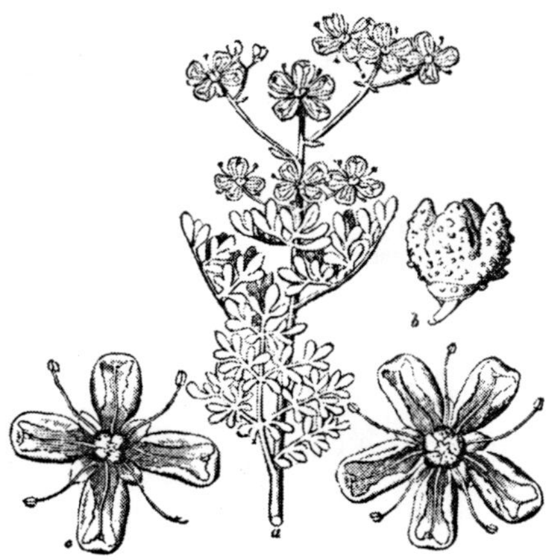

Rue (*Ruta graveolens*)

a. Stem, b. fruit, c. flower with 8 stamens, d. flower with 10 stamens.

Marigold is a native of Southern Europe and is cultivated by us. Time of flowering: July to September. Marigold salve is excellent for skin disease and marigold tea is very good.

Rosemary is cultivated by us in pots and gardens. It grows wild in Italy, Southern Switzerland and Tyrol. It blossoms in April and May.

Sage is cultivated in gardens but also grows wild on chalky hills. It blooms in June and July.

Yarrow thrives everywhere in meadows and grass plots and as a weed in the fields. Time of blooming: June to October.

Cowslips, (the perfumed) the opposite of the common ones grows in dry meadows and woody glades and grassy slopes and blossom in April and May.

Spikenard or lavender thrives on dry unfruitful mountain slopes but can be planted anywhere, and also grows wild here and there. From the plant, the so-called lavender oil is prepared. This oil is good for the stomach and is employed for the relief of epilepsy.

Ribwort is a very well-known plant; it grows in dry meadows on the sides of roads and in grass plots. It blooms from April to October. The extracted juice of ribwort is used for healing wounds.

Centaury is most excellent in its effects. It grows in sunny but not arid spots, especially in thin wooded places on sandy and light chalky soil, in fields and wooded pastures. It blooms in July and August.

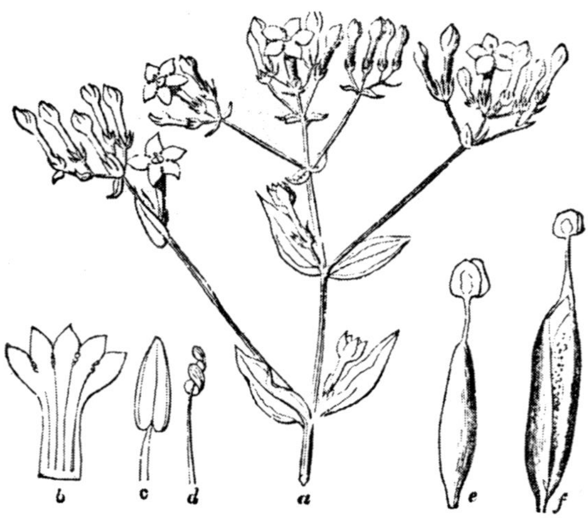

Centaury (*Erythraea centaurium*)

a. flowers, b. cut and unrolled flower, c. young stamen, d. old stamen, e. pistil, f. fruit.

Tormentilla root is found in damp places in the woods.

Bloodwort or fine crab grass, by which name this plant is known to the people, forms a good remedy for bleeding and the tincture is excellent for poverty of blood.

Violet everyone knows and who has not enjoyed its perfume? Not only does it refresh one's sense of smell, its leaves and blossoms are most useful as tea. It blossoms in March and April.

Knotgrass grows wild in paths, pastures and grass. It blossoms from July to the autumn. Knotgrass tea is most beneficial in kidney and bladder diseases.

Juniper berry, the fruit of the juniper shrub is an excellent remedy for the stomach and helpful to dropsical people. The bush grows in light woods of fir and pines and on mountain slopes, it is very well known. It blooms from April to May.

Mullein thrives on all kinds of soil and under all conditions, but it is most prolific on railway embankments. It blooms in July and August. The flowers are used as a tea for sweating and for a gargle.

Shavegrass grows wild on every kind of soil and is well known to the good housewife. The fruit time is March and April.

Gentian, either alone or with some other tea, is good for the stomach, but only a small portion must be taken, at most one gram, for it is sharp.

I have now said all that is most necessary to know about the plants and I desire earnestly that men should come to regard them with more honor than they have hitherto done. They have so much curative power; certainly our ancestors kept their health by the use of herbs and plants and knew no other medicines. To cure or prevent death no little herb has yet been found, for it does not grow; we are all destined to die once and to enjoy in Eternity the fruits of our labors.

—Kneipp, *My Will* *

---

*At this point I wish to draw attention to the book published by Jos. Koesel, publisher in Kempten, called *Father Kneipp's Plant-Atlas*; wherein the medicinal plants collectively mentioned in Kneipp's books are pictorially represented, true to nature and provided with clear and explanatory text, so that by it every novice is placed in a position, even without special botanical knowledge to seek for himself in field and wood the plants recommended by me, enabling him and his family to collect a small medicine chest for the carrying out of my prescriptions. This Atlas has appeared in two editions; the first edition, in ordinary clear print, contains twenty plates. Price: bound in cloth, $2. The second edition printed in colours contains forty-one plates. Price: bound in cloth $3.85. The *Plant-Atlas* has also appeared in French, Spanish, Bohemian, Polish, German, Hungarian and Dutch. —*Benedict Lust.*

1901

Care Of The Teeth

Benedict Lust

How To Heal Wounds Quickly By Natural Methods

Benedict Lust

Okic's Woerishofen Specialties.

OKIC' WOERISHOFEN GOUT CURE

is a remedy which cures rheumatism and gout without fail. It has been used with the same success in thousands of cases. The gout cure is prepared according to the theories of the late Rev. Father Kneipp and is no patent medicine. It is legally protected against imitation.

Large bottle, ... **$3.00**
Small " **2.00**

(Can only be sent by Express.)

TESTIMONIALS.

I suffered by gout for fully 14 years. Knobs formed on my hands and feet in the length of time which were very painful especially when the weather was about to change. On March 3rd, 1897, I was so bad that I had to seek my bed. The knees commenced to swell so much that my feet were stiff. The same took place with my hands. My fingers were swollen so much, that I was unable to make the slightest movement with them. My wife had to feed me like one would feed a baby. What pains I had to stand only one knows who has suffered by gout. I had to be carried on a linen sheet from one bed to the other. Such I spent 11 weeks. All remedies which I tried proved of no value to me, they were without effect. Then I heard that Mr. I. B. Okic, editor of the *Kneipp-Blätter* in Wörishofen, had invented an effective remedy for gout. I decided to try this one as a last resort and, what a surprise, the paines stopped 15 minutes after I had applied this remedy, I could move my fingers and use my hands to eat my breakfast the next morning. The same success I had with my feet after applying Okic's Gout Cure. The knobs and swellings disappeared and to-day I am as well as I ever expected to be. Nobody will think for one moment that I ever suffered by gout. I had spent a little fortune for remedies to cure gout without any success, the small amount I paid for Okic's Gout Cure brought the result looked for in a short time.

Wörishofen, July 14th, 1898.

Johann Georg Bader,
Proprietor of Restaurant "Krone".

I had the gout in my hands and feet. I tried every remedy and improved a little once in a while for a short time. Last winter I grew worse and worse, when a friend, who had spent the summer before in Wörishofen, advised me to give Okic's Wörishofen Gout Cure a trial. I did so and was cured. A little while after applying the remedy the paines ceased, the knobs disappeared and I could hope to get rid of this painful sickness. I recommend this remedy to all sufferers by gout or articular rheumatism.

Peter Bayerl, Tailor,
Weilheim, Bavaria.

Last week I treated one of my patients with Okic's Wörishofen Gout Cure. The effect was excellent. Inside of one hour the pains stopped and did not return so far. Now he is able to leave the room on crutches.

Milwaukee, Wis., November 15th, 1898.

C. Keintz,
Director of Dr. Rhode's Kneipp Sanitarium.

I recommended your Gout Cure to a friend of mine, Mr G., who ordered a bottle to try it. This gentlemen suffered by gout since a few years, and that so much that he had to stay in bed. I learned all about the Gout Cure in the *Kneipp-Blätter*, of which I am a subscriber. I applied the cure at the request of the patient and his wife, and according to your instructions. In 24 hours the gout was gone and my friend cured. Kindly send one bottle of your Gout Cure to Mr. J. B. in Ulm.

Hall, Württemberg, September 12th, 1898.

Rothmaier,
Bookkeeper, Royal States Prison.

OKIC' WOERISHOFEN MOSQUITO CURE.

Last summer an adherent of our system sent a communication to me, containing amongst others the following: I used your Tormentil-soap with the best success against the very fastidious and sometimes poisonous insect stings, therefore I should advise you to make similar experiments, and should they prove successful, it would be advisable to manufacture and put on the market a salve out of your soap."

I followed this advice and found that the above indication was thoroughly correct. I made experiments with other materials and arrived at the surprising result that the new stuff is a most valuable remedy for fresh wounds.

The **Mosquito Cure,** as I call my invention, will now be an indispensable companion for everybody. Principally for cyclists, tourists, and men working outdoors, who are greatly molested in the warm season by Mosquitoes and other insects the salve will be most useful. But of even more importance my invention will be as a remedy against wounds. Even a small wound is often the cause of blood poisoning and dead, then my salve will be a preservative. It is packed in plated tin boxes, nearly two inches long, and can be preserved for years. Along with each "Salve" a piece of English court-plaster and the directions for use are given. The extremely low price puts it within the reach of all. The "Salve" is patented in all civilized countries, every piece bearing on the inner envelope my name (Okic) as trade mark.

10 cents a piece, box of 5, 45 cents, postpaid.

Only Representative in the United States and Canada:

THE KNEIPP HEALTH STORE CO., *111 East 59th Street, New York.*

Wholesale and Retail. **Agents wanted.**

Products obtained from Wöerishofen, the home of Father Kneipp, were found in Benedict Lust's store, The Kneipp Health Store in New York City.

Care Of The Teeth

by Benedict Lust

The Kneipp Water Cure Monthly, II (9), 224. (1901)

To the teeth is assigned a very important part in the household of the human body: we use them for talking, and for masticating our food. For this reason we should pay great attention to their special care.

People with a faulty set of teeth or who have lost all their teeth by some cause or other can only talk very indistinctly, and are not able to pronounce some particular sounds at all.

If the food is not thoroughly masticated it cannot of course be thoroughly permeated by the saliva. The consequence is a bad digestion arising therefrom and the subsequent insufficient nutrition of the individual. From this it will be seen how necessary the care of the teeth really is.

For the maintenance of our teeth, cleanliness of the mouth is an important factor. The food remnants which get stuck between the teeth begin to putrefy sooner or later, if not removed at bedtime, causing not only a bad odor from the mouth but also attacking the teeth themselves and causing them to decay.

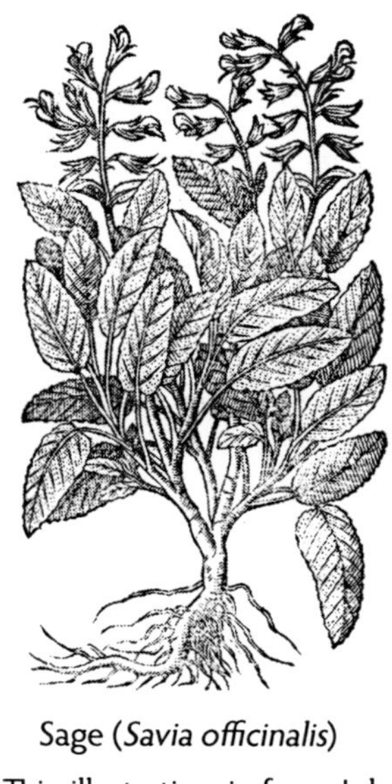

Sage (*Savia officinalis*)

This illustration is from John Gerard's *The herbal, or Generall historie of plantes* (1633).

To prevent this evil, one should never omit to wash out one's mouth after every meal, and especially before going to bed. However, the teeth should also be cared for and kept clean. All the innumerable tooth powders, advertised ever so much as the acme of perfection, are all deleterious to the teeth because they contain ingredients which are harmful to the enamel of the teeth, because they injure it more or less and thereby render the teeth more prone to decay. The very best tooth cleaning remedy is the common garden sage, i. e., its green leaves. Sage not only cleans the teeth but it also purifies the breath by removing bad smells from the mouth.

During the cold season, when fresh sage leaves are not to be obtained, you may take sage leaf powder and finely ground linden wood coal in equal parts, mix them well together and clean the teeth therewith. This powder does not hurt the enamel and purifies the mouth very nicely.

Wet bread crusts are also a very good although cheap tooth cleansing remedy.

The chewing daily of a few juniper berries is also very beneficent for the preservation of the teeth.

One of the best remedies for the preservation of the teeth is the hardening of the system by often repeated water applications, especially to the lower parts of the body, in order to regulate the blood circulation.

Persons who always have warm feet will never have any toothache.

Sage not only cleans the teeth but it also purifies the breath by removing the bad smell from the mouth.

The chewing daily of a few juniper berries is also very beneficent for the preservation of the teeth.

One of the best remedies for the preservation of the teeth is the hardening of the system by often repeated water applications, especially to the lower parts of the body, in order to regulate the blood circulation.

Persons who always have warm feet will never have any toothache.

How To Heal Wounds Quickly By Natural Means

by Benedict Lust

The Kneipp Water Cure Monthly, II (11), 300. (1901)

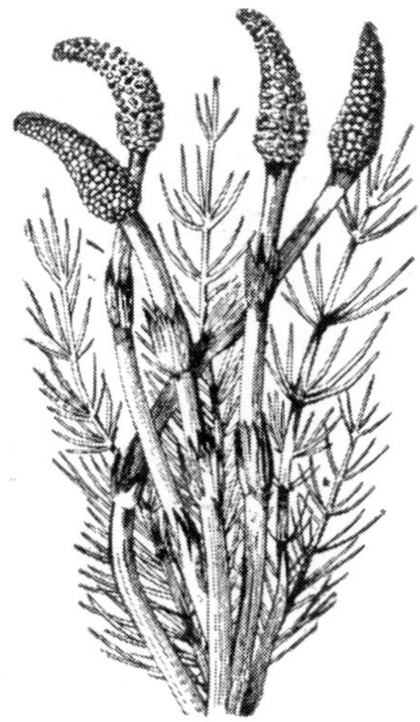

Shavegrass
(*Equisetum arvense*)

Wounds of a light or even a grave character are of frequent occurrence. The former ones heal up as a rule without needing any other aid except one's own natural healing power; but the latter need more or less aid in order to heal up perfectly and without any ill after effects. The greatest importance should be paid to keeping the wound perfectly clean.

One of the best of Nature's cleansers is a decoction of shavegrass. A daily ablution, mornings and evenings, with a shavegrass decoction is quite sufficient to keep any wound clean.

The healing act is accelerated by a decoction of arnica or tincture of arnica. The latter should be diluted with water, either in equal parts, or two parts of water to one part of tincture. Repeated applications of tincture of arnica, if undiluted, may cause arnica poisoning. Further healing remedies are: juice of ribwort, whey and coltsfoot.

To remove foreign bodies, i. e., small splinters, thorns, etc., one may apply Kneipp's *Pitch Plasters*, prepared from shoemakers' pitch and rosin. This plaster readily draws out all the foreign matter, and thereafter the wound should be treated as described above.

In case of larger wounds caused by bits of glass, large splinters, broken pieces of metal, etc., which are liable to cause blood-poisoning, the utmost care should be taken to remove these substances as quickly as possible. If there are any symptoms of blood-poisoning one should at once have recourse to hay flower compresses, or still better bathe the part of the body in question in a decoction of hay flowers. The latter should be very warm, as hot as the body can stand it. As soon as it cools off a second decoction should be ready, etc., etc. This should be continued until the pain gets less and the wounded place loses its peculiar bluish-red tinge. One may, as already said, apply hot hay flower compresses, but still the decoctions of hay flower are preferable.

The ensuing wound fever is best combated by repeated cool ablutions of the entire body.

One of the best of Nature's cleansers is a decoction of shavegrass. A daily ablution, mornings and evenings, with a shavegrass decoction is quite sufficient to keep any wound clean.

The healing act is accelerated by a decoction of arnica or tincture of arnica. The latter should be diluted with water, either in equal parts, or two parts of water to one part of tincture.

If there are any symptoms of blood-poisoning one should at once have recourse to hay flower compresses, or still better bathe the part of the body in question in a decoction of hay flowers.

1902

Kneipp's Popular Healing Remedies And Their Application

Benedict Lust

Kniepp's Apotheca

The Late Mgr. Sebastian Kniepp

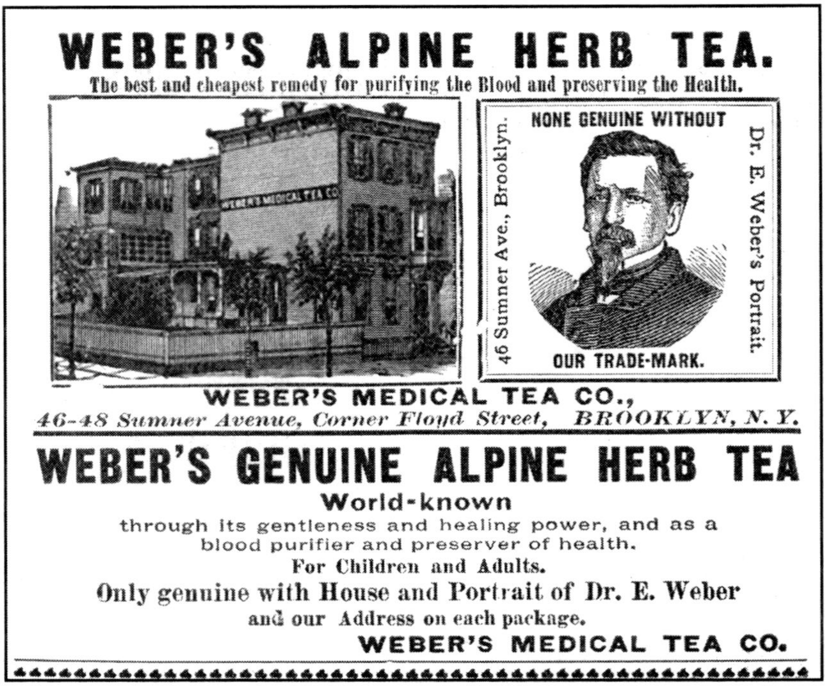

1901 advertisement in *The Kneipp Water Cure Monthly*.

Kneipp's Popular Healing Remedies And Their Application

by Benedict Lust

The Naturopath and Herald of Health, III (8), 348-349. (1902).

Eye Strengthening Remedies

As a general rule it is always advisable, in any case of accident or serious disease of the eyes, to consult a capable naturopathic physician; in slight cases, however, the following remedies will be found sufficient to meet the case in question:

1. Honey-water to purify and strengthen weak and sore eyes.

   Mode of preparation: 1 teaspoonful of pure honey is boiled in ½ pint of water for five minutes. After this has cooled, this honey-water is applied to the eye by dipping a linen cloth into the solution which is then gently pressed out and placed moist upon the eye; repeat as soon as the linen gets warm. The eyes may also be washed several times during the day with this solution.

2. Eyebright: Take as much of this tea as can be held between three fingertips, immerse in ½ pint of water, let it come to a boiling point two or three times, and then pass it through a cloth as sieve. This solution, when cold, may be applied the same as honey-water, it cleans the eyes and strengthens the eyesight.

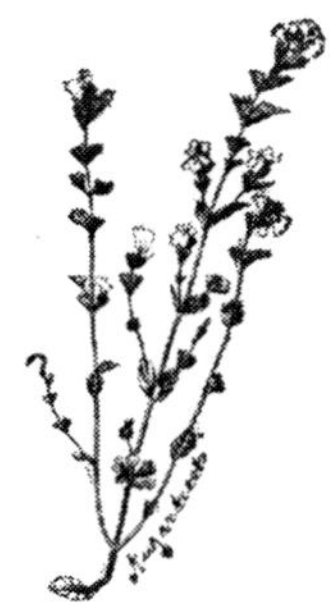

Eyebright
(*Euphrasia officinalis*)

3. For lachrymose (watering) eyes, a solution of aloe-water applied in connection with an internal depurative treatment is very good.

   Mode of preparation: 1 ounce of aloe powder is placed in a tumbler of water and ¼ of a pint of hot water (not too hot, else the tumbler will crack) should be well stirred into this. After all has dissolved, and the water has cooled off the eye should be bathed with this solution internally as well as externally—whenever practicable.

4. A very good eye-strengthening remedy is also made from fennel tea.

   Mode of preparation: Half a tablespoonful of fennel powder should be boiled in half a pint of water, but not long—and then strained through a linen cloth, left to cool off. With this fennel-water (when cold) wash the eyes repeatedly during the day.

For weak eyesight, Kneipp especially recommends repeated short cold water eye-baths.

Remedies For Healing Sores And Ulcers

Among some of the foremost remedies that may be nearly always applied with success may be counted the following: Alum, agave, lime-charcoal powder, sage and shavegrass, all of which have been often and successfully used by the old-school physicians and country doctors.

For the cleaning of wounds, and as decoctions for compresses may be used; alum-water (1 ounce of alum to 66 ounces of water) and agave-water (1 ounce of agave to 50 ounces of water) i. e., a large handful of either of these herbs is boiled for some time in a quart of water, which is then passed through a sieve. The compresses can better be borne cold than warm.

These four remedies are applied successfully for spongy, richly suppurating sores and ulcers, for old pus-containing wounds, painful leg—thigh and other sores, and here, the decoctions of sage and shavegrass are especially beneficial.

The new formation or new growth of the cuticle is accelerated by a sprinkling of agave powder over the sore and thereafter careful wrapping up to prevent contact of the air.

In especially bad cases of suppurating and bad-smelling ulcers, the new formation of the skin is stimulated by sprinkling lime-charcoal powder over the wound, which absorbs and dries the bad matter.

In mortifying, cancerous and lardaceous sores, as well as in caries of the bones, the old-school physicians used lint sprinkled with calamus root powder, which was moistened with a little spirit of wine and placed upon the wound, and this was repeated two or three times a day. In cases of acute sores accompanied by fever, leaves of coltsfoot deaden the pain considerably. Kneipp's pomade of marigold may also be applied to advantage in these cases.

Gout Remedies

In those cases of gout which have been caused by foods containing too much rich and nitrogenous condiments and by a too plentiful absorption of heavy wines and beer, in conjunction with insufficient bodily exercise, the ordinary causes must first be combated.

In cases of so-called irregular or atonic gout, however, the patient should be well nourished—the latter case mostly befalls poor people who are very much exposed to the inclemencies of the weather and are nourished insufficiently and live perhaps in damp dwellings. Especially laborers, working either in or beneath the water, and having similar occupations, are great sufferers from this latter disease.

In cases where (common) gout has been caused by too rich a living, a corresponding diet should at once be observed, and the following articles must be completely eschewed: Eggs, cheese, legumes, heavy farinaceous foods, too rich and especially heavily spiced meats; then also: wine, beer, coffee, chocolate, spices of all kinds, sour fruit and acid foods.

In both forms of gout, however, those remedies which are depurative (blood purifying) and act upon the kidneys, are most to be recommended, to which, always considering the individual circumstances, gentle purgatives may be added.

Especially to be recommended are ground juniper berries, further dwarf elder, parsley, common nettle root; and there should be added from four to six tablespoonful of a mixture of the above remedies to a quart of water, and the lot be boiled until only ¾ of a quart remain.

This tea should be taken two or three times a week for some length of time.

The secretion of uric acid from the blood, which is most essential, is also greatly favored by drinking for some length of time daily one to two cups of tea made from a decoction of ground juniper berries, shavegrass and knotgrass, to which finally, some wormwood should be added. This tea must be taken on an empty stomach in the morning, and warm; and also in the evening, several cups at bed time.

For outward appliance in gout, I would recommend rubbing the joints with oil of camphor; the very best of results, however, may be derived from warm hay flower compresses round the joints. Another excellent remedy, which almost always gives great relief, is *Kneipp's Embrocation of Gout and Rheumatism*, which is rubbed into the sore joints.

Kneipp's Apotheca

by the late Mgr. Sebastian Kneipp

The Naturopath and Herald of Health, III (2), 384-386. (1902)

Among all the things which I abhor and hate, the proprietary drugs, the trading with remedies which are kept as a secret by their inventors, hold a prominent place.

No one shall ever reproach me with such a thing. Therefore, in this second part, I open all the drawers and cases of my apotheca and let everyone look into them even to the last little tea-box and the smallest oil bottle.

Every druggist's shop contains a great many expensive things; but in mine, there is not much of the extraordinary to be found. This I own quite willingly, and instead of a defect, I consider it a great recommendation for my apotheca.

Nearly all my teas, extracts, oils and powders are prepared from medical herbs which are to be had for a trifle, and which our dear Lord has planted in our own garden, in the fields, many of them around our houses, many on remote, unfrequented spots, so that we can gather them free of cost.

I have written my little book first of all for poor sick people, for whose benefit, keeping before my eyes the heavenly reward. I also carry on this troublesome business, or, if you like to put it so, to spoil other people's trade. It was for them that I purposely inquired after the likewise poor old acquaintances, the herbs setting aside many things. For long years I have examined and experimented, dried and cut up, boiled and tasted. There is not one little herb or powder, which I have not myself tried and found good. My only wish is that my old acquaintances may be respected again, at least by one class of people, the poor.

I have long deliberated before I resolved to add this apotheca to the applications of water, which in themselves are sufficient, lest these remedies which assist the water by acting inwardly, could be looked upon as a vote of mistrust in the water.

But there are patients who, from unconquerable fear of water, would have great difficulty in resolving to make a course of water applications, often necessary for some considerable time. I wished to facilitate the cure for them, in other words, to reduce the water applications, to simplify them, and shorten their duration. This can and will be done by giving assistance to the exterior cure (with water) by an interior cure (with remedies).

Those who inspect all the articles of my apotheca will see at once that they, like the water applications themselves, have a threefold aim, i. e., to dissolve morbid matters in the interior, to evacuate them and then to strengthen the organism. Regarding this, I believe I may justly affirm that both cures, the interior and the exterior, harmonize and work together with perfect unity. I caution people against an illusion.

Whoever thinks that the water applications ought to be used very rigidly and harshly is mistaken.

Whoever is of the opinion that he ought to use interior remedies often and in great quantities, is likewise mistaken. Always and in all cases, keep to the golden principle: the gentlest application, be it exterior or interior is the best.*

Plants with doubtful effects, like althea, licorice wood, etc., with the least unfavorable effects, e.g., on the stomach, like senna leaves, hops, etc., above all, poisonous plants, I have put aside on principle.**

How good is God! I cannot help saying it from my heart. He not only makes the earth, He brings forth all that is necessary for the support of life, for our daily bread. He, who in His infinite wisdom has created everything according to measure, number and weight, makes in His paternal love numberless little herbs spring up from the earth in order to bring comfort to man in days of sickness, mitigation and healing to his body convulsed with pain.

How good is God! Oh, that we could recognize it! Let us search for the little herbs, which announced themselves by the smelling bottles attached to them by the Creator, the aromatic wholesome scent; and let us, when gathering them, glorify with filial gratitude our infinitely loving Father, who is in Heaven!

Our house apotheca must consist of four chief divisions, and some smaller compartments.

In the four chief divisions we put the extracts, different teas, powders

---

*Editorial by Kneipp: There are many patients who think that a great number of medicines, pills, etc., must cure them. I remember well a very able physician who ordered as little medicines as possible, and often complained of the foolishness of persons who, against the verdict of the physician, are always crying out for medicines. "When such intolerable fools came and tormented me," he once said, "I gave them pills made of bread with a small, indifferent mixture, simply to give them the smell of chemistry. They took the pills, and when I saw them again, I was sure to learn that these pills, the best they had taken in all their life, had cured them."

**Editorial note by Kneipp*:* One word about sweets and dainties. When I hear of men, tending to such childish things, it makes me feel quite annoyed; if I hear the same of children I pity the poor creatures, and deplore the shortsightedness or want of watchfulness of the parents. To offer such things to a sick person would be an inexcusable offence. I absolutely and decidedly condemn all these dainties, whatever their name or reputation may be! The stomach and other parts can be entirely ruined by them.

and oils. In the smaller compartments everything not belonging to one of the said four divisions, is to be arranged in good order. Also the linen pieces for bandages (always clean and fresh), the cotton wool, etc., may be put in one of the smaller compartments.

The extracts and oil must be kept in bottles; the different teas and powders either in strong paper bags or, which is better, in boxes. (If you order new ones, let them be oval and proportionate, though of different sizes. And put them in ranks like soldiers.) This makes the apotheca a pleasure to look at and gives it a good appearance and that is due to it, too. Keep all in cool but not damp place (to prevent moldering), and not in a remote part of the house.

Every bottle, every box, or paper bag must have the name of its contents written very legibly on it. The best way is to put the different medicines of every division in an alphabetic order.

Above all, great order is to be kept in the apotheca. Any one going to it for the first time, must be able to find in a moment every bottle, every tea, etc. Moreover, great cleanliness is required. There must never be found, I will not say a layer of dust, but not even an atom of it on any box; there must not be any stain of dirt or oil hanging down like carelessly combed hair on any bottle, not even on the oil bottle.

Nothing is more dishonorable to a house than uncleanliness. Mark well as a rule; the estimation of a house rests on the condition of two things. If those things are in good order, the conclusion is that everything else is in order, too. If the contrary is the case, a less favorable judgment of the inhabitants of the house must be given.

Will you know what things I mean?

They are: apotheca and closet.

The best way to keep the apotheca in good order will be for the mother or a diligent son, or the most cleanly and orderly daughter to take the care and responsibility of it.

They will look upon it as a matter of honor to keep the strictest and most conscientious cleanliness, and will always have a duster close at hand. If they hold this office well, which will be a benefit to the whole house, to all its members, they may joyfully remember the words of our Savior: "Inasmuch as you have done it unto one of the least of my brethren, you have done it unto Me."

At the end of this second part, I have mentioned what should generally be found in such a small apotheca.* Do not keep unnecessary things; by and by one or the other remedy may be added.

Here I wish to say a word about the preparation of extracts, teas and powders.

---

* With every medicine it is precisely said in which form it may be used, whether as extract, powder, tea, oil, etc. —*Editorial note from Kneipp.*

Extracts

The interior virtues, the healing juices of a plant can be drawn out in various ways. We get the best and strongest in the real so-called extract.

It is prepared as follows:

> Choose from the herbs, berries, etc., of which you wish to get an extract, the very best, the ripest, the most perfect ones, and dry them on a wooden board in the open air, but (remember this well) always in the shade, never in the sun. The drying will show you which are not quite perfect for use.

After having well dried the herbs, berries, etc., cut them into pieces, if necessary, and put them in a bottle (wine bottle.) This is to be filled with real corn brandy—which I prefer to everything else—or, if you cannot get it, with pure spirit or other brandy, closed hermetically, and kept for some time on a moderately warm spot.*)

I have sometimes kept such bottles standing for a year and longer still; and only then poured off the juice of the herbs soaked with the spirit as extract. In case of necessity, you may use it even if it has only been mixed a few days before.

The extracts are taken by drops, in some cases (it is always expressly said) a teaspoonful is given as the smaller dose, and a tablespoonful as the greater one.

Teas

The weather being dry, you may perhaps on your way home from the fields, or when going out to look at your standing crops, take a ramble to gather here one medicinal herb, and there another. Those growing on dry ground or on the sunny hillside, are to be preferred; the plants gathered in their best blossom will bring you the most excellent, and in your sufferings the most beneficial fruit. Many of the herbs are growing in your meadow or kitchen garden, near your house or your barn. You need only show your ten-year old boy or your little girl what to do then you will not lose any time by gathering the herbs, and will give pleasure to your children.

The garden and field herbs are to be renewed every year, i. e., fresh ones gathered and the old ones thrown away.

Every mother knows how to prepare tea. For one cup she takes as much of the dried herbs as she can hold with three fingers, pours boiling

---

*All the herbs, berries, etc. used for extracts, may also be put in wine, as is said at the place relating to them. This wine, however, is only fit for immediate use, not for long keeping. —*Editorial from Kneipp.*

water into the little pan upon the tea leaves or blossoms, and lets it boil for some minutes, then she pours out the prepared tea.

Prepared in this way tea has the finest taste with the best aroma peculiar to every plant; but it is not the strongest tea.

In my own apotheca the herbs are really decocted for a longer time, thoroughly stewed, so that **not a particle of the healing power is lost, but all is caught in the water.**

How it is to be taken, either by cupfuls or spoonfuls, is said with every disease.

Powders

The powders are prepared by grinding, or by crushing in a mortar the dry roots, leaves, grains, or berries of the medicinal herbs.

Many patients find it easier to take the powders than the teas. The prescribed powder is strewn like a spice (pepper, cinnamon) on the food or mixed with a drink, so that the patient does not perceive it.

The vessels in which the different powders are preserved must be very carefully closed in order to prevent the dust from getting in.

Oils

The preparation of oils which are not bought at the druggists is specially given with every disease for which they are to be used.

It is precisely by the clean appearance of the oil bottles that the sense for order, cleanliness, etc., makes itself known.

For long years I have examined and experimented, dried and cut up, boiled and tasted. There is not one little herb or powder, which I have not myself tried and found good.

Those who inspect all the articles of my apotheca, will see at once that they, like the water applications themselves, have a threefold aim, i. e., to dissolve morbid matters in the interior, to evacuate them and then to strengthen the organism. Regarding this, I believe I may justly affirm that both cures, the interior and the exterior, harmonize and work together with perfect unity.

Whoever is of the opinion that he ought to use interior remedies often and in great quantities, is likewise mistaken. Always and in all cases, keep to the golden principle: the gentlest application, be it exterior or interior is the best.

Those [herbs] growing on dry ground or on the sunny hillside, are to be preferred; the plants gathered in their best blossom will bring you the most excellent, and in your sufferings the most beneficial fruit.

1903

Falling Out Of The Hair

Benedict Lust

Free Hair Food

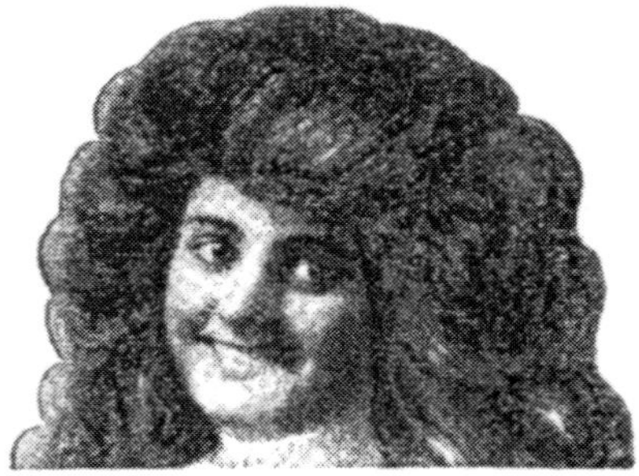

The ONLY WAY to tell the cause of falling hair in men and women is to make a MICROSCOPIC EXAMINATION of the hair. When the DISEASE is KNOWN the CURE CAN BE PRESCRIBED. Send a few hairs to Prof. J. H. Austin, the 30 years' Bacteriologist and Specialist in Diseases of the Hair, Skin and Scalp, and receive ABSOLUTELY FREE, a diagnosis of your case, a booklet on Care of Hair and Scalp and a box of the Remedy which he will prepare for you. Enclose 2 cent postage and write to-day

PROF. J. H. AUSTIN, 1238 McVicker's Bldg., Chicago, Ill.

LUXURIANT HAIR

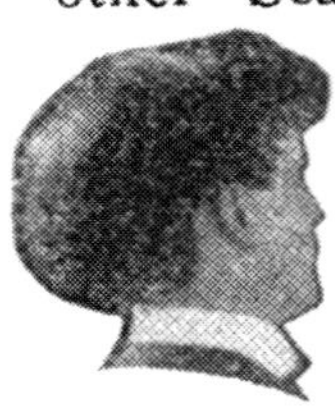

Freedom from Baldness, Falling Hair, Dandruff and other Scalp Ailments may be yours, if you will adopt the methods by which I saved my own hair. No drugs, Tonics, Torturous Exercises, Fasting, Dieting, or Fads. Full personal course, with personal letter advice, covering your special needs with my richly illustrated book, "HARMONY & HEALTH" all for $1.00. Results guaranteed. EARL WARD PEARCE, The Pearce Studio, Dept. 4, Los Angeles Cal., U. S. A.

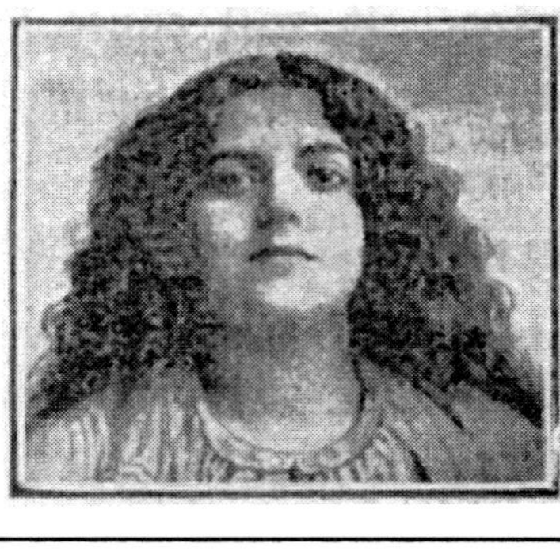

HAIR Like THIS

FREE Let me send you a remarkable treatment for Baldness, Dandruff, Gray Hair, etc., at my own expense. It will surprise and delight you. Write to-day to

WM. CHAS. KEENE, Pres't
LORRIMER INSTITUTE
DEPT. 3004, BALTIMORE, MD.

Falling Out Of The Hair

by Benedict Lust

The Naturopath and Herald of Health, IV (10), 301. (1903)

Father Kneipp's Nettle Hair Water And Nettle Hair Oil

Why the hair falls out is still an unsolved problem to all mankind; and yet there are very few diseases which are so much studied and for which there are so many remedies. Not only physicians but also druggists; not only do barbers and perfumery manufactures prepare remedies which they praise as being excellent; but almost every interested person has his waters or spices, his pomades or oils, which not only fail to give the desired success, but hasten the falling out of the beautiful gift of Nature, and in nearly every case affect the health.

Whence comes this disease? And what are the means of its proper treatment? This disease does not originate from microbes, nor from perspiration as many people erroneously believe. That would mean mistaking the product for the producer, as perspiration and microbes are products of the disease.

If one finds that his hair is falling out, he says: "My head perspires so much! I have so much dandruff and this makes it come out!" And then he goes to the druggist or barber asking what remedies they can recommend.

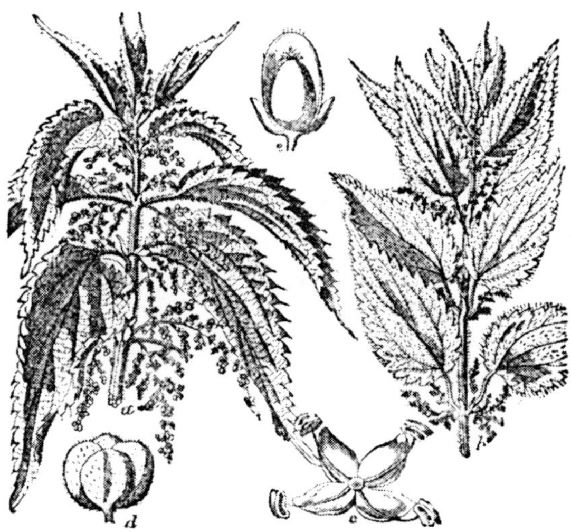

Nettle (*Urtica dioica*)

a. Male plant, b. female plant, c. male flower, d. female flower, e. female flower open.

The druggist or barber picks out a bottle from his closet and says: "This is the best in the market."

The customer buys it and pays for it, without noticing the bald head of his philanthropic furnisher.

His hair continues to fall out. It is time for us to say that the hair disappears owing to insufficient nourishment; the perspiration is not real because it is too greasy; it is the nourishment which is discharged through too widely opened pores.

The real question is how to prevent this discharge and at the same time to give the hair the lost nourishing substances and to contract the pores of the skin so that these substances can be better retained.

Father Kneipp recognized this fact and discovered the right medium. He found the substance in nettles, as they contain the producing properties for the hair. He extracted the oil as nourishment for the hair and uses the nettle-water as a preserve for it.

If both are applied at the same time—especially when the hair is short, as this facilitates the application and effect—the trouble will gradually disappear, and Father Kneipp will always be remembered as a benefactor.

1904

Knotgrass

Benedict Lust

THE PURE HERBAL REMEDIES

OF OUR GRANDMOTHERS

Kubara Tablets are composed entirely of pure herbs, that's all. Perfectly harmless, pleasant to eat, and absolutely free from any narcotics.

If you have a fullness in the stomach after meals, belching of gas or sour stomach, chew up a Kubara Tablet and swallow it, and the relief will be instantaneous.

Kubara Tablets sweeten the breath, prod the sluggish liver, relieve constipation and dyspepsia.

Kubara Tablets invigorate natural digestion, regulate palpitation, throbbing and bloating after meals. Headache caused by nervousness or a deranged stomach is relieved almost immediately. Kubara Tablets are made to be eaten, are palatable and perfectly harmless; can be used in conjunction with all Naturopathic treatments.

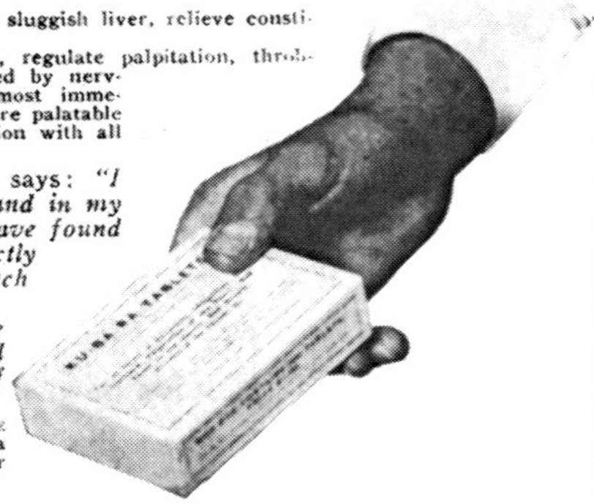

DR. CARR, *Columbus Medical Journal*, says: *"I have used Kubara Tablets in my family and in my practice for over twenty-two years, and have found them the most prompt, effective and perfectly harmless tablet ever devised for all stomach disorders."*

DR. LUST, your Editor, says: *"I have tested Kubara Tablets and can recommend them as a harmless herbal preparation of great practical value."*

Send ten cents to-day and mention THE NATUROPATH magazine, and we will send you a trial package Kubara Tablets postpaid, also our book, free, "How a Doctor Cured Himself."

ADDRESS:

KUBARA TABLET COMPANY, COLUMBUS, OHIO

Genuine Imported

Alpine Vegetable Soap.

—Made in Germany.—

This is one of the most hygienic and yet most agreeable scented soaps imported into this country. It was adopted with great success in the Kneipp-Institute, Hospital and Nursery at "Woerishofen", and is used in numerous Naturopathic Sanitaria and Institutes in Germany and many other foreign countries.

"Alpine Vegetable Soap" may not only be used as a toilet-soap, but also for all ordinary domestic purposes. Its ingredients are chosen and compounded with utmost care, and are mixed with essences of several medicinal herbs growing in the "Alps of Switzerland", which are recommended by the Very Rev. Father Kneipp for their curative properties. These also give to the soap its delicious lingering perfume which characterises it.

Impurities of the skin are entirely removed by the use of **"Alpine Vegetable Soap"**, giving it at the same time a brilliancy and freshness which is lasting.

"Alpine Vegetable Soap" is astonishingly effective for removing pimples, freckles and other skin impurities. Under action of this soap, the pores of the skin are opened and disinfected, thus removing the root of the impurities in question, and the skin is restored to its normal, healthy functions, at the same time contributing to the general improvement of the users health.

This soap is guaranteed to remove naturally all uncleanliness of the entire body.

"Alpine Vegetable Soap" is not like other toilet soaps, which attract the sight by their brilliant coloring and their artificial temporary perfume. It is put on the market in a simple and modest form. But after one trial only, every user will acknowledge that this soap covers most appreciable qualities under its comparatively plain exterior.

As there is practically no waste in the use of it, this peculiarity makes it lastingly superior to those, so-called, "Toilet-soaps" of similar size. For this reason it is practically a cheap soap.

Each cake of this soap bears the trade mark (L'arrisoir) Manufacturer & Exporter: F. Schulein, Kochel in Germany.

Price per single cake 25 Cents, with postage 30 Cents; price per box of 6 cakes $1.25, with postage $1.50.

Address all orders to:

BENEDICT LUST, 124 East 59th Street, New York.

Knotgrass

by Benedict Lust

The Naturopath and Herald of Health, V (6), 137. (1904)

From a lecture by Father Kneipp:

Knotgrass is one of the most excellent healing plants. It is of very great service for stones and diseases of the kidney and bladder. Although shavegrass is also very good remedy for bladder troubles, the application of knotgrass is to be preferred. In cases of stones in the kidneys and the bladder, it separates them into small particles so that they can be easily discharged.

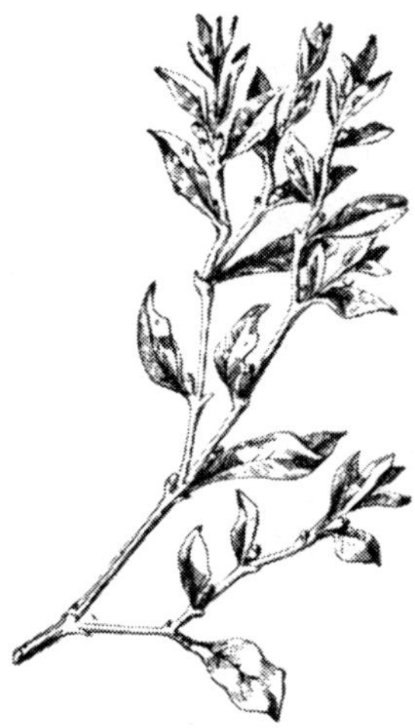

Knotgrass
(*Polygonum aviculare*)

Knotgrass is further very good for colic. If one has colic a cup of tea, from this herb, if taken as hot as possible, will at once give relief. Besides, knotgrass is a safe and effectual remedy for dysentery. In early ages it was much used for this terrible disease. It was cooked with a mixture of water and red wine (in equal parts) and was given to the patient as hot as he could stand it; the diarrhoea usually disappeared at once.

If a person has eaten anything which the stomach cannot digest, knotgrass will render splendid services. One cup of tea of this herb will put the weakened stomach into a normal condition.

It can also be applied with success in cases of poisoning caused by improper foods.

It is also very beneficial for irregularities of the liver. Diseases of the liver may be considered as among the most serious of complaints.

The tea of this plant opens the gall canals of the liver if they are closed, cleanses them, and puts this organ into good working order. People who suffer from ulcers of the stomach should use this tea. It destroys bad substances which may have accumulated in such a stomach and at the same time has a healing effect on the wounds. It can also be successfully applied for ulcer in the intestines.

This tea cures external as well as internal ulcers. The most excellent results have been obtained with old and external ulcers. Such wounds should be washed out with a decoction of knotgrass.

[Knotgrass] is of very great service for stones and diseases of the kidney and bladder. Although shavegrass is also very good remedy for bladder troubles, the application of knotgrass is to be preferred.

Besides, knotgrass is a safe and effectual remedy for dysentery. In early ages it was much used for this terrible disease. It was cooked with a mixture of water and red wine (in equal parts) and was given to the patient as hot as he could stand it; the diarrhoea usually disappeared at once.

If a person has eaten anything which the stomach cannot digest, knotgrass will render splendid services.

The tea of this plant opens the gall canals of the liver if they are closed, cleanses them, and puts this organ into good working order. People who suffer from ulcers of the stomach should use this tea.

1905

Birch Leaf Tea

Allopathic Thinking And Naturopathic Thinking

Father Kniepp's Curative Herbs, Angelica

Benedict Lust

Birch Mountain Tea

A Most Wonderful Discovery of Herbs on the Birch Mountains of Bohemia, which, when made into Simple Tea

Cures Consumption, Asthma, Catarrh and all Lung Diseases

So wonderfully efficacious has Birch Mountain Tea been in the cure of these terrible diseases in Europe that it has received the official endorsement of the Emperor of Austria, highest awards from Hygienic and International Expositions at Rome, Paris, Vienna, Florence, London and Liege; and the discoverer himself decorated with Papal Cross, by H. H. Pope Leo XIII.

Consumption is curable—can be cured, has been and is being cured every day of the year by the simple use of Birch Mountain Tea in the home.

This Tea having been brought to the attention of the President of the Amertcan Anti-Tuberculosis League, he, after satisfying himself of its great curative qualities, has requested an exhibit to be made at the annual convention, which was held at Atlantic City, June 1-4, 1907, before eminent physicians, mayors and governors. This alone speaks more than volumes of the virtue of this wonderful nature remedy. Package, $1. Literature on application.

Bohemian-American Herb Remedy Co.

BAYSIDE, N. Y.

BLACK-FOREST PINE AND FIR-TREE SPECIALTIES

RECOMMENDED BY NOTED AUTHORITIES

Black-Forest Pine Needle Extract, per bottle 30c Best Bath Supplement in cases of Rheumatism Scrofula, Nervous Prostration, etc.

Black-Forest Lohtannin Extract (containing Quebracho, Sumach Oak, Pine Extract.) Electri Baths. 30c. p. b.

Black-Forest Pine Needle Oil (pini sylvestris), p. b. 50c.; p. lb. $3.50.

Black-Forest Fir Needle Oil (pini pumilionis), p. b. 50c.; p. lb. $3.50.

For Massage, Inhalation and for general medical purposes.

Black-Forest Fir Ozone (Edeltanneduft), p. b. 25, 5[illegible] and 90c.

Disinfecting. Sick-, Sitting- and Bathroom Perfume.

Black-Forest Fir Wool in Sheets (Anti-Gout Wool), 50c. p. sheet.

For various medical purposes, also healthy material for stuffing cushions.

Black-Forest Pine Needle Oil Soap, 25c. p. cake.

Black Forest Pine Needle Extract Soap, $2.50 p. doz.

Used for most tender skin. Nothing superior.

Special prices for quantity lots. Correspondence solicited. Goods shipped C. O. D. if payment does not accompany order.

Guaranteed pure natural high-grade products under pure food and drugs act, June, 1906.

SOLE AGENTS:

Trute Brothers, 130-2 Pearl St., NewYork

European herbal teas and products were much favoured in the early 20th century.

Birch Leaf Tea

by Benedict Lust

The Naturopath and Herald of Health, VI (1), 7. (1905)

An Excellent Remedy For Kidney Diseases

Professor Dr. Winternitz writes about this remedy in his journal as follows: "Some time ago a young lady, Countess M. from Posen, came to my Sanitarium in Kaltenleutgeben. She told me she was seriously affected with kidney trouble and had been dropsical, that she had consulted the most celebrated specialists of Berlin and had tried all possible cures and medicines, but that she finally had been declared as incurable and had been given up. Then the manager of her estates brought her a certain kind of tea asking her to try it. This she did. She drank two, three and more cups of it daily and within a short time entirely recovered. According to a statement of the patient, the leaves of the birch trees must be collected in the spring. They are spread out in thin layers in a dry, airy, dark room and allowed to dry. As soon as they are thoroughly dried out, they are put in bags or boxes ready for use. For preparing one cup, take about 25 to 30 grams of leaves, pour 150 to 200 grams of boiling water over them, let it boil for a few moments and keep it 1 to 2 hours to steep in the infusion. Then strain the tea which is now ready for use. One can also prepare the whole daily portion (2 to 3 cups) at once and drink the strained tea at various times between meals cold or lukewarm. The tea has not a very strong, but a somewhat bitter taste." According to Professor Winternitz the effect of the birch leaf tea is a powerful one, without in any way stimulating the kidneys.

(Birch leaves are also sold at the Kneipp Store, 124 East 59th Street, New York City)*

. . . the leaves of the birch trees must be collected in the spring. They are spread out in thin layers in a dry, airy, dark room and allowed to dry.

For preparing one cup, take about 25 to 30 grams of leaves, pour 150 to 200 grams of boiling water over them, let it boil for a few moments and keep it 1 to 2 hours to steep in the infusion.

According to Professor Winternitz the effect of the birch leaf tea is a powerful one, without in any way stimulating the kidneys.

---

*At various time in his career, Benedict Lust occupied several dwellings that served as school, clinic and store. This was his second location in New York City, where he operated his school and a store selling Kneipp health products. —*Ed.*

Allopathic Thinking And Naturopathic Thinking

by Benedict Lust

The Naturopath and Herald of Health, VI (2), 36. (1905)

Many Allopaths are quite surprised when they observed occasionally that Naturopaths do sometimes think. They have the foolish idea that we do not do any thinking at all. The Naturopath makes his pack, that is all, with that he heals everything. Nowhere in the healing art is thinking more necessary than in our method of procedure. We should therefore not experiment. There is one point in which the difference in allopathic thinking and naturopathic thinking is observed, namely in the treatment of heart disease. The heart diseases are almost always treated with ice and *Digitalis* by the Allopaths, as I know myself other instances in a number of cases in which the Allopath did not even know that *Digitalis* causes a slowing of the heart beats, and accompanied by low temperature put the ice bag over the heart and are generally surprised when the patient gets worse. They do not think that cold applied to the slow-going heart cannot do less than enliven it. If we wish to strengthen a weak heart we can rub vigorously the locality of the heart with cold water until the skin reddens. Also give the body several times a day a treatment consisting of cold water ablutions, and a sponge bath, thus getting the blood out of the congested condition. The same we can do with hot food and health baths. I have always benefited a weak heart by the natural method of healing and not by injecting poisons into the system which only make the patient's condition worse.

Especially do the Allopaths like in lung diseases to give *Digitalis*. By applying packs and bandages we regulate the action of the heart. What injury the application of *Digitalis* can do I had recently the occasion to observe. In a small town, where no Naturopath is located an adherent to the natural method of healing, treated his sick wife who suffered from pneumonia, with packs. Everything went well. On the ninth day some weakness appeared and he called an allopathic physician; he gave *Digitalis*. After the first powder the woman became uneasy; after the second, her breathing became difficult because the heart was going too slow. She became blue, and vomited. With vigorous cold water ablutions, cold water washings and friction, the man brought his wife again to herself so far that she could stay out of bed. The slowing of the heart, however, kept on and respiration was difficult and the patient asked for help and her husband brought her to the Naturopathic Health Home, where she was perfectly cured.

Father Kneipp's Curative Herbs, Angelica

by Benedict Lust

The Naturopath and Herald of Health, VI (6), 164-165. (1905)

> "The Lord makes the herbs grow, and whoever has common sense does not despise them." Sirach, 38, 4.

For this favorite curative herb people have various names as angel's root, aerial root and so forth. This plant has large, radical leaves; greenish-reddish, many-flowered, fastigiated umbels, and a thick root-stalk, which is grey-brown outside and white inside. The angelica favors the neighborhood of brooks where its roots may be permeated with humidity; it is also met with on meadows which are not too sour, and on forest soil where the trees have been cut down, but where grass and shrubs are still growing. The stalk is hollow, and reaches a height of 1½ or 2 meters. Boys are fond of these stalks, of which they make whistles. Many a wise housekeeper in country districts gather these roots, take them home, cut them into small pieces, dry them in the air, and preserve them. Then if anybody in the house should be overtaken by cramps, she will prepare a strong tea out of these roots and the disturbance in the stomach will be cured.

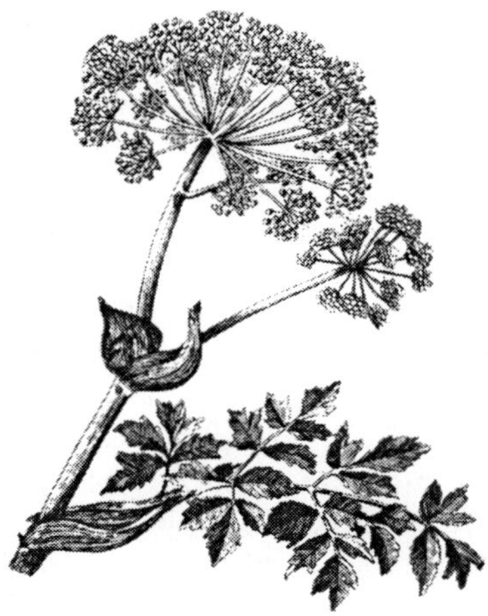

Angelica (*Angelica silvestris*)

This tea is an excellent remedy for gripe and indigestion. In olden times this root was believed to be a preventive against the plague. The nurses who had to attend these patients used to chew it to ward off contagion, or carry it on their persons as a disinfectant against noxious exhalations.

Angelica root cleanses the stomach, expels all impure matter, dissolves accumulated gases, and is an excellent antidote against decayed or half-poisoned food. It will also prove useful in cases of congestions, whether of the throat, the windpipe, or in the whole body; it will clear any obstructions of phlegm and cure headaches, if caused by indigestion. Many diseases may be traced to poor circulation of the blood; this, too, will be regulated by this root. On account of all these good qualities we ought to take pains to gather and prepare the angelica root; the more so, as the druggists do not carry it any longer.

Not only tea, but powder may be made out of this root; this is very convenient for use on journeys, as it may be carried in a little box in the waist-pocket. All who, in the course of their business or occupation have to inhale impure air should take a pinch of this powder; its aroma will warm the stomach. As it promotes digestion it would be wise to throw a knife-point-full of the powder on the food. The tea is best taken three times a day; that is, one cup full in three portions.

Not only powder and tea may be made from this root, but also tincture or drops. For this purpose the roots are cut into small pieces and put into a glass up to one third part of it, while the remaining space is filled with the best spirits of wine. If left to stand for a few days, the finest tincture will be produced.

The cases to be treated by this herb have been already mentioned. No one who takes too much need be frightened, for the greatest evil that will befall him, may be a too free excretion, and this never does any harm. In cases of poisoning, life will be saved by taking one spoonful of angelica tincture in three or four spoonful of water; instant relief will be given.

All these qualities will make angelica root valuable. The best time to gather it is in the beginning or middle of August, before the meadows are mowed. Roots, leaves and seeds are alike useful. The seed, ground to powder, is as good as that gained from the roots. This fact has to be borne in mind: the kernel is the finest, the root the sharpest, and the leaves and blossoms are the weakest parts. Of course it is important that those who gather these plants, should know them accurately; else they may take herbs similar in appearance but altogether different in the qualities and effects.

The French, famous as cooks and confectioners, preserve the tender stalks and roots in sugar, like other fruits or berries; and they are said to be great dainties.

Angelica root cleanses the stomach, expels all impure matter, dissolves accumulated gases, and is an excellent antidote against decayed or half-poisoned food. It will also prove useful in cases of congestions, whether of the throat, the windpipe, or in the whole body; it will clear any obstructions of phlegm and cure headaches, if caused by indigestion. Many diseases may be traced to poor circulation of the blood; this, too, will be regulated by this root.

In cases of poisoning, life will be saved by taking one spoonful of angelica tincture in three or four spoonful of water; instant relief will be given.

The best time to gather it is in the beginning or middle of August, before the meadows are mowed. Roots, leaves and seeds are alike useful. The seed, ground to powder, is as good as that gained from the roots. This fact has to be borne in mind: the kernel is the finest, the root the sharpest, and the leaves and blossoms are the weakest parts.

1906

Kniepp's Medicianal Herbs, Arnica Montana

The Effect Of Hay Flowers, Heublumen

Benedict Lust

KNEIPP'S MEDICAL HERBS, ARNICA MONTANA

by Benedict Lust

The Naturopath and Herald of Health, VII (1), 9-10. (1906)

The *Arnica montana* is of the most varied uses. It is especially found on mountains, fields, clearings, also on plains and near the border of forests where the wood has been cut down. In many, and wherever the arnica is in full bloom, the meadows glitter like gold. Of this plant, the root, stalk and flower are used. The stalk has least value; the best part consists of the flowers.

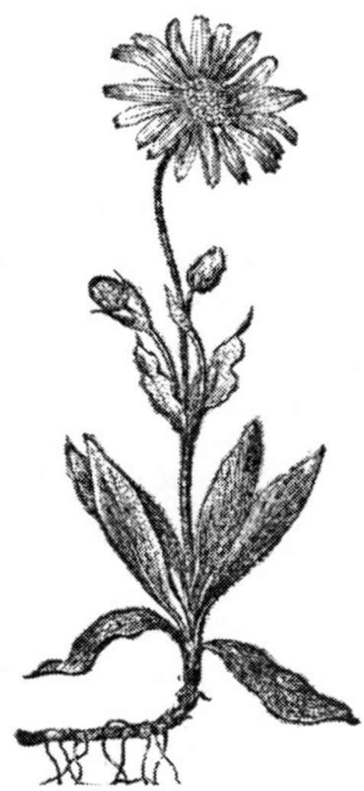

Arnica
or German Leopard's
bane (*Arnica montana)*

The curative power of this plant has long been known to physicians. The tincture prepared from arnica is of great value, well known to the common people, and continually applied to bruises and contusions.

Once, a girl had cut her finger to the bone on the bread machine. The surgeon advised sewing up the wound, but a plain woman insisted upon the application of arnica. Every particle of dust and dirt was removed, the flesh was pressed together as it had been before, covered with a wad which had been soaked in arnica, and then dressed with a linen rag. The pain subsided. Next morning the bandage was removed and the wound was closed; only a small streak, the trace of the cut, was visible. The wound was again moistened with a few drops of arnica and dressed with a wad and linen. For two days the bandage was not touched. On the third day it was opened to see if there was any formation of purulent matter; but the finger was in good order. It was dressed again in the same way, and after three more days the bandage was removed and the finger was completely healed.

I had another case. A horse had been kicked so violently by another horse that it had such swellings on one hind foot as to be unable to stand on it. The owner thought best to have it killed. Then a trial with arnica was made. The wound was washed with a mixture of arnica and water. This was repeated several times at short intervals, and the horse soon began to feel comfortable. These washes were repeated for several days and the horse's foot was healed.

Anything that is good, taken externally, must also be good internally. Arnica is good for stomach troubles and abscesses. In all cases, arnica has to be diluted with water. If taken internally, fifty to sixty drops should be taken diluted in half a pint of water, and then taken in small doses during the day. In colic, packs of arnica may be put on the abdomen. For this purpose, the whole plant with its root is boiled in water and vinegar.

But physicians have discarded this plant and replaced it by carbolic acid, a poison. Is not a harmless remedy of equal healing power preferable to a poison?

Tincture of arnica is thus prepared: the whole plant, with roots and flowers, is dried in an airy place, and put into a bottle. Alcohol is poured on it, and the bottle closed with a stopper. After letting it stand for a few days, it should be strained through a sieve. Arnica tincture thus prepared will keep for years.

A bottle of this tincture should always be at hand in every household.

The tincture prepared from arnica is of great value, well known to the common people, and continually applied to bruises and contusions.

Arnica is good for stomach troubles and abscesses. In all cases arnica has to be diluted with water. If taken internally, fifty to sixty drops should be taken diluted in half a pint of water, and then taken in small doses during the day.

In colic, packs of arnica may be put on the abdomen. For this purpose the whole plant with its root is boiled in water and vinegar.

Tincture of arnica is thus prepared: the whole plant, with roots and flowers, is dried in an airy place, and put into a bottle. Alcohol is poured on it, and the bottle closed with a stopper.

The Effect Of Hay Flowers, Heublumen

by Benedict Lust

The Naturopath and Herald of Health, VII (1), 40-41. (1906)

A well-known and very popular application recommended in Kneipp's works are hay flower compresses, hay flower shirts, as well as the addition of hay flowers to baths and steam baths. According to Kneipp, hay flowers are understood to be the waste products of hay and aftermath, such as stems, leaves, flowers and seeds, and even hay and aftermath themselves. This waste, which otherwise has no value and receives little attention, has been taken up as a healing power by Kneipp who esteems it very highly. Kneipp has been the pioneer of the treatment by herbs which had fallen into discredit. Kneipp has drawn the attention to the healing properties of many herbs which are frequently looked upon as weeds, and therefore useless. As he admits himself, he has experimented for a large number of years, has examined, tried and cut up, steamed and cooked them, and thus invented many useful remedies, and given us good ideas in regard to the usefulness of the different herbs.

Kneipp uses hay flowers for treating different diseases. However, he never uses them as an exclusive remedy but always in connection with water applications. In the first stages of blood poisoning, of frozen limbs, of symptoms of diseases of the abdomen, etc., scalded hay flowers have never failed to give relief. In rheumatism gout, scrofulous symptoms, wrappings and shirts that have been dipped in hot hay flower decoction, do excellent service. However, it would be useless to use hay flowers alone for such diseases.

The good effect of hay flowers has been frequently mentioned in this publication, and references have been made to many cures. We will add a few more cases which this excellent remedy has benefited.

1) Farmer D., in spreading manure, injured his left foot by treading on a manure fork. He paid little attention to the wound and covered it up without cleaning it thoroughly, as he should have done. The next day the wound caused some pain, the foot became swollen and inflammation of the sore part increased. Red stripes, inflammation of the lymph ducts, ascended to above the knee and the swollen glands of the hip joints caused a painful sensation on pressing them or moving. When the swelling and the pain further increased, the assistance of a physician was called. He ordered the leg to be wrapped to beyond the knee with scalded hay flowers, as hot as the patient could stand it, and left directions to renew this procedure as soon as the wrapping had cooled off. Only a few hours afterwards the pain had diminished considerably and the swelling of the leg commenced to decrease. The fever, which up to that time had reached a high stage, moderated.

On the sole of the foot a soft boil formed, which was cut, discharging matter in considerable quantities. After that the improvement by applications of wrappers, washings and baths was a rapid one. To keep the fever down several cold wrappings and washings of the entire body were used.

2) Mrs. G., while attending to the duties of her household, had inflicted a small injury to her right hand. The hand rapidly became swollen and caused considerable pain, which went as far as the armpit. As the swelling and pain greatly increased, a physician was consulted. The right hand as well as the right forearm up to the elbow were greatly swollen and had a dark red appearance. The pain was so severe that the woman had not slept for two days, and one night; her temperature being 124° F/51° C [sic]. The glands of the armpit were also swollen and very sensitive when touched. The arm was wrapped with scalded hay flowers and in a very few hours after this application, the pain had diminished. The swelling went down, and the fever disappeared gradually too. Around the injured part a swelling formed that discharged some matter later on.

3) Mrs. M., had injured her left little finger at the base while cutting ham and did not pay much attention to the slight wound. Several days after, however, she felt a peculiar burning and aching in the hand. It began to swell rapidly and gave her much discomfort. The physician called in prescribed wrappings with sublimate and when the inflammation continued up the forearm, he lanced it. When the symptoms of inflammation still continued and pain increased another physician was called, who was a Kneipp follower. He at once recommended the use of hay flower wrappers. After much persuasion, a trial was made and after they had been applied during the night Mrs. M. became quieted and the pain could be endured. After this favorable effect it was decided to continue the wrappings. The wound was protected by covering it with iodoform gauze. Matter discharged from the wound in the forearm in considerable quantity and then the healing process went on rapidly. A stiffness of the hand, which remained for some time, was finally overcome by hand baths and massage.

I have known many cases of less serious inflammation, which had been caused by infection, and in every case hay flower wrappings led to a decrease of the inflammation and the reduction of the swelling. The sooner the wrappings were applied the more effective they proved to be. The hay flowers must be put on as hot as one can stand them and in rather thick layers. This treatment must be a little inconvenient, and requires some perseverance, but when a favorable turn in the sickness can be expected, the relatives of the patient should be glad to do anything necessary.

WILL ALFALFA RENEW LIFE?

A Scientific Discovery of Importance to Every Seeker for Health and Beauty

How far will the wonderful Alfalfa Plant go in solving the mystery of life is the question scientists are now asking themselves. This marvelous plant has proven a wonder in building up tissues and nerve strength, rounding out the form, purifying the blood, stopping stomach, kidney and liver troubles and brain fag. Robinson's famous Alfalfa Nutrient gives you the very "soul" of the Alfalfa. Send 4 cts. for a 35-cent 10-day treatment of Alfalfa Nutrient with 56-page book, "Health and Beauty," to Alfalfa Chemical Co., 759 Unity Bldg., Chicago, Ill. It's a revelation. Also an exceptional money-making opportunity for agents.

How can we explain the effect of the hay flower wrappings? Hay flowers themselves are of no special value, unless they are scalded and applied hot. The continuous effect of the damp heat hastens the forming of the matter in the inflamed parts. The poisonous substances, which by accidental injuries have entered the blood, are thus made harmless and discharged. In the three cases mentioned above, it also caused a relatively quick formation of matter. After the breaking open and discharging of the matter the fever decreased and an improvement was at once observed. How far the aromatic properties of the hay flowers were responsible for the healing has not yet been fully ascertained. Dr. Martin asserts that they have an antiseptic effect.

This simple treatment after Kneipp's method has saved many and prevented many from being cripples for the rest of their lives. But, notwithstanding this success, medical science still ignores this simple remedy and prefers to resort to heroic, even though almost hopeless, operations because it refuses to condescend to use so simple a remedy, the beneficial effects of which science so far has not been able to explain.

A refreshing sponge bath will reduce any fever quicker than bottles full of drugs.

Kneipp has been the pioneer of the treatment by herbs which had fallen into discredit. Kneipp has drawn the attention to the healing properties of many herbs which are frequently looked upon as weeds, and therefore useless.

In the first stages of blood poisoning, of frozen limbs, of symptoms of diseases of the abdomen, etc., scalded hay flowers have never failed to give relief. In rheumatism gout, scrofulous symptoms, wrappings and shirts that have been dipped in hot hay-flower decoction, do excellent service.

I have known many cases of less serious inflammation, which had been caused by infection, and in every case hay flower wrappings led to a decrease of the inflammation and the reduction of the swelling.

The hay flowers must be put on as hot as one can stand them and in rather thick layers.

This simple treatment after Kneipp's method has saved many and prevented many from being cripples for the rest of their lives.

1907

Medicinal Virtues Of The Oak Tree

Timely Talks

Medicinal Virtues Of Shavegrass

Medicinal Virtues Of The Common Elder

Medicinal Virtues Of The Mint Plant

Medical Values Of Fennel

Bogbean, Menyanthus Trifoliate

Benedict Lust, N.D.

EFFICIENT AND TRUSTWORTHY

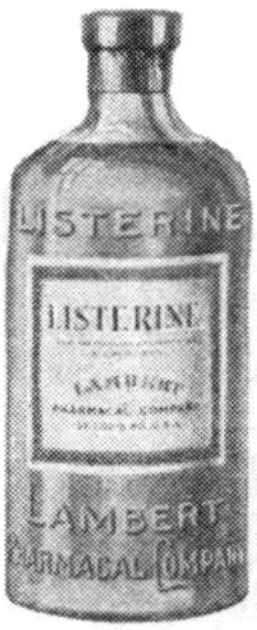

¶ As an efficient, non-toxic antiseptic of known and definite power, LISTERINE is unsurpassed. It is prepared in a convenient form for immediate use.

LISTERINE

is a saturated solution of boric acid, reinforced by the antiseptic properties of ozoniferous oils. It causes no irritation, even when applied to the most delicate tissues, nor does it coagulate serous albumen.

¶ It is generally accepted as the standard antiseptic for use where a poisonous or corrosive solution cannot be safely applied. LISTERINE may be freely and continuously used without prejudicial effect either by injection or spray, in all the natural cavities of the body.

¶ LISTERINE is advertised to the laity for the promotion of personal hygiene, and in case of accidents as "the best first aid until the doctor comes"—not as a *specific*, but as a *prophylactic*.

¶ The circular around the bottle warns against self-treatment of disease—even with LISTERINE.

¶ There is no possibility of poisonous effect through the absorption of LISTERINE.

Manufactured only by

LAMBERT PHARMACAL COMPANY, St. Louis, U. S. A.

Sagine WOLFRAM

"A Doubting Thomas"

"I have been with the best of physicians and several specialists, but no one could help me, consequently I have lost faith in doctors and their medicines. Now you claim that you have remedies which heal, where doctors fail—how can you explain this? I have suffered for years and have grown worse and worse."

This is very easy to explain. Most doctors don't believe themselves any longer in the medicine which they prescribe, and often give absolutely nothing. The remedies of the old school have proven to be worthless. Even today a lady sent us a label, where they had given her strychnine—rat poison.

SAGINE ANTISEPTIC is a pure Kräutermittel, made of herbs only, and as harmless as a weak tea, but *germs of disease cannot live in it.* Inflammation, swelling, pus and disgusting odor disappear very quickly after SAGINE ANTISEPTIC is used. Can anyone say this of any other preparation? Every day we are bringing proof that SAGINE HERB REMEDIES heal where the prescriptions of the doctors fail.

Sagine Antiseptic	$.50
Sagine Catarrh Remedy	1.00
Sagine Throat Chips	.10
Sagine Constipation Capsules	2.00
Wolfram Maltum	.25

SAGINE COMPANY
6-8-10 E. Chestnut St.
Columbus, Ohio

Top: Listerine, invented by Dr. Joseph Lawrence and Jordan Lambert in 1879 as an antiseptic for bad breath, contained four essential oils: eucalyptol, menthol, thymol, methyl salicylate. Below: Sagine, a pure herbal antiseptic from Germany claiming to be gentle and powerful, did not divulge its plant sources.

Medicinal Virtues Of The Oak Tree

by Benedict Lust, N.D.

The Naturopath and Herald of Health, VIII (3), 67. (1907)

Editor's Note: Each month the editor intends to take one of the various medicinal plants to be found in the Kneipp pharmacopeia and treat it in a popular way. By following these articles closely the student of Naturopathy will be able to become acquainted with the use of herb remedies in treating disease.

Quercus Sessiflora SM, Quercus Pedunculata EHRH*

The oak is the strongest of all trees. Often enough I have thought the single parts of the oak tree might be turned to good account for humanity; and I have attained the following results.

First of all, the fruits may be used. The acorns are roasted and ground for coffee, which is not only free from poison but rich in nourishing substance. This statement was proven by experimenting on a baby who had come to life seven weeks too early. I advised the mother to bring it up on acorn coffee with milk. And oh joy, the child grew up strong and healthy. Also adults, when run down in health, may be benefited by acorn coffee. I really am uncertain, if I shall prefer malt or acorn coffee.

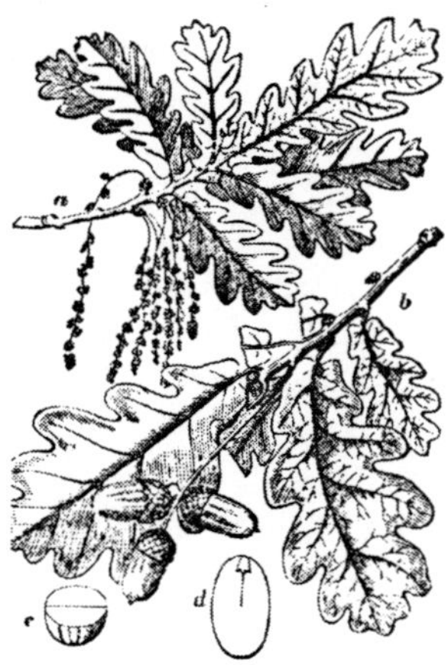

Oak (*Quercus pedunculata*)

a. Branch with male blossoms,
b. fruit bearing branch,
c. cross section of the germ,
d. germ cut lengthwise.

We may also make tea from the oak. This tea is prepared of acorns and is not only of value as a remedy, but also a nourishing food.

Tea prepared of oak leaves, may be recommended to people whose organism is totally run down. This tea has to be taken sparingly, that is, in the morning and in the evening, each time three tablespoons.

I tried the bark; of course, not the thick, old, brown one, but the young, fresh, green bark, which is of curative effect on the abdomen and on the rectum.

---

*These initials SM and EHRH appeared in the original text that refer to botanical authorities that coined the Latin naming of the different Oak subspecies. —*Ed.*

The tea of oak bark is to be recommended against goitre and swollen throats; it may be applied outside as well as inside. If applied externally, a cloth is wetted in the decoction and put around the throat. If used internally, from two to three teaspoons are taken in the morning and in the evening. As long as the goitre is not too hard, it may be cured by tea made of oak bark.

These throat ailments are often caused by too tight collars, which impede the circulation of the blood.

Once a sixteen year old girl, which had a slight enlargement of the thyroid gland, called on me. I prescribed poultices of a decoction of oak bark; but this failed to cure her. Then I had her take the tea internally; every day two or three teaspoons. Within three weeks the swelling had abated, and after two weeks more it had altogether disappeared. Oak bark has an astringent power. The tea contracts the organs and the water is forced out.

Once a gentleman called upon me, who by applying iodine, had within six weeks lost 75 pounds in weight. His blood was totally vitiated. He was treated with packs and washed of water and vinegar, and had to take every day two spoons of olive oil. He was fully restored to health.

Finally, I have tried the effects of oak sawdust. I have boiled it to a good brown broth; when fed to cows they will yield more milk. An ox, I had exclusively fed on oak sawdust, received a premium at a cattle exhibition.

Tea prepared of oak leaves, may be recommended to people whose organism is totally run down.

The tea of oak bark is to be recommended against goitre and swollen throats; it may be applied outside as well as inside.

Oak bark has an astringent power. The tea contracts the organs and the water is forced out.

---

*The title of the original article was "Healing Herbs From Nature's Laboratory". —*Ed.*

Timely Talks

by Benedict Lust, N.D.

The Naturopath and Herald of Health, VIII (4), 101-103. (1907)

The Advent Of Spring

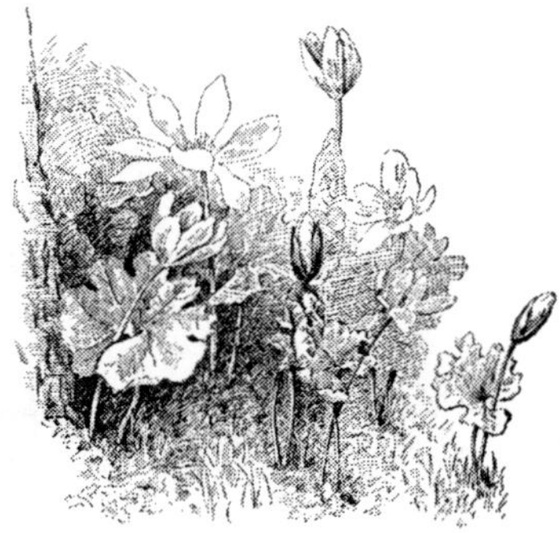

Bloodroot
(*Sanguinaria canadensis*)

And now cometh the goddess Eostra, mistress of the beautiful springtime*, and as she lifts her fairy wand, lo! The dark, dispiriting days, and the rough winds and the snow flurries of March are compelled to sullenly retreat and in their places are ushered in the soft south wind, the rare days of sunny stillness and the pleasant April showers! Many of the early harbingers of spring are already here. We can hear the noisy conclave of the blackbirds in the woods dinning the air with their hoarse yet welcome jargon, and here and there we catch sight of a stray robin or a bluebird bringing with it a message of warmer days. There is joy and gladness and awakening in the very air we breathe, in the songs of the birds, in the shouts of little children, in the mother soil and in the first burst of early blossoms at this time of the year. It is Nature's strange rebirth and God, Himself, the Great Creative Principle of Life, is stirring deep within the vast and depths of His own being.

The First Early Wild Flowers

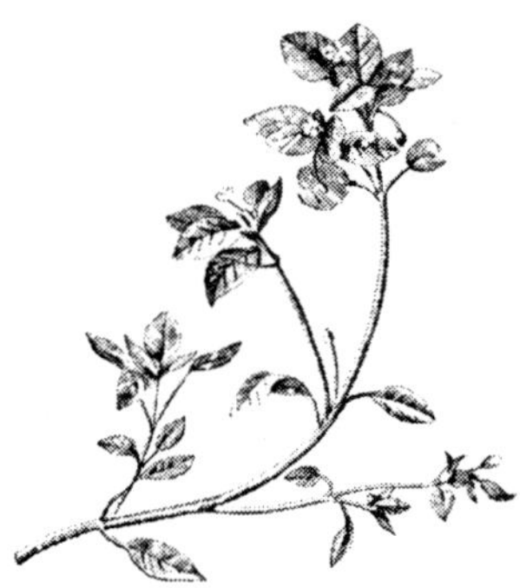

Chickweed (*Stellaria media*)

To the lover of Nature and of outdoor life, there are no more pleasurable days than these early days of springtime. Out where the little gurgling brook has commenced to sing its way once more among the rocks, the hepatica, earliest of our spring flowers, has put forth its tiny head, thrown back its silvery, furry hood and is beaming in the first warm sun of the year. If our fancy leads us to a stroll in the woods we will be able to find the lungwort, the silverweed, the trailing arbutus and

---

*Eostra or Ostara was the German Goddess of Spring. —*Ed.*

the dearly prized violet, and in the fields, so long covered with a shining white, we can find the hardy little dandelion, the shepherd's purse, the bloodroot, the twin-leaf [*Jeffersonia diphylla*], the marshmallows and the exquisite tiny blossoms of the chickweed and mouse ear [*Hieracium pilosella*]. Almost all of these *little friends*, who come to us by the grace of a Divine agency, come with a message of two-fold service to us. If we take the trouble to glance through the Kneipp pharmacopeia we will find that they are listed there as valuable herb medicines. The tiny yellow blossoms of the silverweed plant, though little known as a therapeutic agent, is one of the best remedies in cases of tetanus, and where promptly employed invariably results in a permanent cure of this trouble. The leaves of the common nettle possess healing properties that act beneficially upon the lungs and kidneys. The roots, dried and ground, are used in the form of a tea, and are excellent in the cases of dropsy. Cooked in water that has been slightly perfumed they make an excellent hair food. Marshmallow leaves and roots are dried and used largely as a tea in cases of chronic coughs and colds. The tiny blossoms of the shepherd's purse are used as a tincture in cases of blood hemorrhages, especially in hemorrhages of the stomach and lungs and in cases of profuse menstruation. The blossoms of the tiny mistle*are used for the same purpose. The blossoms and leaves of the chickweed, lungwort and sweet basil are valuable in cases of chest catarrh. The therapeutic value of the dandelion is too well known to need further reference here. The blossoms and leaves of the mouse ear are good in diseases of the liver, dropsy, gall stones, spleen, etc. And last, but not least of these, is the little violet, dearest of all the early spring flowers. The tea of dried, crushed violet blossoms is one of the best known remedies for whooping cough, and is excellent in cases of sick headache, head fever, hot blood to the head, asthma and consumption.

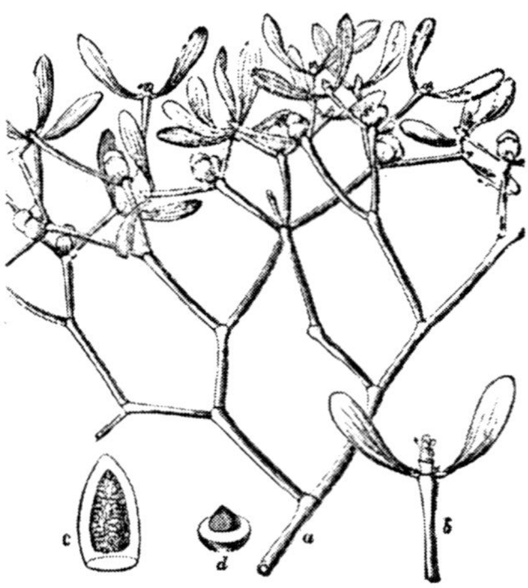

Mistletoe (*Viscum album*)

a. Branch, b. flower, c. seed, d. section of berry, smaller than its natural growth.

*Mistle is used in the original text and refers to mistletoe. —*Ed.*

If you prize early spring flowers, why not choose a sheltered, sunny spot of the garden, facing south and plant seeds of some of the early varieties. An early spring garden is certainly a garden of delight. The ground will soon be starred with a burst of exquisitely colored blossoms; crocuses, snowdrops, daffodils, pansies, violets, star-flowers, winter sweet, Jessamine [*Carolina jessamine]* and the bush honeysuckle; all of these are easily raised and you will be able to gather a bouquet of flowers very soon after the last snow disappears. And be assured they will give you as much pleasure as the choicest blossoms you can buy from the most expensive florist. The various spring catalogues of the seed men referred to in another part of this magazine will be of help to you in choosing your favorites.

Rebirth Of The Body

The same profound and mysterious creative force that is working outward constantly through all Nature and that seems to become quickened at the time of the year, operates within the body in the same strange and wonderful way. In every one of the millions of tiny, living, breathing, sentient cells that go to make up our bodies, a change is taking place. Cell activity and cell reproduction are going on more rapidly. Daughter cells are born in phenomenal numbers and the parent cells that sacrifice their lives in this process are being eliminated as fast as possible from the system. This explains the various s*pring ailments* so prevalent at this time of the year. Among those who are subject to these spring attacks there is a feeling of something wrong within the body and ill-defined, uncomfortable sensation and a feeling of weakness known best perhaps as *that tired feeling*. If the system is unable to eliminate properly, its dead cell matter and whatever other impurities there may be, the blood becomes surcharged with the poisons and an ailment sets in. Usually the symptoms are dull headache, slow blood circulation, dull eyes, tongue coated, appetite poor, constipation, extreme lethargy and mind and inactive life. This condition is further aggravated by the patient persisting on a winter diet of heavy, heating foodstuffs that the system neither desires, nor is capable of assimilating. Consequently most of the food eaten becomes waste matter in the system and very often becomes actual poison to the body.

The Spring Tonic

At this stage the real mischief usually begins, instead of intelligently assisting Nature in the wonderful process of renovating and rebuilding the body by adopting a restricted diet and employing such other natural methods as the occasion may require, the patient invariably goes to the corner druggist, buys one of the widely advertised patent medicine poisons labeled *Spring Tonic*, or perhaps something just as good which the druggist may have prepared in anticipation of the coming of just such fools as this one is, and foolishly takes the concoction, only to add another poison to a system already freighted with poisons of its own.

It is now universally known that patent medicines which brace up the system are for the most part composed of alcohol, and furthermore that the alcohol is of the cheapest and rankest kind. Most of them contain from 25% to 35% alcoholic spirits, whereas whiskey contains only 15% and beer 5%. The formula of some of the most widely advertised medicines on the market today is about as follows: flavoring matter, 5%, usually obtained from some varnish factory; coloring matter, 5%, usually burnt sugar; water, 65%, and to these are added the chief constituent of the medicine—alcohol, 25%. This fraud concoction is placed in bottles, attractively labeled, and wonderful metamorphosis, we have "Blood, Iron and Wine", "Nervine", "Vegetable Compound", etc., etc.

Spring Ailments Must Be Remedied By Natural Means

Not one of the patent medicines commonly advertised is of benefit in any cases of spring ailments. The alcohol in the medicine may stimulate the system momentarily, but that is all—and anyone who wants stimulation can, we should think, follow the example of the tippler who goes to the dram shop and there at least gets his *bracer* pure and undisguised by injurious coloring matter.

If we expect to avoid spring ailments, we must look to purifying our blood by simple, natural means. Almost any of the various herbs mentioned in the beginning of this article will be found effective for this purpose. Then, too, we must look to our diet and bathing habits. A most important thing in meeting the change within the system at this time of the year is to adopt a suitable diet. It must be remembered that the system now calls for less food. If we persist in eating the same heavy kind and quality of food as during the winter months we must expect that our system will become clogged, our spirits depressed and, as is very often the case that the poisons within the body will break out in disagreeable forms of skin eruption. On the other hand, if a carefully restricted diet is adhered to the body will be helped to accommodate itself to the changes going on among the cells, and none of the disagreeable symptoms due to a poisonous condition of the body will be evident.

Let us remember also that the system is in need of plenty of water at this time. There is no better and less expensive medicine for purifying and thinning the blood and cleansing the body internally than this inexpensive and invaluable therapeutic agent. In almost every instance as dull skin and poor complexion can be remedied by drinking plenty of pure water.

Therapeutic Value Of Fasting

Possibly the greatest help in keeping in good condition at springtime is a short fast. In the same way that clean people renovate their households in the spring, clean people ought to renovate their bodies for a brief time. Of course, the longer the fast is the purer the circulation of the blood will become, but in every instance the eyes become clearer, the skin fairer, the breath sweeter and the entire body improved in health. Fasting will likewise remove every possibility of pimples that are liable to break out on the skin at this time of the year. In fact, it is the simplest and most effective means of assisting the cellular life of the organism in reproducing new, large cells and in aerating, purifying and cleansing the system as a whole. If adopted in connection with other simple natural methods of keeping the body in health there will be no necessity for taking medicine of any kind at this time of the year.

The tiny yellow blossoms of the silverweed plant, though little known as a therapeutic agent, is one of the best remedies in cases of tetanus, and where promptly employed invariably results in a permanent cure of this trouble.

Nettle roots, dried and ground, are used in the form of a tea, and are excellent in the cases of dropsy. Cooked in water that has been slightly perfumed they make an excellent hair food.

The blossoms and leaves of the chickweed, lung wort and sweet basil are valuable in cases of chest catarrh.

The blossoms and leaves of the mouse ear are good in diseases of the liver, dropsy, gall stones, spleen, etc.

The tea of dried, crushed violet blossoms is one of the best known remedies for whooping cough, and is excellent in cases of sick headache, head fever, hot blood to the head, asthma and consumption.

Possibly the greatest help in keeping in good condition at springtime is a short fast.

HEALING HERBS FROM NATURE'S LABORATORY

BY THE EDITOR.

Editor's Note: Each month the editor intends to take up one of the various medicinal plants to be found in the Kneipp pharmocopeia and treat of it in a popular way. By following these articles closely the student of Naturopathy will be able to become acquainted with the use of herb remedies in treating disease.

Medicinal Virtues Of Shavegrass

by Benedict Lust, N.D.

The Naturopath and Herald of Health, VIII (5), 135. (1907)

This is the season of the year when you can go out into the open and gather the fertile stems of the shavegrass plant in almost every field and along the roadside. It is a matter of regret that this humble plant which is so easily procured is not better known and better appreciated in this country. In Germany, thanks to popular education along herbotherapy lines, shavegrass is one of the most popular of the Kneipp household remedies. It is used externally and internally. It is excellent as a cleansing solution in cases of old or putrid wounds, gangrenous ulcers, running sores and caries. In these cases, it serves in an extraordinary manner, in washing out, dissolving and burning out, as it were, the impurities that may exist in the wound.

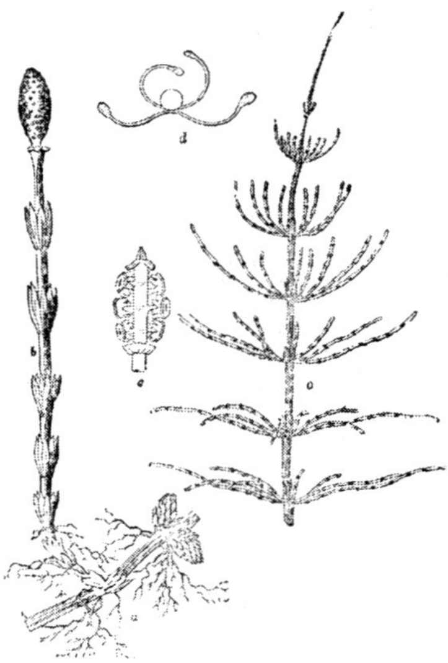

Shavegrass (*Equisetum arvense*)

a. root, b. fertile stem, c. cone, d. spore, e. upper part of the sterile stem.

Shavegrass can be used either in the form of a wash solution, or tea or for external application. If intended for the latter purpose it is made into a decoction and applied as an ablution or in connection with compresses, bandages, etc. It can also be applied in connection with a wet cloth in which a quantity of the shavegrass has been placed and this is laid over the wound or painful part.

Used as a vapor for inhaling purposes, shavegrass has a marvelous healing effect upon the lungs and throat and upon the inner membranes of the nose. It also clears the head effectively and for this reason is invaluable for relieving colds and catarrh in the head. Shavegrass vapor is likewise a complexion beautifier. It opens and cleans the pores of the skin and at the same time heals.

Used as a tea, shavegrass is even still more useful and we can only mention some of the uses to which it can be put in this direction. An occasional cupful will tend to purify the stomach and intestines and keep them in good condition. Taken daily, shavegrass tea will relieve urination ailments, kidney troubles and will ease pain in cases of stone and gravel disease. It is the best tea to be taken in cases of hemorrhage, blood vomiting and excessive menstruation. In instances of this kind one or two cups should be taken daily. I have had cases under my personal observation where profuse bleeding ceased entirely four or five minutes after the tea had been taken.

In cases of violent nasal bleeding, a decoction of the tea is snuffed up gently through the nostrils. The tea has the effect of contracting the blood vessels involved and it is only a matter of a few moments before the blood flow ceases.

I sincerely hope that every Naturopath will become interested enough in shavegrass to gather some of it and give it a trial. I have had illustrations made and they are presented on opposite page, so that the plant may be easily recognized when you go out to find it.

It is excellent as a cleansing solution in cases of old or putrid wounds, gangrenous ulcers, running sores and caries. In these cases it serves in an extraordinary manner, in washing out, dissolving and burning out, as it were, the impurities that may exist in the wound.

Used as a vapor for inhaling purposes, shavegrass has a marvelous healing effect upon the lungs and throat and upon the inner membranes of the nose. It also clears the head effectively and for this reason is invaluable for relieving colds and catarrh in the head.

It is the best tea to be taken in cases of hemorrhage, blood vomiting and excessive menstruation. In instances of this kind one or two cups should be taken daily. I have had cases under my personal observation where profuse bleeding ceased entirely four or five minutes after the tea had been taken.

MEDICINAL VIRTUES OF THE COMMON ELDER

by Benedict Lust, N.D.

The Naturopath and Herald of Health, VIII (7), 199. (1907)

In the good old days, in the eastern states, the elder bush was a typical part of every farm. It grew up alongside of the low stone walls that surrounded each farmer's property, in many instances completely hiding it, and lent a green, picturesque appearance to the place. To an extent, the elder bush can still be found on eastern farms, but it is not as frequently met with as in years gone by. The modern barbed wire fence has displaced the old stone wall and the elder bush has gone with it. Its growth seems limited now to the highways or byways and even here it is rooted up to make room for road improvements. It seems a pity that this plant is not valued more highly since every part of the elder bush, leaves, blossoms, berries, bark and roots are all efficacious or valuable as remedies.

Six or eight elder berry leaves, cut up into small pieces and allowed to boil like tea for about ten minutes, are an excellent spring remedy for purifying the blood. Take a cup each morning an hour before breakfast until the blood has been thoroughly cleansed of all impurities. The leaves can be dried and carried over until the winter when they will make an excellent tea for purifying purposes.

Elder flowers purify the blood in like manner. They can be gathered and dried and stored away as a valuable medicinal remedy during the winter months. In cases of colds, tea made from the flowers will induce proper perspiration thus assisting in removing the impurities.

Who has not eaten the delightful little suabian cube made with elderflowers as a principal ingredient.* It is said that these cubes are an excellent protection against ague and fevers. Elder root, prepared in the form of tea, is recognized as the most powerful medicament in dropsy [edema] known in the Kneipp pharmacopeia.

The berries, gathered in autumn, are usually boiled and eaten as porridge or marmalade. If people who travel great distances to undertake the *grape cure* would procure elder berries that are so easily procured, they would have a more effective and less expensive remedy than is found in eating grapes.

The berries, boiled down with sugar, or better still with honey, make an excellent syrup for all medicinal purposes. A spoonful stirred in a glass of water makes a splendid, cooling or refreshing drink, operating beneficially on the kidneys, lungs or other organs of the body.

---

*Refers to a historical region of southwest Germany and one of its famed confectionary from this district. —*Ed.*

An illustration of the elder plant is herewith given and I sincerely hope that this valuable plant will grow into esteem with the friends of herb therapy in this country.

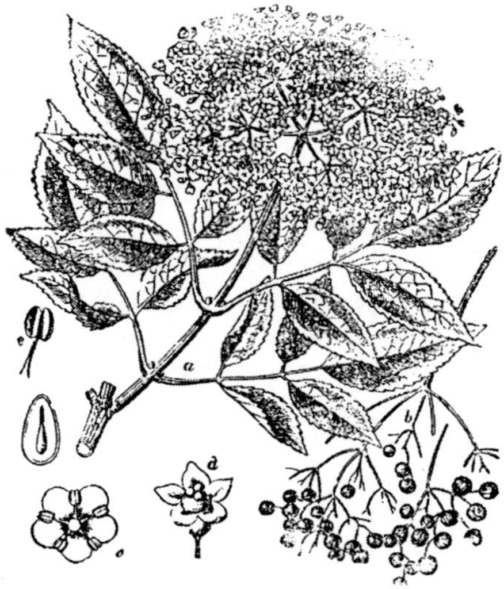

Elder (*Sambucus canadensis*)

Six or eight elder berry leaves, cut up into small pieces and allowed to boil like tea for about ten minutes, are an excellent spring remedy for purifying the blood. Take a cup each morning an hour before breakfast until the blood has been thoroughly cleansed of all impurities.

In cases of colds, tea made from the flowers will induce proper perspiration thus assisting in removing the impurities.

Elder root, prepared in the form of tea, is recognized as the most powerful medicament in dropsy [edema] known in the Kneipp pharmacopeia.

HEALING HERBS FROM NATURE'S LABORATORY

BY THE EDITOR.

Editor's Note: Each month the editor intends to take up one of the various medicinal plants to be found in the Kneipp pharmocopeia and treat of it in a popular way. By following these articles closely the student of Naturopathy will be able to become acquainted with the use of herb remedies in treating disease.

MEDICINAL VIRTUES OF THE MINT PLANT

by Benedict Lust, N.D.

The Naturopath and Herald of Health, VIII (8), 231. (1907)

MENTHA PIPERITA, L. AND MENTHA AQUATICA, L.

Peppermint and watermint are among the most delightful of all the pleasant plants in herbo-therapy. It is to be regretted that, like other common plants which the Creator has so liberally provided for the healing of diseases, we do not appreciate it enough to make it a valuable remedy. While both of these plants exert a similar beneficial influence upon the system, the watermint is usually preferred owing to the slightly stronger effects produced.

Mint is counted among the principal herb remedies for strengthening the stomach and assisting the digestion. A cupful of tea taken every morning and evening stimulates the digestive juices and purifies the blood so that a fresh, clear, healthy appearance is produced. In powder form, mint renders the same service if one or two pinches are taken daily in the food or in water. While of course, mint is a harmless and indeed, beneficial remedy we should always remember that other natural means must be taken to strengthen the system and restore the normal digestive functions.

In violent headache and in pain across the eyes relief and ease will be experienced immediately by binding mint across the forehead. Persons weakened by protracted illness, or who are seized with palpitations at the least disturbance to them, as well as in cases of nausea and frequent vomiting, will find relief by frequent use of mint tea and mint powder.

A preparation of mint tea prepared with equal parts of water and grape juice, using a cupful daily will remove bad breath and strengthen the entire system. Added to milk and sipped warm, it speedily removes abdominal pains. Mint decoction, prepared with vinegar, stops blood vomiting.

Let us see to it that this valuable little plant is not forgotten in planting the garden. It takes up small room, imparts a pleasing perfume about the place and person and is found handy as a simple home remedy.

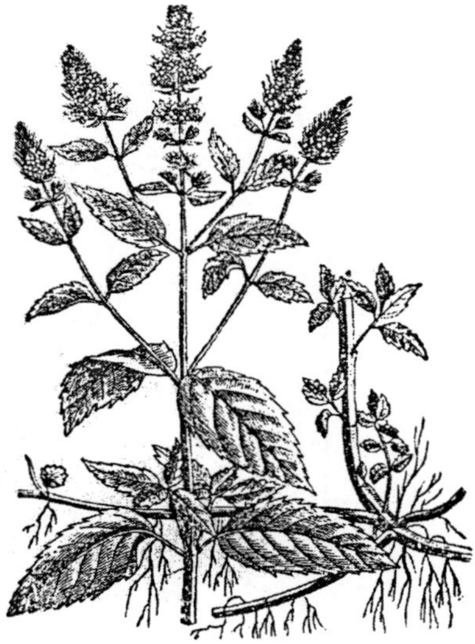

Peppermint (*Mentha piperita*)

Mint is counted among the principal herb remedies for strengthening the stomach and assisting the digestion. A cupful of tea taken every morning and evening stimulates the digestive juices and purifies the blood so that a fresh, clear, healthy appearance is produced.

Persons weakened by protracted illness, or who are seized with palpitations at the least disturbance to them, as well as in cases of nausea and frequent vomiting, will find relief by frequent use of mint tea and mint powder.

Mint decoction, prepared with vinegar, stops blood vomiting.

HEALING HERBS FROM NATURE'S LABORATORY

BY THE EDITOR.

Editor's Note: Each month the editor intends to take up one of the various medicinal plants to be found in the Kneipp pharmocopeia and treat of it in a popular way. By following these articles closely the student of Naturopathy will be able to become acquainted with the use of herb remedies in treating disease.

Medical Virtues Of Fennel

by Benedict Lust, N.D.

The Naturopath and Herald of Health, VIII (9), 263. (1907)

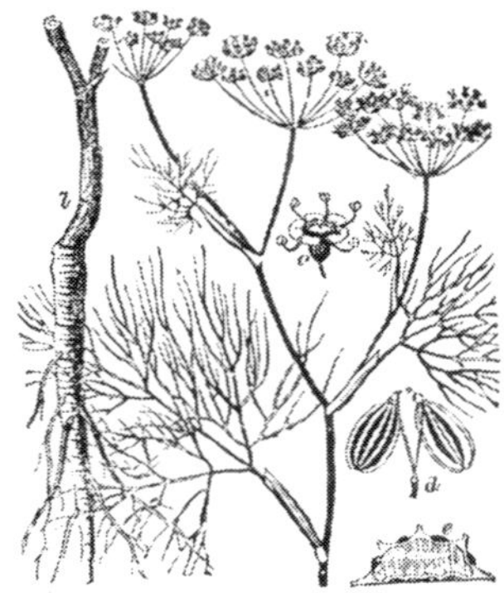

Fennel (*Foeniculum vulgare*)

The time is coming when the study of plant life will assume an ever widening sphere in the curriculum of public school studies. Natural methods of instruction must and will take the place of much that is artificial in our present educational system. Most of the public schools now devote a part of the class time to nature study. The children are requested to bring leaves of trees and plants into the class room and these are used in the study of botany. Leaves are dissected, drawings are made, and in other ways the child is taught the wonders connected with the life and growth of a single leaf. On occasion, an entire class makes an expedition to the woods, there to study plant life at first hand. All this is as it should be. We cannot introduce too much of Nature into school studies. Observation of plant life is the most delightful way of supplying the youthful mind with material for intellectual development. The child acquires powers of observation, reflection, discernment and memory in a natural and normal manner instead of having these faculties developed by artificial drill work. Nature study also serves to develop interest in horticulture. We need more Burbanks* to give us wonderful creations and new combinations of plant life to please the eye and improve man's food. A boy acquires by such studies a love of Nature that he does not lose when, in after years he goes into the turmoil of active business life. We have many instances of professional and business men who make nature study their hobby. President Roosevelt, tied down as he is with the burdens and cares of the busiest nation on earth, finds time to take an active interest in nature study and at present, in the newspaper accounts, we read how he starts out in the early morning with his boys camps in the woods and there gives them the best schooling in the world, the schooling in God's out-of-doors, the study of animals and birds and plants we find in the woods.

---

*Luther Burbank (1849-1926) was an American horticulturalist and an inventor that developed over 800 varieties of plants over his 55 year career. —*Ed.*

But the most significant factor in connection with natural instruction of this kind is the fact that it will revive interest in a therapeutic art that has almost been lost today. Herbotherapy, which the ancients knew, which the Indians knew and which our grannies practiced to perfection, has been made almost an obsolete science by a profession that has adopted poisons and the knife to cure patients by killing them off. There is more virtue in the homely herbs that the old granny will recommend than in all the prescriptions of the learned medical practitioner.

In this issue the value of fennel is described.

In cases of colic, with its attendant spasms, a spoonful of fennel boiled in a cup of milk from five to ten minutes and taken by the patient as warm as possible, never so hot as to cause discomfort, will quickly abate the trouble. A warm compress of water and vinegar may be applied to the stomach in connection with this treatment.

Fennel powder, sprinkled on the food, removes the gases from the stomach and the lower regions.

The powder is made by drying the corns in a pan over a fire and then grinding them in an ordinary coffee mill. Fennel oil can be obtained at the druggist's.

A good eye wash, healing in its effects, is made by taking a half tablespoonful of fennel powder and boiling in water. The eyes may be washed with this three times a day. Another effective method is to use the steam of this concoction by throwing a towel over the head. A similar effect is obtained by using ground anise or caraway. Frequently these three kinds of seeds are mixed and are used together for the vapor bath.

Herbotherapy, which the ancients knew, which the Indians knew and which our grannies practiced to perfection, has been made almost an obsolete science by a profession that has adopted poisons and the knife to cure patients by killing them off.

In cases of colic, with its attendant spasms, a spoonful of fennel boiled in a cup of milk from five to ten minutes and taken by the patient as warm as possible, never so hot as to cause discomfort, will quickly abate the trouble. A warm compress of water and vinegar may be applied to the stomach in connection with this treatment.

Another effective method is to use the steam of this concoction by throwing a towel over the head. A similar effect is obtained by using ground anise or caraway. Frequently these three kinds of seeds are mixed and are used together for the vapor bath.

HEALING HERBS FROM NATURE'S LABORATORY

BY THE EDITOR.

Editor's Note: Each month the editor intends to take up one of the various medicinal plants to be found in the Kneipp pharmocopeia and treat of it in a popular way. By following these articles closely the student of Naturopathy will be able to become acquainted with the use of herb remedies in treating disease.

Bogbean, Menyanthus Trifoliate

by Benedict Lust, N.D.

The Naturopath and Herald of Health, VIII (10), 295. (1907)

Medicinal Virtues Of The Bogbean (Water Trefoil), Menyanthus Trifoliate

For ages the delicately scented clover has been theme for poets. Bliss Carmen speaks of the "sea of clover" over which the "roving bee sails his way". Keats, Milton, and indeed all the poets of name and fame have had a good word for this humble flower.

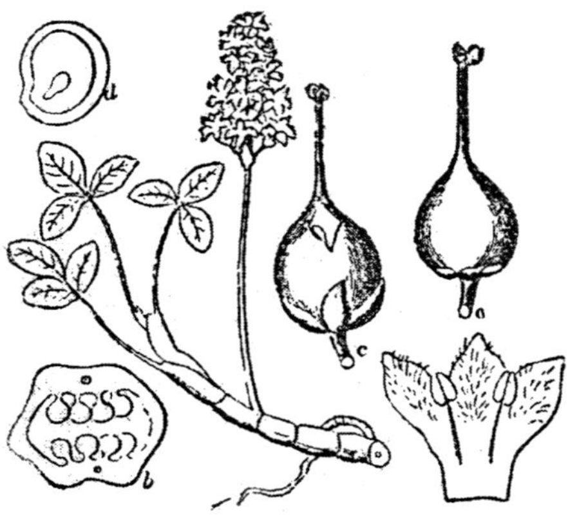

Bogbean (*Menyanthra trifoliata L.*)

a. ripe fruit, b. cross-section, c. ripe fruit bursting (2-6 times magnified), d. cross-section of the seed (6 times magnified), e. part of the flower.

There are different kinds of clover the most common of which is the popular red clover, which is indeed a delicacy much enjoyed by the cattle and without doubt beneficial to them. Another variety is the hare's foot trefoil, so-called, because hares are known to be fond of it; at least those that live in forests. The writer has frequently eaten this clover while roaming through the woods and considering its delicacy as a food, it is surprising that it is not gathered and used as a salad.

A third kind of clover is the marsh, or water trefoil. While this variety is not suitable as a food, it plays a great role among the healing herbs. It has a bitter taste like the centaury and wormwood plants and in Germany is called, on this account, *Bitterklee* or better clover.

You can find the water trefoil growing on marshy banks, in meadows and in ditches. It may be gathered at any time and dried in the shade for use during the winter months for the same medicinal purposes that wormwood is mostly used. The greatest medicinal value of water trefoil is in connection with stomachic troubles. Its bitterness excites the humors, removes morbid matter, strengthens the digestive organs, and, consequently, aids the process of digestion. It is excellent for children who have overloaded their stomachs. Water trefoil has also been used among the Germans, from time immemorial, for blood cleansing purposes. In connection with the general hardening of the body by means of Kneipp water treatment, water trefoil is valuable in remedying anemia of the blood. For strengthening the whole constitution this plant, prepared as a tea, is beneficial.

Water trefoil can also be mixed with other herbs. Two or three leaves of water trefoil, one leaf of wormwood and a centaury flower will produce an excellent combination that will strengthen and improve the stomach.

Water trefoil is an excellent remedy for liver complaints. Many people who have been troubled for years have been benefited in a remarkably short time by this single herb remedy. Its effect upon the kidneys is also beneficial. Like almost all the other herbs in the Kneipp pharmacopeia, it is a beneficial remedy to the system in general. Gather it now while you can; the possibilities are that an occasion may arise during the winter months when you will be glad that you have some of this valuable herb in the house.

A third kind of clover is the marsh, or water trefoil. While this variety is not suitable as a food, it plays a great role among the healing herbs. It has a bitter taste like the centaury and wormwood plants and in Germany is called, on this account, Bitterklee *or* better clover.

It may be gathered at any time and dried in the shade for use during the winter months for the same medicinal purposes that wormwood is mostly used. The greatest medicinal value of water trefoil is in connection with stomachic troubles. Its bitterness excites the humors, removes morbid matter, strengthens the digestive organs, and, consequently, aids the process of digestion.

In connection with the general hardening of the body by means of Kneipp water treatment, water trefoil is valuable in remedying anemia of the blood.

1908

Herbs For Stomach Troubles

Dr. Alfred Baumgarten

The Science Of Herbotherapy

Benedict Lust, N.D.

Phytotherapy (Plant Cure)

Dr. Karl Kahut

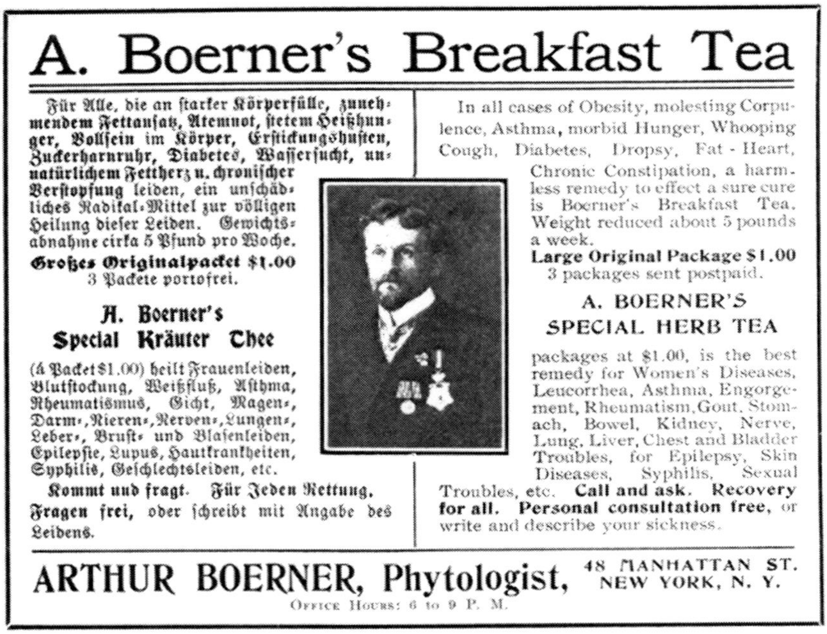

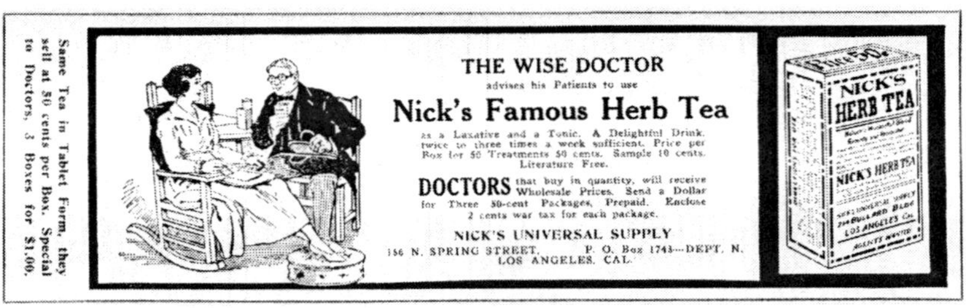

Herbal tea continues to be a popular beverage and remedy for many health complaints.

Herbs For Stomach Troubles

by Dr. Alfred Baumgarten

The Naturopath and Herald of Health, IX (2), 40-41. (1908)

Recently we have had a discussion about the diseases of the stomach. We have heard something about digestion and have come to the conclusion that, in order to have a good digestion we must know how to eat and how much to eat. First of all, we have to study our own special organism. In order to properly maintain the activity of the digestive organs, God has given us certain herbs about which we ought to know.

As stomach herbs the bitters rank highest. Their flavor stimulates the mucous membrane of the stomach; they strengthen the stomach itself and consequently the digestion. The very best remedy of this kind is wormwood; it is the cheapest and always at hand. It may be used as tea, as tincture, as powder, in a word, in all forms.

Wormwood

The best way to make wormwood tea is to take a quantity of wormwood; pour boiling water over it and drink it at once, in order to have the full effect of the flavor and to neutralize the bitter taste. Fresh green wormwood is the best; it is one of the first spring plants, and if one takes good care of it, one may keep it green till the fall. If dried, it is good enough; this drying should be done in the shade, and never in the sun. One may also make the tea of half fresh and half dried leaves. The powder is made of dry leaves, pestled and strained through a sieve. This powder may either be taken in water or in a wafer. This wafer is moistened in the water; the powder put on it, then folded and swallowed with the assistance of a draught of water.

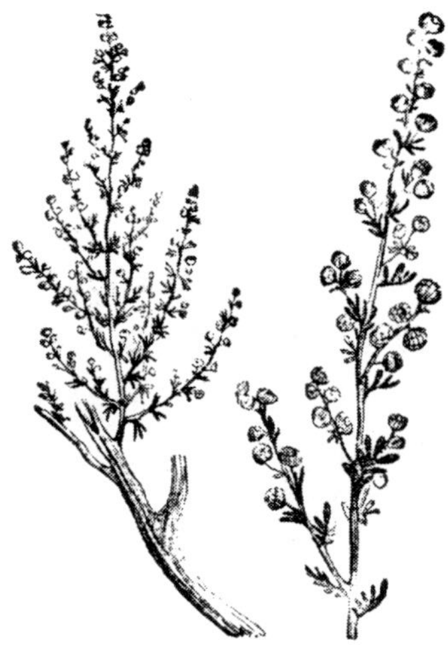

Wormwood
(*Artemisia absinthium*)

Wormwood is also used as a salve for the eyes. This salve must be made very carefully. One must take fresh leaves, pestle, rub them, boil the juice and by constant stirring mix it with honey. Then you get the correct wormwood salve for the eyes.

The tincture, as all tinctures, must be put in spirits of wine. Wormwood wine is also a good thing. People living in the wine countries and accustomed to the daily use of wine, cannot easily give it up; these should take wormwood wine. For this composition, the southern wines ought to be taken; the sugar they contain assimilates best with the flavor of the wormwood. A tablespoonful of this wine taken three times a day is an excellent tonic for the stomach.

GENTIAN ROOT

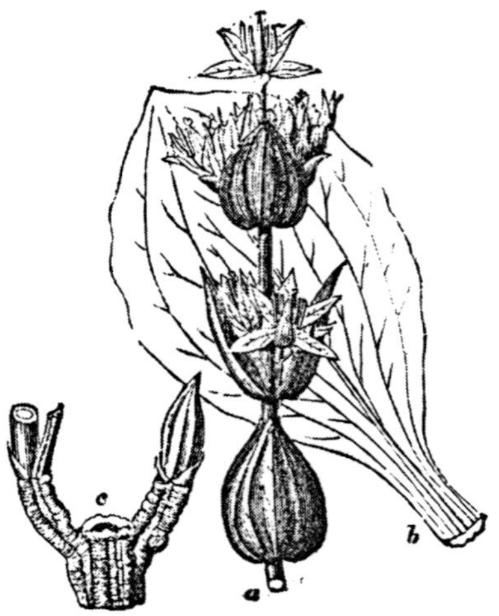

Gentian (*Gentiana lutea*)

a. Top of the stem with flowers (half its natural growth), b. leaf, c. part of the root (very much smaller than its natural growth).

The next best remedy I can recommend is gentian. Gentian grows on mountains, under stones and rocks. From these and the soil it extracts valuable elements out of the earth. It is only the root that benefits humanity. Gentian is well known to mountaineers. A flask of gentian brandy is never missing in the knapsack of a tourist or a mountaineer; this brandy with a piece of bread and cheese is all sufficient for these plain people. Though the use of brandy is, as a rule, not [generally] allowed. In excessive bodily exertions and intense cold a dram of gentian brandy can do no harm.

The gentian root is very bitter; mixed with wormwood and shavegrass, we have an excellent tea for strengthening the digestive organs. Men, who suffer from involuntary loss of semen, will be cured by taking a knife-point full of gentian powder four or five times a day.

SHAVEGRASS

Then we have the shavegrass or common horsetail. In many a household it is used to polish tin, dishes, bottles, glasses and so forth. But Father Kneipp promoted it to a remedy. There are many species of shavegrass; they vary from the smallest weeds, not higher than a finger to tall and gigantic shrubs, under the shade of which a rhinoceros may hide; they are [found] in the arctic zones as well as in the tropics. Shavegrass can be used in the most various ways. First of all, it may be added to any tea, as wormwood and gentian, thereby contributing to their strengthening and cleansing effect.

Shavegrass, especially, affects the kidneys and bladder. Anyone who takes shavegrass will notice that it stimulates the activity of the kidneys. Besides, it is of good hemostatic effect; whenever loss of blood takes place it is wise to drink shavegrass tea. It is well known that nose bleeding may be stopped by snuffing shavegrass powder. Then it also acts as purgative; though it would not be of any service in cases of chronic constipation; people suffering from diarrhea would only increase the evil by using shavegrass. But chronic stomach catarrh* may be cured by a tea composed of wormwood, gentian and shavegrass.

A cup of shavegrass tea is always preferable to a cup of chocolate. There are people who try to do their very best, and yet fail in their endeavors. Once I called upon a lady who, according to her own ideas, fully [followed] Father Kneipp's cure, but she failed in one thing. She consumed a great deal of sweetmeats, candies and other similar things. Consequently, she fell short of her aim, the attainment of perfect health.

Rosemary

There is scarcely one cottage in any village that has not a rosemary on the windowsill. With the common people it is a plant of great value and importance. It has its special meanings at weddings. It is a remedy of great value, especially for old people. Rosemary dissolves the congestions in the body, first of all, those brought on by slow circulation of blood, the so-called edematous swellings. Rosemary may be taken in various ways. It is most popular in wine. Rosemary wine is an excellent remedy, especially popular with old people. This wine is prepared in the following way. Into a bottle of common white wine put a rosemary twig; let it draw for a short time, according to the strength desired. During this process the wine must remain in a warm room. After five or six days the twig is taken out and the wine is ready for use.

---

*Stomach catarrh is the inflammation of the mucous lining of the stomach with excessive mucus. —*Ed.*

DWARF ELDER

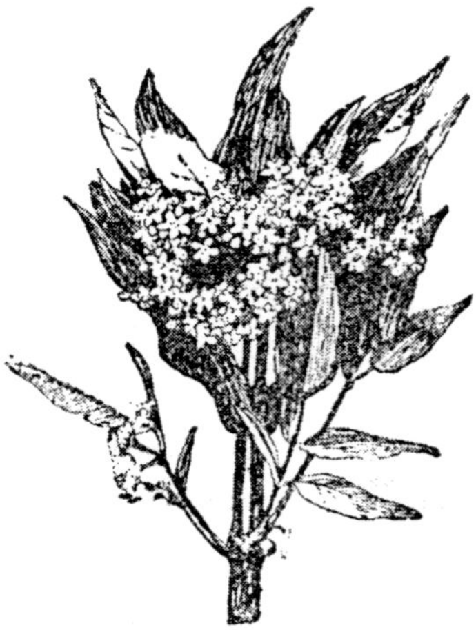

Dwarf Elder
(*Sambucus ebulus*)

Another strong herb is the dwarf elder. It grows on sloping grounds. The root of the dwarf elder produces urine in a far greater degree than rosemary or shavegrass. A composition of dwarf elder, rosemary and shavegrass is of great efficacy in dropsy.* If it is desired to strengthen the digestive organs, a pinch of agave should be added to the dwarf elder. This herb must be carefully cleaned and dried, but never washed; it should be cleaned with a cloth, cut into small pieces and then dried in the shade. All herbs must be dried in the shade. Although the sun dries better and more quickly, it also draws out the powerful ingredients of any plant while by drying in the shade this power is preserved.

BUCKBEAN

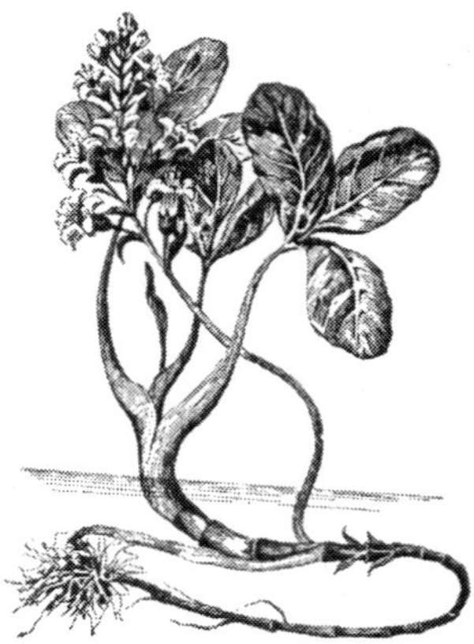

Buckbean
(*Menyanthes trifoliata*)

Another very valuable herb for the stomach is the buckbean, which grows in swamps and owes its name to its excessive bitter taste. It resembles common clover, though it has a stronger stalk and a larger and more beautiful leaf. These buckbean leaves are gathered, dried in the shade, and added to other stomach invigorating herbs. In order to prepare an excellent tea, the following points should be borne in mind: the more buckbean leaves are used for making tea, the worse it will taste; the fewer leaves and the less time steeped the better. The buckbean is also taken in the form of tincture; in fact, this is the best way to take it. Ten drops of this tincture taken two or three times a day will usually affect a good cure.

*Dropsy refers to edema. —*Ed.*

Peppermint

Finally, I must draw the reader's attention to peppermint. It is good for cramps, fainting spells and stomach troubles.

Ribwort

Of ribwort, I will only say that its juice is of great value in pulmonary troubles. The preparation of the juice is rather complicated, and for this reason it is better to buy it at a Kneipp store.

At last I must remark that all these herbs growing in our subalpine climate are better than the same species growing in other latitudes, therefore orders for these herbs ought to be sent to Wőerishofen.

The best way to make wormwood tea is to take a quantity of wormwood; pour boiling water over it and drink it at once, in order to have the full effect of the flavor and to neutralize the bitter taste.

One must take fresh leaves, pestle, rub them, boil the juice and by constant stirring mix it with honey. Then you get the correct wormwood salve for the eyes.

The gentian root is very bitter; mixed with wormwood and shavegrass, we have an excellent tea for strengthening the digestive organs. Men, who suffer from involuntary loss of semen, will be cured by taking a knife-point full of gentian powder four or five times a day.

Then it also acts as purgative; though it would not be of any service in cases of chronic constipation; people suffering from diarrhea would only increase the evil by using shavegrass.

Rosemary dissolves the congestions in the body, first of all, those brought on by slow circulation of blood, the so-called edematous swellings.

A composition of dwarf elder, rosemary and shavegrass is of great efficacy in dropsy. If it is desired to strengthen the digestive organs, a pinch of agave should be added to the dwarf elder.

The root of the dwarf elder produces urine in a far greater degree than rosemary or shavegrass. A composition of dwarf elder, rosemary and shavegrass is of great efficacy in dropsy.

The Science Of Herbotherapy

by Benedict Lust, N.D.

The Naturopath and Herald of Health, IX (6), 167-173. (1908)

Its Unlimited Value In Connection With The Natural Method Of Healing Disease

The application of single curative plants in single diseases is confirmed by the original instinct of nations in the early stages of history and safely transmitted for thousands of years. This method is the simplest, and it will have effect in slight cases of acute diseases, because it influences, accelerates and even produces single prominent symptoms of the disease, especially excretory processes which remove the poisons of the disease.

The proper systematic phytotherapy works in a different way. If we examine the non-poisonous plants, we find out that each one has a certain relationship to some organ of the body and that it excites and increases the metabolism in this organ as well as its special function by supplying the cells of the corresponding organs with its proper food. The poisonous plant may increase its function also, not by supplying with necessary food, but by irritating the resistance of the cell against itself. This resistance, this reaction, however, is accomplished by the cell at its own expense; it loses a part of its strength. Thus, the poisonous substances cause a real and continually weakened activity of the cells; such is not the case with non-poisonous plants.

In plants which are related to the same organ, the effect is by no means identical; there are slight differences which can hardly be pointed out, but which are shown by the fact that the effect of a single plant is greatly behind that of a mixture of a larger number from the same group. On this account, in cases in which the fight is of long standing and is more obstinate, especially in the course of chronic diseases, a mixture of more or less remedies is to be preferred, because then the active material is many-sided and is more appropriate to satisfy all the parts of the diseased organ, while a single plant is rather one-sided and acts only upon single tissue elements and as soon as the proper cell is satisfied it loses its action, while other cells are still undergoing pathologic changes.

There may be different prescriptions as to the selection of single plants and their quantities. It does not depend entirely on the form or the name of the disease; but the same disease may require different mixtures for different people. Influenza sometimes attacks the lungs, sometimes the secretions of the intestines or the stomach and requires either lung remedies or those of the other organs affected. It must first be settled which organ is affected, whether a limited part of any organ, or the poison of disease spreads in the blood and consequently over the whole body; and, secondly, it must be observed which way the body will remove the excreted morbid matter.

The selection of curative plants which are at our disposal is by no means easy. A great number of these are classified according to their principal action as follows:

I. Plants Which Raise Metabolism In General, Raise The Activity Of The Blood

Artemisia absinthium, wormwood plant; *Cochlearia officinalis*, scurvy grass; *Erythraea Centaurium Persoon*, common European centaury plant; *Matricaria chamomilla,* German chamomile flowers; *Fragaria vesca*, strawberry leaves; *Juglans regia,* common European walnut leaves; *Achillea millefolium,* milfoil [yarrow] flowers and leaves; *Quercus robur*, English oak bark; *Rubus fruticosus*, European blackberry leaves; *Viola tricolor,* pansy plant.

II. Plants That Strengthen Metabolism, Lymphatics And Liver

The following act with more strength on metabolism, activity of the lymphatic glands and the other large glandular organs, as the liver. They are good in severe general disturbances of nutrition, chronic poisoning, cachexia, scrofula, syphilis, gout, sugar in the urine:

Guaiacum officinale, guaiacum wood; *Smilax medica schlechtendahl,* sarsaparilla root; *Vaccinium myrtillus,* bilberry or huckleberry fruit and leaves; *Capsella bursa pastoris,* shepherd's purse plant; *Equisetum arvense*, horsetail plant, shave grass; *Urtica dioica*, stinging nettle plant; *Menyanthes trifoliate,* buckbean; *Arctostaphylos uva ursi, Sprengel,* bearberry leaves; *Tussilago farfara,* coltsfoot leaves; *Salix peutaudra* willow bark and leaves; *Spirea [Filipendula] ulmaria,* meadowsweet flowers; *Arnica montana,* arnica root and flowers.

III. Plants Acting Upon The Nervous System

Archangelica officinalis hoffman, [Angelica archangelica], lingwort root; Arnica montana, arnica root and flowers; *Capsella bursa pastoris*, shepherd's purse plant; *Mentha piperita*, peppermint leaves; *Melissa officinalis*, [lemon] balm leaves; *Valeriana officinalis*, valerian root; *Humulus lupulus*, hops strobiles; *Thymus serpyllum,* thyme plant; *Chenopodium ambrosioides var. anthelminticum*, American wormseed plant.

IV. Plants Acting Upon The Skin

Tilia parviflora and *grandiflora,* European lime tree flowers; *Sambucus nigra*, elder flowers; *Juglans regia,* walnut green shell of the fruit;

Guaiacum officinale, guaiac wood; *Viola tricolor*, pansy plant; *Ononis spinosa*, restharrow root; *Salvia pratensis*, sage leaves.

V. Plants Acting Upon Kidneys

Juniperus communis, juniper fruit; *Levisticum officinale,* lovage root; *Ononis spinosa*, restharrow root; *Quercus robur*, oak bark; *Petroselinum sativum hoffman*, parsley seed and root; *Arctostaphylos uva ursi*, bearberry leaves; *Betula alba,* birch leaves.

VI. The Digestion Herbs

Artemisia absinthium, wormwood plant; *Acorus calamus*, sweet flag rhizome; *Cnicus benedictus,* St. Benedict thistle; *Erythraea centaurium pers.*, European centaury plant; *Mentha piperita*, peppermint plant; *Matricaria chamomilla*, German chamomile flowers; *Marsdenia condurango nich.*, condurango bark; *Foeniculum vulgare mill.*, fennel seed; *Gentian lutea, purpurea*, gentian root; *Origanum vulgare* [oregano]; *Melilotus officinalis desr.,* melilot plant; *Achillea millefolium*, milfoil [yarrow] flowers and leaves.

VII. Lung Activity

Althaea officinalis, marshmallow root; *Arnica montana*, arnica flowers and root; *Pimpinella anisum*, anise seed; *Chondrus crispus*, Irish moss; *Tussilago farfara*, coltsfoot leaves; *Inula helenium*, elecampane root; *Verbascum thapsus*, mullein leaves; *Cetraria islandica*, Iceland moss; *Glycyrrhiza glabra*, licorice root; *Symphytum officinale*, comfrey root; *Pulmonaria officinalis,* lungwort plant; *Plantago major* and *media,* plantain leaves; *Polygala amara*, bitter milkwort plant, flowers and root.

This, of course, is not the full list of useful plants. There are no definite rules for the selection of remedies in any given case, but art and experience teach us how to give the right treatment. It is to be mentioned that essential mistakes cannot be made, for the simple reason that we deal not with different, strongly acting or even poisonous plants and that in a mixture of numerous plants but a small quantity of each produces some effect.

If one defines the seat and the kind of the disease, he will be able to use those plants which act upon the corresponding organ, and also remedies which raise the general metabolism, because there is hardly one disease which should settle locally independently from the general organism. It happens even quite frequently the opposite that local troubles are the result of general illness. On the other hand, every local focus of disease [affects] the whole organism because the products of the diseased process must enter the circulation.

Finally, we consider also the activity of the excretory organs, because these are very important for the removal of morbid products, and prescribe remedies which act upon these organs. Mostly, the body itself gives us the necessary indications, because Nature takes up the fight against the virus (poison) of disease, and in the symptoms (signs) of disease, as coughing, sputum, vomiting, diarrhoea, sweat, urine, rash, etc., show the course by which the dangerous substances are best excreted.

Plant cure has its chief object to accelerate or to bring out the natural effort within the body to heal.

We could then in every single case decide on a certain mixture. But this is not practical. Experience has shown that for every symptom a separate mixture is to be taken and then these different mixtures to be used interchangeably. Thus it is easier to follow the changing requirement of the course of the disease. For one suffering with neurasthenia or disease of the spinal cord, combined with diarrhoea, we have to prescribe first remedies which act on general metabolism and which improve the blood (group I), then such remedies as act on the nervous system (group III), and finally such as regulate the activity of the digestive apparatus (group VI). We make one mixture, then the second, the third, afterwards the first again and so on, one more, the other less, according to the change in strength and importance of the symptoms. Thus, it is generally seen that the foundations of this method are quite simple, and that its practical application requires experience and skill to consider every case and to individualize it.

It is to be mentioned particularly: the stronger the symptoms of disease are which must be considered as a curative effort of Nature, the more carefully the curative plants must be used and in a smaller dose, because in these symptoms, as during fever, the efficiency of the body has certain limits which cannot be overstepped without harm. The simplest form in which curative plants are used is that of infusion. The dried plants are dipped in boiling water or boiled in water a certain length of time according to their properties, and then used. This is generally done in slight cases. Glunicke also received strong concentrated extracts by boiling.

Those extracts proved most active which were made according to my directions. I let the dried plants stand in cold water under the pressure of a few atmospheres and thus obtain extracts very similar to the juices of the fresh plants. The use of these extracts is to be recommended in all severe, obstinate, wearisome, chronic cases of disease.

The quantity of the dried constituent parts of the plants to be used is different with different individuals. For children one year old 1-3 grams (15-45 grains) of an infusion; for older children 4-12 grams (1-3 drams); for adults 15-20 grams (3 ½-5 drams) are sufficient on the average. An experienced practitioner will occasionally exceed these limits.

How many plants and how much of each shall be taken depend on the action and especially on the taste of each and every plant. About ½ gram (8 grains) to 6 grams (1 ½ dram) of each drug shall be taken for one day and about 10-15 plants be mixed, i. e., the extracts from such an infusion to be used daily.

The action which curative plants exert on the body depends on the quantity of the different substances and their combination. To ascertain and to give the chemical definitions of these substances is hardly possible, except cases of a very few of them. Notice is also to be taken of the fact that the substance isolated from the plant by itself may have a prominent action, and that this does not correspond to the action which it produces when combined with all the other active substances. The plants themselves, or rather their extracts, produce a milder and more uniform action, while single isolated substances frequently cause strong and at times poisonous results. This is based on the fact that such substances are greatly diluted in the cells of the plant and besides are chemically combined with other constituents which prevent its action above the physiological limit.

In regard to this point, a number of substances can be classed as active which will be mentioned here in short.

The first group of these substances contains organic acids, such as valerianic, formic, citric, malic, tartaric, succinic, oxalic, and salicylic. All these acids are strong poisons, if used chemically pure and in concentrated form. In the plant, they are contained in the form of highly important sources of power and health in the human body. The same is with tannic acid which is found in the plants in many different forms. And just tannic acid, combined with the mentioned organic acids, forms a uniform action. The one or the other factor, used separately for a longer period, may produce trouble in the organism; both combined strengthen their favorable action and neutralize their somewhat harmful properties.

The mineral salts which are present in the plants in organic form are highly important, as Lahmann's and Strasser's works show. These minerals are: potassium, sodium, calcium, magnesium, iron, phosphorus, sulphur, silicon and chloride. These are the same substances which play an important part in the composition and in the normal activity of the human body.

Here may be shown an example in which the chemical analysis at times confirms the historically transmitted use of some plants in certain diseases. The leaves of the walnut are a remedy which was successfully used for generations against rickets. This disease is recognized by softness and brittleness of the bones as a result of deficiency in calcium. The analysis of the leaves gives 53.6% of calcium in the ashes; thus the action is explained.

Here is to be repeated that the mentioned minerals chemically pure are of no use to the body, at times even dangerous poisons, and in the organic form, prepared by the plant, they form the most important foundation in the building up of the forces in the human body.

Furthermore, we have to consider also from the same standpoint the ethereal oils which influence the nerves, the mucous membranes and the kidneys and act as antiseptics, and the bitter substances which also hinder fermentation and thus act perhaps as febrifuge; but they are essentially important owing to their action on the digestive organs.

The remarkable peculiarity of the plant cure, at least in the form taught by Glunicke, is the application of injections [enema] into the intestines for which decoctions or extracts of curative plants are used.

The large intestine, especially its lower end, is an important excretory organ for the refuse of metabolism and poisons of disease. This excretory activity is increased by the injections. The increased activity of the intestinal wall is combined with a stronger flow of blood. This results in a derivation from the proper focus of disease, as in the chest or in the head and the occurrence sometimes of dangerous congestion in the organ as well as subjective complaints, such as pain and difficult breathing are lessened. Finally, the injections remove the products of decomposition in the intestines; this may become a source of disease by poisonous products of decomposition entering the circulation.

Plants which can be used for injections [enemas] are as follows:

Plants Rich In Acids Aiding Secretions:

Rumex acetosa, common sorrel; *Oxalis acetosella,* wood sorrel; *Valeriana officinalis,* valerian; *Saponaria officinalis,* soapwort; *Achillea millefolium,* milfoil [yarrow]; *Vitis vinifera,* grape leaves; *Cochlearia officinalis,* scurvy grass; *Taraxacum officinale,* dandelion; etc.

Plants Rich In Tannic Acid And Are Invigorating Tonics:

Quercus rubur, oak bark; *Juglans regis,* walnut leaves; *Salvia officinalis,* sage leaves; *Ruta graveolens,* rue.

Anti-spasmodic And Sedative Plants:

Valeriana officinalis, valerian; *Tilia europaea,* lime tree flowers; *Verbascum thapsus,* mullein; *Matricaria chamomilla,* chamomile; etc.

Antiseptic:

Quercus robur, oak bark; *Mentha piperita,* peppermint; *Melissa officinalis,* [lemon] balm; *Eucalyptus globulus*, blue gum tree; *Thymus vulgaris*, thyme; *Origanum vulgare*, marjoram; etc.

If the patient suffers with constipation or diarrhoea, one has to select more plants from one or another group.

Finally, it is to be mentioned that for different external applications, as eye washes, gargles, injections, treatment of wounds and abscesses, compresses, etc., the non-poisonous plants offer abundant choice and give excellent results.

Definite quantities of the infusion or an extract of the plant, made with water, sugar and fruit juice into lemonade, may be taken internally. Injections into the intestines may be made 1-3 times weekly, in exceptional cases only daily, as in diarrhoea.

Generally, the course of the cure is marked at first by a certain feeling of relief which comes on, the appetite is increased and the patient's temper is improved. It is caused by the foreign substances in the body being loosely combined and easily thrown off and washed away. Now the older and deeper layers in the focus of disease begin to undergo resolution gradually. This is accompanied by more or less sudden symptoms which we call crises. These crises produce symptoms in the focus itself which are noticed generally by pain, then by special symptoms of the activity of the corresponding organ, as cough and sputum from the lungs, vomiting from the stomach, convulsions from the brain, etc.; these are mostly the same symptoms that the disease itself produces. Plant remedies act in the same way which Nature herself shows and takes up. At the same time the other organs of excretion, as the skin, the kidney, the intestine, by their activity assist in the removal of morbid matter.

After such a crisis, which is always sudden and which lasts a longer or a shorter period, a period of rest and of relatively good health comes till a new crisis follows again. Thus, the crises are repeated at greater or smaller intervals till the poison of disease disappears. If the crises occur more rarely and become weaker, the quantity of the remedies which is taken daily may be reduced gradually. It is remarkable that if the patient recovers completely, he frequently dislikes the plant juices; it is also noticed in very strong crises, and it is then advisable to obey the signal given by the body and to reduce the daily dose because otherwise too strong crises may occur which will exhaust the patient.

The action of plant remedies proves sufficiently that phytotherapy belongs to Nature Cure. This view is based on the theory of crises which Nature Cure received from behavior of disease, and by no other method of cure is treatment of disease by crises better explained than by plant cure.

It has already been mentioned many times that the plant cure is not a separate system. It is to be strongly emphasized that it is but a part and, of course, a very valuable part of Nature Cure. Thus, it is understood that plant cure is supplemented by the other factors of Nature Cure, as light, air, water, gymnastics, massage and mental influence which grow on the same common footing, act in the same direction and handle the body in different situations.

The number of diseases in which herbotherapy is applied successfully is unlimited. Though slighter diseases, in spite of every treatment and even without any treatment may heal of themselves by the aid of the internal healing powers, the plant cure warrants a more rapid and more radical cure because it produces and supports the healing power within the body more than another method, and because it takes care that the foreign substances and those that produce disease shall not remain in the body, as it often happens in the allopathic treatment of internal diseases. On this account it is also very important in the treatment of acute diseases, especially if the high fever temperature is suppressed and the symptoms of disease become weakened. If at this time and especially during convalescence, the morbid matters are not removed completely sequelae and relapses occur very frequently. This is always prevented by the timely use of non-poisonous plants. Yet, not only the natural poisons of disease are removed by this method, but also all the artificial remedies with which the allopathic system poisons the body, are again driven out and their harmful actions put aside. Therefore, the plant cure finds the application of plants after any kind of poisoning with medicine successful, as after febrifuge (against fever), hypnotic (to sleep) medicines, vaccination, poisoning with anti-toxin, tuberculin injections, but especially in poisoning the body with iodine and mercury. Mercury, however, is given, according to the allopathic prescription books in use, in 62 different diseases either pure or under disguise.

But if a severe chronic disease has been already developed, then the plant cure is called upon to raise the powers within the body and to excite them to fight against the disease. Even when medicine has been unable, till now, to fight the germs of disease, the plant cure may do wonders:

- in severe diseases of the blood and of the body in general, such as scrofula, rheumatism, gout, diabetes mellitus, obesity, etc.;
- in disease of different systems in the body and in severe diseases of the brain and the nervous system such as nervous headache, migraine, inflammation of the brain, epilepsy, convulsions, general nervous debility, neuralgia, sciatica, etc., and in diseases of the spinal cord;
- in severe chronic catarrh, consumption of the lungs, etc;
- in heart diseases; in disturbances of the circulation due to valvular disease;
- in calcification and dilatation of the arteries; in inflammation of varicose veins;

- in stomach troubles, as catarrh, dilatation, ulcers, cramps;
- in inflammation, catarrh of the intestines, colic, hemorrhoids, etc.;
- in inflammation and swelling of the liver and kidneys (dropsy);
- in venereal diseases (syphilis);
- in diseases of the male and female organs, as inflammation of the prostatic gland, of the testicle, womb, ovaries;
- in skin diseases, as rashes, eruptions, boils; and
- in inflammations and abscesses of the ear and in diseases of the eye.

Even some surgical diseases, as caries, tuberculous inflammation of the bones which were cut with the knife with no help to the patient, plant cure can do much good.

It is self-evident that not every patient in whom vitality is greatly destroyed can be saved. Yet this method, especially if combined with the other factors of Nature Cure, can cure many so-called incurable cases. Even in cases that it cannot cure, it gives comfort and proves that in harmony with Nature's laws it is the best and most effective method of cure. Extraordinary improvement of general health is reached also in many incurable cases.

Preventive And Cooling Cure

From what was told about the non-poisonous curative plants follows that they can be used to prevent, improve and cool the patient. Even without getting a severe disease the body gradually takes in foreign and disease-producing substances by overwork, by harmful mode of living, as staying in narrow, badly-aired rooms, hard work for a long time, insufficient exercise, eating irregularly, using wine and beer, smoking tobacco, and etc. If they are not removed from the body, the foreign and disease-producing substances find the place prepared to get any kind of disease. A cure with non-poisonous plants, especially in spring after the hardships of winter, and also in fall from two to six weeks, according to the circumstances, rids the body from all mischief, washes through all its canals, restores the normal activity of all the organs, lungs, stomach, nerves, skin, kidneys, liver, and purifies the blood.

This method is to be especially recommended for all those that, not being sick, yet are attacked by exertion and mode of living, and that are always in the house and at the desks as mental occupation requires, scholars, public officers, and office workers.

Such a cure with non-poisonous plants invigorates the body, enables it to renew activity and strengthens it against disease. Such a cure, if undertaken every spring, removes the harmful substances which have been stored up during the year in the body and also the foreign bodies and the germs of new disease. Finally it is to be stated that such cure may be accomplished without any interference with regular duties.

The poisonous plant may increase its function also, not by supplying with necessary food, but by irritating the resistance of the cell against itself. This resistance, this reaction, however, is accomplished by the cell at its own expense; it loses a part of its strength.

If one defines the seat and the kind of the disease, he will be able to use those plants which act upon the corresponding organ, and also remedies which raise the general metabolism, because there is hardly one disease which should settle locally independently from the general organism.

Finally, we consider also the activity of the excretory organs, because these are very important for the removal of morbid products, and prescribe remedies which act upon these organs.

Plant cure has its chief object to accelerate or to bring out the natural effort within the body to heal.

Notice is also to be taken of the fact that the substance isolated from the plant by itself may have a prominent action, and that this does not correspond to the action which it produces when combined with all the other active substances.

Here is to be repeated that the mentioned minerals chemically pure are of no use to the body, at times even dangerous poisons, and in the organic form, prepared by the plant, they form the most important foundation in the building up of the forces in the human body.

Now the older and deeper layers in the focus of disease begin to undergo resolution gradually. This is accompanied by more or less sudden symptoms which we call crises.

cont'd

It is remarkable that if the patient recovers completely, he frequently dislikes the plant juices; it is also noticed in very strong crises, and it is then advisable to obey the signal given by the body and to reduce the daily dose because otherwise too strong crises may occur which will exhaust the patient.

It has already been mentioned many times that the plant cure is not a separate system. It is to be strongly emphasized that it is but a part and, of course, a very valuable part of Nature Cure. Thus, it is understood that plant cure is supplemented by the other factors of Nature Cure, as light, air, water, gymnastics, massage and mental influence which grow on the same common footing, act in the same direction and handle the body in different situations.

Though slighter diseases, in spite of every treatment and even without any treatment may heal of themselves by the aid of the internal healing powers, the plant cure warrants a more rapid and more radical cure because it produces and supports the healing power within the body more than another method, and because it takes care that the foreign substances and those that produce disease shall not remain in the body, as it often happens in the allopathic treatment of internal diseases.

Even without getting a severe disease the body gradually takes in foreign and disease-producing substances by overwork, by harmful mode of living, as staying in narrow, badly-aired rooms, hard work for a long time, insufficient exercise, eating irregularly, using wine and beer, smoking tobacco, and etc. If they are not removed from the body, the foreign and disease-producing substances find the place prepared to get any kind of disease.

Phytotherapy (Plant Cure)

by Dr. Karl Kahut, of Berlin

The Naturopath and Herald of Health, IX (8), 233-235. (1908)

Phyto-therapy (from the Greek phyton—plant and therapy—cure) or plant cure, is called the systematic treatment with curative plants which are free from poison, i.e., such plants the active parts of which become completely assimilated to generate this substance in the body. These substances can be of such kind only as has existed in the body as its normal constituent and with which every active life is connected. The healthy body normally takes these substances from the food. The curative plant supplies the sick body with pure and concentrated forms. Thus, it is clear that Plant Cure belongs also to Nature Cure.

The old physiatric Nature Cure School knew only external natural applications, as light, air, water, movement and massage; it therefore was considered as a method of cure with external applications and without medicines. This definition is wrong, because the word "medicine" is not taken in its right meaning. Medicine generally means a curative substance which becomes a part of the body, to act together with the blood. If the medicine consists of substances which are different from those in the body and which are poisonous, it is not used by Nature Cure, but if it contains exclusively substances which are similar to the body and which can be assimilated by it, such medicine is used and agrees with the nature of the human body. This point must be emphasized in opposition to the assertion which is frequently made by Allopaths that poisons like arsenic, mercury, strychnia, etc., are given to us by Nature.

Not everything that is given by Nature is used in Nature Cure; but that which is according to the nature of the human body, i.e., which can be transformed into energy and material in the human body. Thus, it is proved that plant cure is a part of Nature Cure.

History

The oldest works of art and literature show that the old nations knew by experience the connection of plant life with human beings, and especially the curative powers of different plants in sick persons. This knowledge has been in existence thousands of years, and is transmitted by the common people from one generation to the other, and is kept even at the present time. Medical science has never taken up this theory because it ignores popular opinions and because experimental manipulation of the substances with exact mathematical results is very difficult. Yet, there were always specialists who by chance or by inclination were led to the study of curative plants. Nevertheless, independent literary works are very hard and very seldom to be found.

The numerous old herbals have described all kinds of plants, even poisonous ones, which were ever used as remedies. They represent especially collections in which everything obtainable is put together without any critical examination. The more known works are the writings of Dicoris, after Matthiolus's commentaries, the popular herbals of Dr. Muller, and of Dr. Hochstetter, as well as of Shimpfky, the different compends on medicinal botany, then the highly valuable work of Dragendorff: *The Curative Plants of all Nations and all Periods*. In all these works the curative plants are explained separately; with each are counted the disease against which it can be used. The whole compilation is considered entirely from the historical and literary point.

The first signs of a peculiar and systematic use of plants in medicine are found with Dr. J. Kampf, who was physician to the elector of Hessen in the eighteenth century. He had compiled a treatise for physicians and patients on a new method to cure the diseases of the hypogastrium and of the hypochondrium, in which are described systematic cures with herbs. Besides the internal use, Kampf recommends enemata (injections into the intestines) which he performs with decoctions of mixtures of certain herbs, in some cases a few times daily. Nevertheless, he does not mention yet systematic rejection of poisonous substances, though he uses mostly curative plants free from poison.

Only lately, though not in word but in real application, the point was emphasized by prelate Kneipp and by the very experienced physician, Dr. Walser, that only plants free from poison shall be used in curing disease.

In an independent standing as therapeutic specialty, phyto-therapy was introduced by the late Martin Glunicke, formerly a lawyer in Berlin. He became a mental and physical wreck after a severe disease. Having looked in vain for a cure by allopathy, homeopathy, hydrotherapy and massage, he tried his own ways to cure himself. Observations that tanners drank tan in any disease successfully, and that in a tan-bath, the first one ever established, enemata were administered with thinned tan, made him try the effect of oak bark on his own body. Though great relief and considerable improvement was the result, yet complete constipation and inflammation of the liver followed the continual use of oak bark. Now he began to use fruit juices, on which he fed exclusively. Having used fruit juices for a long time, he received attacks of diarrhea, anaemia and weakness; thus the middle course was found in the combination of both factors. In the corresponding combination, the dangerous effects are removed, while the curative effects are increased. Later on, when Glunicke, by experience and hard work, increased his knowledge, he took in more and more curative plants gradually, and made a rule that a curative plant must be free from poison to be able to cure.

Together with Glunicke, and especially after his death, the writer of this work has continued to develop the method of plant cure. Glunicke's writings were only to propagate the truth and put a hint at the method itself. The scientific explanation was first made only in my book: *Phytotherapy, a Method to Treat Internally Diseases with Curative Plants Free from Poison, According to the Principles of Nature Cure* (second edition in 1900), by exactly representing the curative plants free from poison, and their application, and by basing their action on theory. Further facts on this subject are given in the monthly journal *Plant Cure*, published by the Society of Plant Cure in Berlin, such as Dr. Strasser's essay, which applied Lahmann's theory on nutritive salts to the effect of curative plants.

In relation to practice, Dr. Klimascewski is to be mentioned who explained different forms of useful application of curative plants. Dr. Ide wrote also a short essay on this subject. He classified the plants according to their more important mineral substances, as calcium (lime), iron, sodium, etc., and then ordered them for certain diseases according to the chief salts contained in them.

1909

Aromatic Powders

Kniepp's Herbs And Their Uses

Contents Of A Little Kneipp Home Dispensary

Benedict Lust, N.D.

Aromatic Powders

by Benedict Lust, N.D.

The Naturopath and Herald of Health, XIV (1), 33. (1909)

Herbs as ribwort, common nettle, violets, and sage are cut in pieces, dried in the shade in the open air, mixed, pestled and strained. This powder will cure any irritating cough, if taken three times a day: a knife-point full in water or in a wafer.

Stomach troubles will be alleviated by a composition of wormwood, mint and gentian, prepared and taken in the same way as the just mentioned herbs.

Hemorrhages from the stomach are cured by: shavegrass, shepherd's purse and mistletoe every hour a knife-point full.

Aromatic powders have to be kept in hermetically closed boxes; if prepared according to the recipe they will be effective for months.

KNEIPP'S HERBS AND THEIR USES

by Benedict Lust, N.D.

The Naturopath and Herald of Health, XIV (8), 482-486. (1909)

WORMWOOD

Tea used as eye-water, has often rendered the best services in eye complaints.

SILVERWEED, POTENTILLA ANSERINE L.

The silverweed grows best, as its German name (*Gansefingerkraut*) implies, where geese like best to be. It is found in the vicinity of houses, on commons, and along the roads.

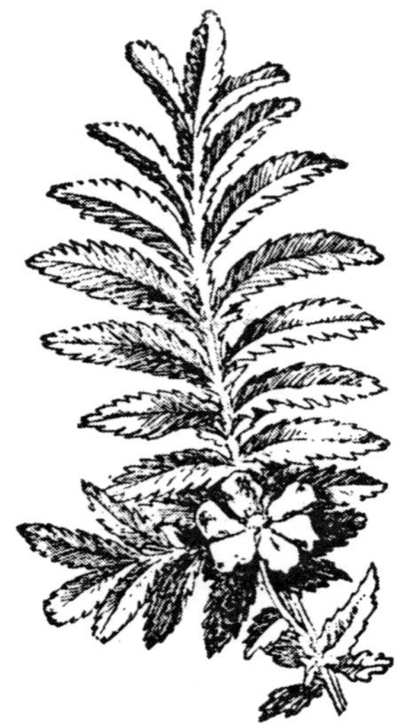

Silverweed (*Potentilla anserine*)

People have named it, after its mode of operating, cramp herb. Tea made from silverweed is an excellent remedy in attacks of cramp in the stomach, abdomen, or elsewhere. Even in cases of tetanus—insofar as this can be worked upon—this little herb renders very good service. At the commencement of the attack, or better still, when symptoms of the cramp first appear, the patient should be given three times daily very warm milk (as warm as possible) in which such herbs (as much as can be picked up with three fingers) have been boiled for tea.

A greater effect may be obtained if at the same time as the tea is taken a poultice is made of the boiled herbs and laid upon the affiliated part.

No mother of a family should omit to gather and dry a sufficient supply of such herbs. She knows, herself, how painful such frequently occurring spasmodic attacks are, and how it gives her still greater pain if she sees her dear ones suffering without being able to help them.

ST JOHN'S WORT, HYPERICUM PERFORATUM L.

St. John's wort, on account of its great effects, formerly bore the name of witch's herb. Nowadays, both it and its services are quite forgotten.

This medicinal herb has a particular influence on the liver; its tea is an excellent remedy for it. A small admixture of aloe powder increases the effect, which can be observed chiefly in the urine; whole flakes of morbid matters are sometimes washed away with it.

Head complaints arising from watery matters or obstructions of phlegm in the head; stomach spasms, slight obstructions of phlegm on the chest and lungs are healed at once by tea made of St. John's wort.

Mothers, who are caused a great deal of trouble and anxiety by their little bed wetters, could tell us much about the strong effects of such tea.

If St. John's wort is not to be had, common yarrow (*Achillea millefolium L.*) may be used in all the given cases.

Succory Or Chicory, Cichorium Intybus L.

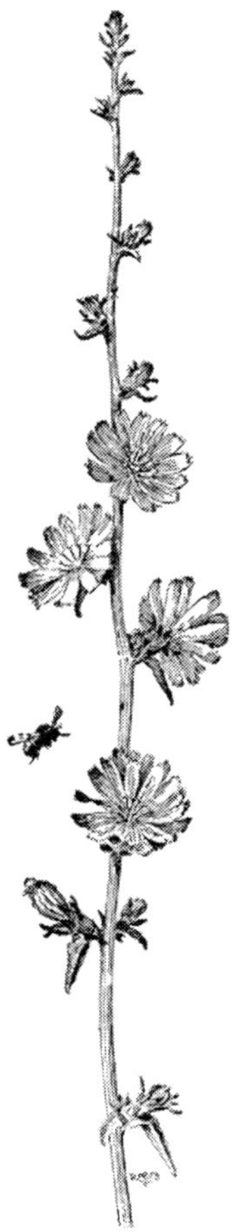

Chicory flowers

The succory (*Wegwart* in German) waits on every path for him who desires to gather it for his dispensary. It is also called *sun-whirl*, as its leaves are always turned to the sun. When you look at it, the good succory, with its half-starved-looking stalks and entangled leaves, it seems like a rough-head among all the other plants. Only the color of its blossom, rather brighter than that of the cornflower, brings it some degree into reputation and respect again.

Appearances are often deceptive; and so it is with the succory, for its interior is golden.

Tea made from succory removes phlegm from the stomach, takes away the superfluous gall, purifies liver, milt [spleen] and kidneys, and leads out the morbid matters through the urine. For this end two cups of tea are taken daily, for three or four days, the one before breakfast, the other in the evening. The same may also be taken in order to restore the stomach when it has been upset by any kind of food, etc., and to assist the digestion.

For cramps in the stomach, also for painful inflammation on the body, a poultice made by boiling the herbs and flowers and then wrapping them up in a cloth, is laid on the stomach or painful places. This is renewed two or three times daily.

The herbs are very often put in spirit [alcohol]. Decaying limbs are restored by this spirit when rubbed well with it about twice a day. The roots as well as the other parts of the plant are useful for the given medicinal purposes. They are rooted up most easily in rainy weather.

Tonic Laxative I And II

Forty or fifty years ago it was customary at an exact given time to be bled, at another, a term carefully noted in the almanac (a certain quarter of the moon), to take the yearly or half-yearly purgative. How times, opinions and people who form them, change!

Even in our days many people will not give up the idea that, from time to time, the stomach needs a thorough cleaning out.

One could laugh if it were not, in all earnestness, most lamentable. In truth, if those of a regular, simple and healthy mind reflect on the conduct of certain people, I feel almost tempted to say, of whole classes of society, and on the food and drink which they take, and then indeed the above idea is not unfounded.

If the dreadfully tormented and sinfully overstrained (because overloaded) stomach could give a sound, it would cry out and call for help against that kind of unreasonable malefactors! But as it is, it must *swallow* all, and thereby certainly be miserably ruined.

Therefore, first of all, I recommend a reasonable mode of life, a worthy treatment of the laborer which lays the indispensable foundation for all further work. Thus only will and can this faithful and diligent worker, the stomach, remain healthy.

Should unexpectedly—it may easily occur—a misfortune happen to it also, I advise most decidedly against drastic (too strong) purging. I reject all purgatives which operate violently, let them be called by whatever name.

By purging surely nothing else is understood than striving to produce a more copious evacuation of the bowels, without injuring the health and bodily strength. But this can be done in so simple and harmless a manner! The herbal remedies do not, so to speak, seize the stomach as an enemy, but as true friends they walk arm in arm with it, supporting it, and raising it, to proper activity. They only offer it their juices as means to assist its own means of digestion (juice of the stomach).

For a long time, I have selected from among the different plants those which having the most excellent particular effects, also exhibit their particular healing virtues by acting collectively *viribus units* (with united powers) and efficaciously to assist the stomach, i.e., when weakening it by thoroughly dissolving and removing all morbid substances, they strengthen it at the same time that it not only does not suspend its work for a single hour, but does not even grumble and complain about it.

I think I have found the remedies and their mixture. Both kinds of tea shall be no secret; on the contrary, I wish that very many use them, and prepare them for the relief of others.

The first recipe is this:

TONIC LAXATIVE I

two tablespoonful of pounded fennel
two tablespoonful of crushed juniper berries
one tablespoonful of *Foenum graecum*
one tablespoonful of aloe powder

Mix them all well together, put the mixture in a box, and keep it in a dry place. The remedy operates after twelve to thirty hours. The tea is taken generally at night before going to bed; a small cupful is a dose. One teaspoonful of the mixture is sufficient for a cupful; it is boiled for a quarter of an hour, then poured off and drunk either cold or warm, with or without sugar.

Strong persons may drink a cup of the tea on two succeeding days. Weaker patients would do better to divide the cupful for two or three days, so that they take four to six tablespoonful [of herbal] medicine every evening. Without any uncomfortable feeling, they will experience its effects.

With many who make use of this tea, it will be entirely without result, although they feel its active work in the interior. The police seek, but sometimes find no thief. The tea seeks; but where there is nothing to find and remove, it leaves all else in peace, and thereby does not cause that great and lamentable weakness which otherwise follows purging.

In the same manner as upon the evacuation of the bowels, this tea operates also on the urine. Even great obstructions of phlegm on the chest are removed by it.

Cases have often occurred to me in which after tedious diarrhoea, difficult to stop, this tea has removed the remainder of the impurities, and the deepest and most lasting peace followed the internal revolution. One small cupful drunk during the day in three portions is quite sufficient.

The second recipe for this tea is the following:

TONIC LAXATIVE II

two tablespoonful of pounded fennel
three tablespoonful of crushed juniper berries
three tablespoonful of powder from dwarf elder roots
one tablespoonful of *Foenum graecum*
one tablespoonful of aloe powder

This tea does not exclude purging effects, still its districts are (instead of the stomach and bowels) more the kidneys and bladder. It drives the morbid matters out through the urine. Those who feel uneasiness in the abdomen (in the vicinity of the bladder), or difficulty in making urine, burning in the bladder and the kidneys, those who are in the first stages of dropsy, may calmly use this second tea. In the application, the same rules are to be observed as with regard to the first recipe.

VALERIAN, VALERIANA OFFICINALIS L.

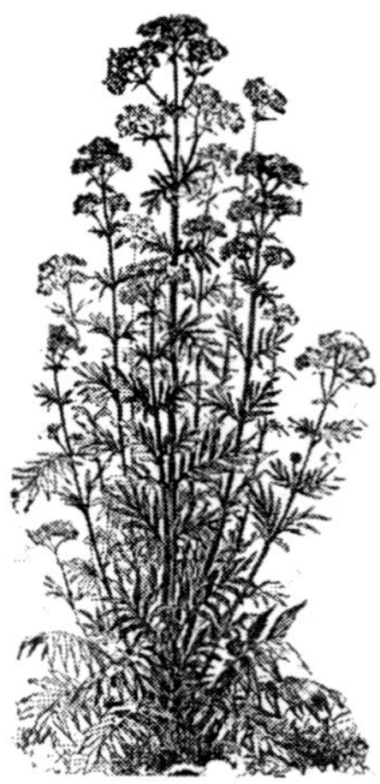

Valerian
(*Valeriana officinalis*)

That something special must be hidden in valerian is proved to us by the cats, which are so attracted by it that they roll themselves among it.

We use only the roots, which are either cut up for tea or pounded for powder, and which (both as tea and as powder) are taken in small quantities only.

Valerian root relieves head complaints, and removes spasms in a similar manner to rue; it operates upon both complaints, as it removes their principal cause, viz., the gases.

WILD ANGELICA

There grows on damp meadows or wet woody places a plant with a stalk from about twenty to forty inches high. The stalks are hollow, and the lads like to make whistles of them. This plant bears the name of angelica. It is, like many others, not known in its sanitary effects on the human body.

If anyone has taken unwholesome or half-poisonous food, tea made by boiling its roots, seeds and leaves is an excellent remedy for removing these injurious matters.

As the blood is prepared from the different kinds of food, and as these are not all good and wholesome for the system, this tea leads the bad matters out of the blood again.

How often does it happen that an uncomfortable coldness takes possession of the stomach! A cup of tea made from such roots, brings more warmth to the stomach again. It is best to divide such a cup of tea into three parts, and to take the first in the morning, the second at noon, and the third in the evening.

If there are morbid matters in the stomach or bowels, or if gripes are caused by gases, this tea is again an efficient remedy, especially if half-wine and half-water are taken for the tea. Thick phlegm on the lungs and chest, heartburn, phlegm in the wind pipes, are by this tea especially and very easily removed.

Angelica can be highly recommended as an excellent home remedy, and country people ought to gather a good quantity of it, for the whole year, in the meadows and woods, dry it in the air, and keep it in a dry place. These roots, seeds and leaves, well dried, may also be made into powder, and a good pinch of such a powder taken twice or three times daily will supply in the place of the tea.

I caution those who have little knowledge of plants against gathering angelica lest they should carry home hemlock (poisonous plant) instead.* I was urged to give this warning by the fact that cases of such dangerous mistakes have repeatedly occurred.

Wormwood

Wormwood ranks among the best known stomachics. It leads the wind out of the stomach, improves the stomach juices, and so affects a good appetite and good digestion, whether it is taken as tea or as powder.

For a bad smell from the mouth, if it proceeds from the stomach, wormwood is of excellent effect. Whoever is suffering from liver complaint (melancholy) let him take the little box of wormwood powder instead of his snuff-box, and put a pinch of its content into his first spoonful of soup, or sprinkle it like pepper on his food once or twice a day. The decreasing yellowness of the skin will soon show the improvement of gall, and the patient, whose breath has been, as it were, laced up by the foul air and often still more foul juices—real dung-hills of the stomach—will breathe more freely again.

Wormwood can also be used as a tincture, which may be preserved for a long time. As a single little corn of incense glimmering on the charcoal will fill a whole room with perfume, so a little leaf of wormwood is sufficient to give a bitter taste to the contents of a whole spirit bottle; a sign of the virtue of the tincture and its effects.

Travelers who are much troubled with indigestion and nausea should never forget to take with them as a faithful companion their little bottle of wormwood tincture.

---

*Angelica and water hemlock can be mistaken for each other. Angelica has thick, purplish and hairless stems and large compound leaves with the veins in the leaflets extending to the tips of the teeth on the margins. Water hemlock has smooth and waxy stem with purple blotches and its glossy leaves are small and fern-like. —*Ed.*

Tea made from silverweed is an excellent remedy in attacks of cramp in the stomach, abdomen, or elsewhere. Even in cases of tetanus—insofar as this can be worked upon—this little herb renders very good service.

This medicinal herb [St. John's wort] has a particular influence on the liver; its tea is an excellent remedy for it. A small admixture of aloe powder increases the effect, which can be observed chiefly in the urine; whole flakes of morbid matters are sometimes washed away with it.

Tea made from succory removes phlegm from the stomach, takes away the superfluous gall, purifies liver, milt [spleen] and kidneys, and leads out the morbid matters through the urine.

Forty or fifty years ago it was customary at an exact given time to be bled, at another, a term carefully noted in the almanac (a certain quarter of the moon), to take the yearly or half-yearly purgative.

For a long time, I have selected from among the different plants those which having the most excellent particular effects, also exhibit their particular healing virtues by acting collectively viribus units *(with united powers) and efficaciously to assist the stomach, i.e., when weakening it by thoroughly dissolving and removing all morbid substances, they strengthen it at the same time that it not only does not suspend its work for a single hour, but does not even grumble and complain about it.*

Valerian root relieves head complaints, and removes spasms in a similar manner to rue; it operates upon both complaints, as it removes their principal cause, viz., the gases.

Wormwood ranks among the best known stomachics. It leads the wind out of the stomach, improves the stomach juices, and so affects a good appetite and good digestion, whether it is taken as tea or as powder.

Contents Of A Little Kneipp Home Dispensary

by Benedict Lust, N.D.

The Naturopath and Herald of Health, XIV (8), 486. (1909)

Tinctures

Arnica, bilberry, gentian, juniper berries, rosemary, succory or chicory, and wormwood.

Tea

Althea, oak bark, bogbean, brier, blackthorn blossoms, chamomile, centaury, coltsfoot, elder, nettle, yarrow, cowslip, dwarf elder, eyebright, juniper berries, lime tree blossoms, lungwort, mallow, mistletoe, mullein, mint, ribwort (plantain), rosemary, rue, sage, St. John's wort, shavegrass (Equisetum), silverweed, strawberries, succory or chicory, sweet woodruff, Kneipp Tonic Laxative, valerian, violet, wild angelica, and wormwood.

Powder

Alum, aloe, coltsfoot, dwarf elder, eyebright, fennel, fenugreek, linseed, mint, sage, sandal, valerian, wormwood, and wild angelica.

Others: bone-dust, chalk, and coal dust.

Oil

Anise, camphor, fennel, juniper berry, and rue.

Others: almond oil, oil of cloves, lavender oil, and salad oil.

1910

Rosemary Wine
Benedict Lust, N.D.

Drugs And Drugs
William Waugh

DECEMBER, 1919—PAGE 614 HERALD OF HEALTH AND NATUROPATH

The following from Dr. Benedict Lust, the well-known author and editor of the HERALD OF HEALTH, speaks for itself:

MY DEAR DOCTOR:

I have lately been using your Flaxolyn, my last order of which was three dozen, in my treatment of a number of my patients at the Butler Sanitarium. I consider it a most modern and natural adjunct, and find it a great help in assisting the process of elimination of irritants from the system. It helps bring the body back to its normal stage. It is certainly a natural food remedy, and complies with the teachings and tenets of the great Father Kneipp, and other authorities of natural healing. I advise every drugless practitioner to give Dr. Luntz's Flaxolyn a fair trial.

Fraternally yours,

B. LUST, N. D., M. D.

Nature's Roots and Herbs Compounded with Baked Flaxseed. That is FLAXOLYN

The Modern Remedy for all Stomach Ailments, Liver Trouble, Constipation, Gall Stones and Kidney Trouble

IT was the open publication of the FLAXOLYN FORMULA that from the very first won the confidence of both physicians and the general public.

When you take a medicine, you should know what you are taking. When you are not told, there is a reason for not telling you.

You do not need to be convinced that the ingredients of FLAXOLYN are absolutely harmless. Your instinct tells you that they are good for you. Here are the sole ingredients of FLAXOLYN, and their use:

1. *Baked Flaxseed*—Relaxes congestion and acts as an astringent.

2. *Vegetable Charcoal*—Aids digestion, sweetens the stomach, overcomes acid and gas, purifies undigested, fermenting food.

3. *Juniper Berries*—Cleanse, purify and stimulate the kidneys and bladder.

4. *African Ginger Roots*—Quicken the flow of the vital digestive juices.

5. *Dandelion Roots* — Purify the liver and blood.

6. *Cardamom Seeds*—Act on the stomach lining as an aromatic, cleansing tonic.

7. *Chinese Rhubarb*—Invigorates the stomach and the liver.

8. *Spanish Licorice Roots* — Remove any foreign mucous that may be clogging and poisoning the digestive organs.

9. *Culver's Roots*—Stimulate the natural flow of bile and so purify the liver.

10. *Gentian Roots* — Create a healthy, normal appetite.

11. *Greek Valerian Roots* — Tone the nerves and induce the restful sleep of health.

12. *California Bark*—Cleanses the colon and removes foreign matter from the intestines.

PRICE, $1.00 PER BOX, POST PAID

Special Price for Physicians

SEND THIS COUPON FOR BOOKLET

Dr. H. H. LUNTZ
1155 St. Johns Place, Brooklyn, N. Y.
Please send me your free booklet containing rules of health.

Flaxseeds have had a long history with Naturopathy.

Rosemary Wine

by Benedict Lust, N.D.

The Naturopath and Herald of Health, XV (5), 291. (1910)

Dropsy, asthma, emphysema, kidney troubles are, though not always cured, but thoroughly relieved by rosemary wine. Tea made of this little herb is excellent, but far more superior is the rosemary wine. This wine is prepared in the following way: young, fresh branches of the rosemary shrub are cut into finger lengths, washed in cold water and a handful of it put into a bottle of genuine, old white wine; kept at a place of medium temperature, and then within a fortnight it is ready for use. According to the degree of the ailment, three spoonfuls of this wine, taken twice a day, will be of beneficial use.

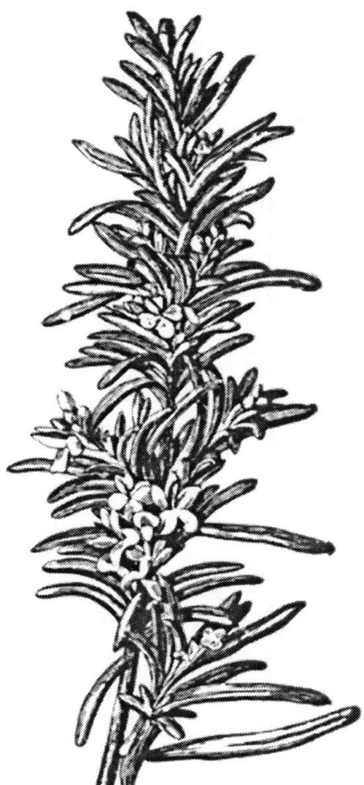

Rosemary (*Rosmarinus officinalis*)

DRUGS AND DRUGS

by William Waugh

The Naturopath and Herald of Health, XV (8), 469-471. (1910)

Benedict Lust's Editor's Note: Above article is something unusual in this magazine. We have always been denouncing drugs strongly and had a number of complaints from respectable old school physicians, and after some correspondence with Dr. W. Waugh, in which I promised to give space and give the other side also a chance to present their arguments. So here it is and our readers are the judges.

It seems that we Americans can never be contented with half-way measures, but we must push an idea to the limit or drop it altogether. The Germans have a proverb that says, "In emptying the bath, we need not spill the baby" and we might well adopt it.

Fifty years ago, the medical profession and the people placed a ridiculous estimate on the values of drugs, and neglected everything else in the treatment of the sick. Reaction began when Oliver Wendell Holmes remarked that it would be better for man but worse for the fishes were all the drugs to be emptied into the sea. The expression took like the measles, and ever since we have had a succession of smart folks who try to say the same thing in other words. We have gotten to the point where many worthy people look on drugs as the work of the devil and their employment as irreligious.

There are some of us who advance the thought that drugs are not essentially evil, but things that possess certain properties that may be utilized by those who know how; and that wholesale denunciation is never quite in accordance with fact. Let us argue the matter a bit.

Drugs are substances which exert some influence over the functions of the human body, increasing the action of some or lessening the action of others. Disease causes an alteration in the vital functions, depressing some or elevating others.

If any certain disease increases one of these vital functions and a drug lessens it, we may give just enough of the drug to balance the irritation of the disease, and the function is restored to that normal exercise or equilibrium we term health. Three things are necessary: the doctor must be able to recognize the departure from health, he must know just what drug will restore the physiologic balance of activity, and he must give just enough and no more. This implies knowledge of the fundamental branches of medical science, such as we spend many years in endeavoring to acquire.

Here we meet the principal difficulty, the source of most of our woes—for drugs do not always accomplish what we desire or expect. The reasons are not commonly appreciated, and may be mentioned.

Vegetable drugs consist of the leaves, roots, seed, or other parts of plants. These are not uniformly active, but consist of woody fibre, coloring matter, and other plant parts or ingredients, none of which exerts any power over the vital functions, and they are hence termed "inert". They are essential to the plant, but only so much encumbering dirt as far as the medical values of the plant are concerned. These reside in a group of substances known as the active principles, because they exert some active influence over the human body when given as medicines. These are known as alkaloids, glucosides, resins, etc. They are the real medical principles on which plants depend for their remedial values, the rest being so much dirt, as has been said. By leaving out the dirt we reduce the dose, render it far less disagreeable, and find that it is more quickly absorbed and gets to work sooner. So, instead of administering the whole plant, we seek to reduce its value to an extract, tincture, infusion or decoction. All these have been found deficient because in all liquid preparations there is a steady evaporation of the fluid parts, the water and alcohol, and a degeneration of the active principles which are altered into inert matters such as the coloring substances. It is this that makes medicines gradually darken with age. In the cultivation of cinchona it was found necessary to wrap the trees with moss to prevent the change of the quinine into coloring matters. Hence the strength of liquids was a matter of uncertainty, since if evaporation was rapid the strength was increased, but if decomposition went on quickly it was lessened.

Another element of uncertainty lay in the fact that many plants develop more than one active principle, and these are often antagonistic. Hyoscyamus [has the property] that induces sleep and calms excitement, another that prevents sleep and arouses delirium. Jaborandi has a group of principles that induce sweating and increase the milk of the nursing mother, and another group that exactly opposes both actions. Gelsemium, the pretty yellow jasmine, has a most valuable soothing agent in it and another that causes constant convulsions. The greater celandine has seventeen active principles; opium has 26; and Peruvian bark no less than 30, no two of which exert precisely the same influence when given as medicines.

We must remember that these are developed in the plant directly for its own purposes and only remotely for ours. Under the varying influences of sun and shade, heat and cold, dryness and moisture, soil, climate and many others, these active principles develop in varying quantity and proportions. Hence the plant may at one time exert one [effect], and another specimen one precisely the contrary, even if they are handled in the same manner by the druggist. Opium may contain a large quantity of morphine and put the patient at rest, or little or none, but much thebaine [alkaloid], and kill him with convulsions. The way to find just what a drug would do was to try it on the patient and this warily, ready to run at the first evidence of peril. Only in this way could we tell just what a drug would do and how much of this effect it would exert. The experimentation had to be renewed each time we used that drug, for we could not be sure no change had taken place in a week or more. The inevitable result was timidity in the use of drugs and the loss of precious time, for the best time to put out a fire is when it is beginning, and disease is a fire that will grow into a conflagration if not extinguished at once.

These considerations have led some of us up to the extraction of each of these active principles and its use in a state of absolute chemic purity, so that we get from it exactly the same effect every time, in exactly the same quantity. These when put up in granules with pure sugar of milk, experience no decomposition as long as moisture is kept away. I have such granules over twenty years old that are as active as the day they were made.

We know precisely what each of these active principles will do, every time the same thing and we are therefore ready to use them at once, and with the boldness that comes from knowledge. We believe we can abort acute disease by treating it at the beginning, before it has had time to make a lodgment in the tissues of the body, because we are doing that every day. The others do not believe this because they do not use these remedies, and that alone make it possible.

Knowledge is power. Confidence comes with the use of certainties and inspires confidence. Frankly, if I had to use only the old trash I would leave the practice of medicine. You cannot say more or worse of it than it deserves, but when you use remedies that are sure to do exactly what you want, that is another matter. We then find that such drugs afford us the readiest and quickest, the most powerful and effective known means of combating disease. I am not saying a word against the use of other than drug means—their value is established too well; but in nine-tenths of the ailments for which we are consulted we get better results from drugs, the right ones, applied rightly. Take two cases—a man told me he had spent $97.00 on non-drug methods and then got more benefit from two cents worth of salts in a few hours. A working man was ill and his employer kindly sent him his own specialist, saying he would foot the bill. After a week of non-drug treatment the sick man dismissed the fashionable adviser and sent for a drug man, saying he could not afford to be away from his work so long.

Moral: Cuss the ordinary misuse of drugs and we add our hearty amen; but we draw the line at the right use of the right drugs, with a clear idea of why we use them and what they will do.

Fifty years ago, the medical profession and the people placed a ridiculous estimate on the values of drugs, and neglected everything else in the treatment of the sick.

We must remember that these [constituents] are developed in the plant directly for its own purposes and only remotely for ours.

These considerations have led some of us up to the extraction of each of these active principles and its use in a state of absolute chemic purity, so that we get from it exactly the same effect every time, in exactly the same quantity.

1911

Naturopath Advocate Offers Elder Blossoms As Blood Purifier

Benedict Lust, N.D.

Our Most Medicinal Herbs, Knotgrass

P. Heinrichs

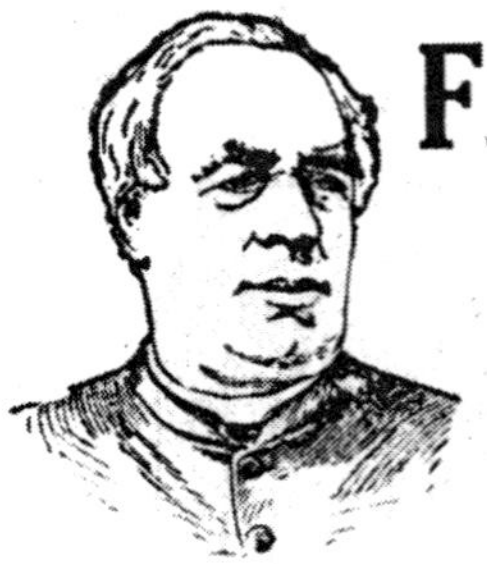

FATHER KNEIPP'S PILLS

They are free from all injurious aperients, being exclusively composed of herbal ingredients, and are universally considered the best for keeping the bowels open without weakening the stomach. These same herbal ingredients were used by Rev. Seb. Kneipp at Wörishofen in his treatments. The pills may be taken for years without injury to the system, and with only beneficial results. It is therefore easily explained why our Kneipp Pills are recommend by celebrated professors. medical men, the followers of the Kneipp treatment, and by the public at large, and that they are preferred to any other pills or laxatives. The Kneipp Pills are the best and most pleasant laxative in the world, on account of their efficiency in most stubborn cases of constipation, indigestion, piles, giddiness, and all complaints of the liver. Pfarrer Sebastian Kneipp has given to Oberhäuser & Landauer, of Würzburg, the exclusive right to denominate same with his name, and to attach his picture and signature, registered as a trade-mark. Price, 50c.; by mail, 52c.

Send all orders to Kneipp Store, 465 Lexington Avenue, New York City, near 45th Street.

Catalog of Kneipp's genuine remedies, herbs, teas, books, underwear, etc.; prospectus of Kneipp Institute and Kneipp Sanitarium "Yungborn," Butler, N. J., mailed free on application.

In 1911, Benedict Lust expanded his store by moving to a new location, 465 Lexington Avenue near the bustle of Park Avenue. Lust continued to import and sell Kneipp's herbs which were also made available in pill form.

Naturopath Advocate Offers Elder Blossoms As Blood Purifier

by Benedict Lust, N.D.

The Naturopath and Herald of Health, XVI (7), 443. (1911)

We quote the following item, which appeared in one of the papers of Los Angeles:

One who claims to know what he is talking about came into our office, and presenting himself to the editor, said:

"Well, Mr. Editor, here I give you a paper sack filled with blossoms of the elder. These blossoms are one of the best blood purifiers of nature. Don't make a tea out of them, for boiling will destroy the best properties they contain. Eat them just as they come, perfect out of the best laboratory on earth and you will derive the best results. Put on a little olive oil and lemon juice. There are a good many other blood purifiers, such as the dandelion (the whole plant), the burdock root, bull thistle root, both of the latter in the first year of existence; the blackthorn blossom, for those who know how to handle themselves the so-called poison oak, and a good many others. In addition to the frequent use of cold water baths, wind, air, and sun baths, correct breathing and correct diet can easily purify the blood. To attempt to do this by the use of chemicals in the form of drugs, pills, tablets, patent medicines, nostrums, or Christian Science, I would advise nobody, for in this way the remedy is all the time worse than the disease.

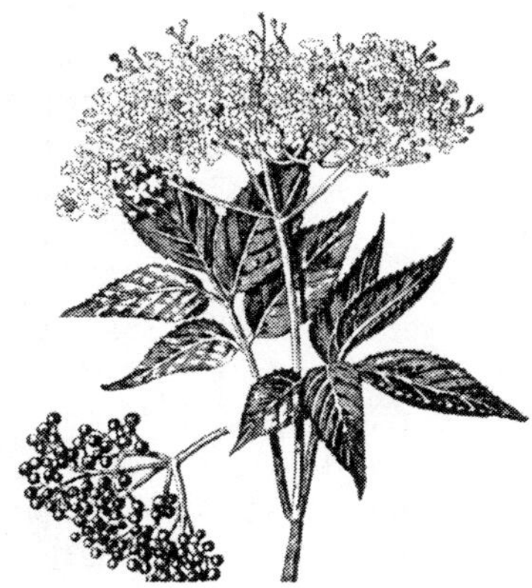

Elder was a valued and indispensable herb.

"Now then, if the blood of a person is clean and pure, it is impossible for that person to get sick even if he tries to."

The editor took the paper sack filled with blossoms of the elder, and said: "I'll try it; good-bye Mr. Buetzenbach."

OUR MOST MEDICINAL HERBS, KNOTGRASS

by P. Heinrichs

The Naturopath and Herald of Health, XVI (12), 786-787. (1911)

BY WAYS AND RIDGES

A Slavic tale relates: "Once upon a time, early of a morn, an old witch set out and went up to the high mountains to practice her witchery and gather herbs there. Towards noon she started on her home journey and met the knotgrass or swine grass that was fleeing to the mountains in great haste. The witch asked it: 'Why! Whither, birdie? What trouble drives you to tread this rough path?' The swine grass answered: 'Alas, mother dear, down there I can stay no longer. Whenever the peasant digs or turns up the soil, he also weeds with all his might, and he chokes and tears and flays me, tries to uproot me and that means I must flee in order to find a little resting place where I can grow in peace and multiply.' Thereupon the witch replied: 'Birdie, up and back to your home! Mark you: wherever they dig and turn up the soil and weed much, there everything thrives more and the roots can spread much better. As the proverb has it: Woe unto the thing that hath no one to take care of it!'" The knotgrass returned and since that time it is found in fields and meadows, in wine plantations and gardens, in short, everywhere where it is not wanted, and it is very hard to root it out thoroughly.

The swine grass is really one of the most widespread of plants and surely there isn't one among my readers who hasn't stepped on the lowly herb a hundred times; for even if the farmer try his utmost to deprive it of its place in field and pasture, it spreads itself so much more on crossroads, on little used places of highways, nay, even between the flagstones of quiet city sections. It loves company of its own kind and often assumes exclusive rule over broad stretches of land. With its thin, almost thread-like stalk, which are from 30 to 60 cm. long, it lies flat upon the ground and with profuse branching spreads out in all directions. It also knows how to adapt itself somewhat to space conditions where there is no room for extension in all directions; e.g., between grass and grain, a portion of its stalks point upward, but even in this case they are generally surrounded on the ground by a wealth of creeping shoots of the same length. The small, oval leaflets which cover the stem quite fully in alternate positions, come to a point at both ends; one can hardly speak here of a stemlet. They are therefore designated as sedentary; with their flat side they cling to the ground. Most of them are bluish-green; some appear to have a reddish tint. On the ground are short, whitish, dry-skinned side leaves, which surround the stalk in the form of a cornet and have a silvery shimmer; they are split and have a ragged edge. From the axils sprout insignificant, minute blossoms.

1912

St. James's Oil

Otto Carqué

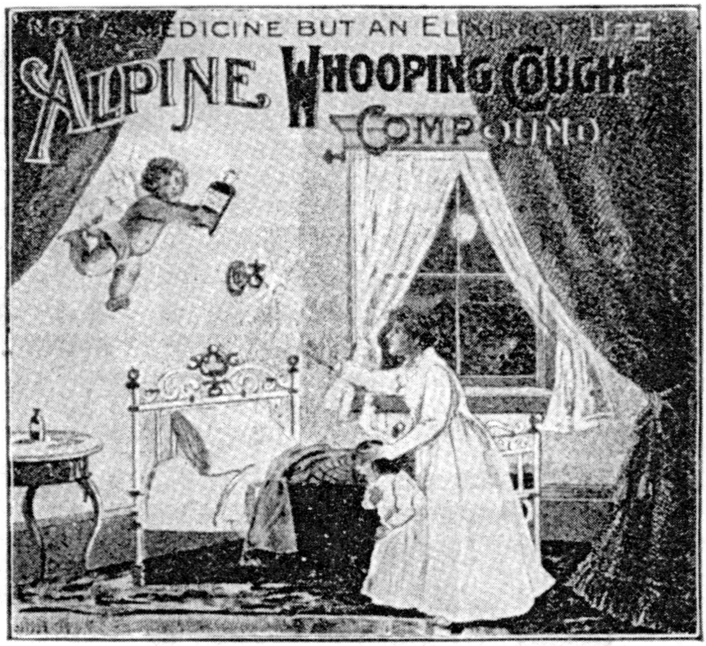

"Alpine Whooping Cough Compound" is a syrup prepared from various plants, which cleanses the lungs (which is most important) and creates an appetite. The narcotic remedies used at present produce mostly opposite effects.

The remedy has relieved hundreds of cases and in no instance has any fatal result occured, nor has any case resulted unfavorably, which fact can be vouched for by certified testimonials.

This remedy is not only beneficial for Whooping Coughs, but can be used as well for all ordinary coughs and colds, which latter it cures more rapidly.

In case not obtainable at your druggist, write to the

ALPINE MEDICAL CO.,

1150 MYRTLE AVE., BROOKLYN, N. Y.

The early Naturopaths treated whooping cough with confidence using herbs and hydrotherapy.

St. James's Oil*

by Otto Carqué

The Naturopath and Herald of Health, XVII (2), 114-115. (1912)

It Radiates Health—A Wonderful Aid In The Rebuilding Of The Body

For thousands of years the oiling of the body has been valued in Oriental countries as a most helpful hygienic measure. The passage in the Epistle of St. James: "Is any among you sick? Let him call for the elders of the church; and let them pray over him, anointing him with oil in the name of the Lord," does not refer to the mere making of the sign of a cross on the forehead with a finger dipped in oil, but to the custom of oiling the whole body. This was usually done after a warm bath. Costly oil, mixed with perfumes, was used for this purpose by the rich.

Inunction is an exceedingly valuable therapeutic measure. It has been far too much over-looked in modern times. It increases the activity of the skin and diminishes susceptibility to cold. By equalizing the temperature it has great power in allaying fever. It soothes the nervous system, produces sleep, and lessens the frequency of the pulse, and thirst. The pulse may be reduced from 120 to 90 in a few hours after a few applications of the oil. It is also very serviceable in lowering the temperature in typhoid and typhus fevers, pneumonia and all febrile disorders. It is particularly valuable in the treatment of smallpox, alleviating the suffering of the patient by soothing the skin and lowering the temperature, lessening the liability of pitting and of communicating the disease to others.

It is, however, mainly in chronic ailments of long standing that inunction is most efficacious. It is of great value in the treatment of consumptives, dyspeptics, diabetic patients, those suffering from anemia, or thin blood, and all classes of invalids whose skin is dry or inactive, and who cannot assimilate much food. It will sometimes produce marvelous results in the cases of infants who seem to be wasting away without adequate cause. It will be found of great service in preventing bed sores in patients long confined to their beds, for which purpose it should be applied once or twice a day.

St. James's oil is also very effective when applied to sprains and bruises.

It is a popular error to suppose that oiling checks the perspiration. This is not the case. Oiling the skin does not interfere with the perspiratory process.

---

*I was unable to determine what St. James's oil was made from. —*Ed.*

Now-a-days people are wisely discarding poisonous drugs which never cure disease, but only suppress the symptoms for a time, adding the poison of the drugs to that of the disease. The old saying is a wise one: "Food for the stomach; medicine for the skin."

St. James's oil has been prepared according to a suggestion made by Harry Ellington Brook, editor of the Care of the Body department of the *Los Angeles Sunday Times* magazine, by whom it is strongly endorsed. It is a combination of three selected oils, one of which is very expensive.

For the present, until arrangements are made for a wider distribution, St. James's oil may be obtained from the St. James's Oil Company, Otto Carqué, Manager, 943 West 12th Street, Los Angeles, California. Eastern Depots: Kneipp-Store, Butler, New Jersey, and Naturopathic Supplies Store, 465 Lexington Avenue, New York City. Price $1 per bottle, expressage 25 cents extra, or six bottles packed in a box will be sent, expressage paid, to any part of the United States for $5.00.

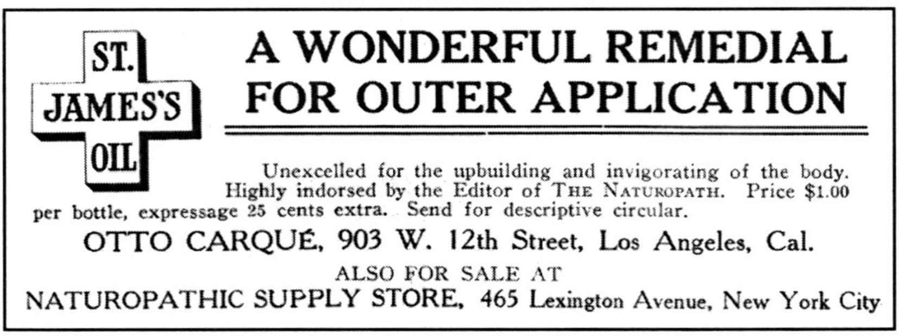

Otto Carqué published several books on dietetics and nutrition and in 1912 established the Carqué Pure Food Company in California, selling health food products. The St. James's oil was one such product.

1913

Curled Leaved Mallow Or Hygeia Plant

George J. Drews

Curled Dock

George J. Drews

Dandelions

George J. Drews

Autumn's Peace, Autumn's Bliss

Benedict Lust, N.D.

A Moral Diet **is the foundation to perpetual health, morality and all reform**

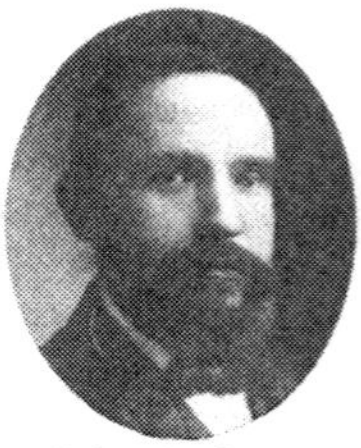

"**Trophotherapeutics**" is the art of curing diseases with natural specific food." (in Nature's own way) without the use of dangerous drugs.

Unfired Food and Tropho-Therapy

— BY DREWS —

A Text Book For Nurses, Physicians, Students and Mothers

It is a book embracing five volumes in one. It contains 325 pages, bound in black cloth and stamped in white foil. It is illustrated with 30 halftones and some etchings. Price $2.00.

PART INTRODUCTORY

The matter under this head points out the snares and delusions in the present, disease breeding, system of diet and introduces a natural disease-preventing and disease-curing diet.

PART I.

UNFIRED FOOD contains 360 recipes for preparing and combining health perpetuating food in such a way as to make it most palatable, delicious, satiating and artistically dainty. It covers drinks, soups, salads, brawnfoods, cakes, pies and confections. This is the first book giving recipes for uncooked soups, flower salads and unfired pies and wedding cake.

PART II.

MATERIA ALIMENTARIA treats on the healing properties and medicinal value of wholesome specific foods. It contains all the American food analyses and European organic salt analyses published to date. The many simplified tables which classify food into specific remedies are most valuable and the first of their kind.

PART III.

TROPHOTHERAPY (Natural Food Cure) and Prophylactic (preventive) Feeding, treats on the cause, cure and prevention of all common diseases. It tells how to remove the cause of disease, how to help Nature to re-establish health and how to perpetuate health by feeding on Nature's Panacean Foods. It also contains a diagram for diagnosing diseases from the iris of the eye.

PART IV.

PROMISCUOUS SUBJECTS treats on hygienics, the value of sunshine, fresh air, breathing, exercise, felicity and serenity of mind, fasting, social dinners, effects of food on morality, refinements and beauty, commercial foods, dairy products, infant feeding and drugs—drugs the cause of chronic diseases.

PART V.

ALIMENTARY BOTANY. Under this head 200 natural foods are described with reference to source, value, wholesomeness, flavor, use and preparation. This covers fruits, esculent flowers, herbs, roots, nuts, cereals, and legumes. This department ends with Cottage Garden Culture and a diagram with directions for an economical arrangement of a city garden.

This book is absolutely original in the style of its recipes. The ingredients of each recipe are arranged in a left marginal, bold faced column. A glance at this column tells you what you want and saves you the time of re-reading, underscoring and memorizing. Each recipe is provided with a column of weights to insure perfect results and save waste of material. This feature will be appreciated most by schools of Domestic Economy. You would be surprised if I told you how few utensils are required for the preparation of Natural food.

If you are interested in "Return to Nature" you cannot do without this book. It teaches the only moral diet known to science and is the most complete Nature Cure food book in print. There is no disease for those who feed on unfired food and the sick will get well by it. Unfired food is the foundation to all reform. If you will try it honestly for six months you will eat no more cooked food.

This is the first Food Book which treats on Trophotherapeutics (curative feeding).

Price, $2.00 By Mail, $2.20

BENEDICT LUST, N. D., "Yungborn Health Home," Butler, N. J.

George Julius Drews, Al.D., D.C. defined Apyrotrophy as the science, art and practice of living on the moral unfired diet for the perpetuation of perfect health and cure of disease. He was the original raw food vegan who wrote *Unfired Food and Tropho-Therapy* (1912) and began a movement of raw food vegetarianism in America.

THE NATUROPATH AND HERALD OF HEALTH'S

Apyrtropher Section

DEVOTED TO

APYRTROPHY—the Science, Art and Practice of Living on the Moral Unfired Diet for the Perpetuation of Perfect Health and Cure of Disease.

It is also the organ of the Apyrtropher (*Unfired-fooder*) Society. Address all communications for this department to its editor.

GEORGE J. DREWS, M.D., D.C., 1910 North Harding Avenue, Chicago, Ill.

Curled Leaf Mallow Or Hygeia Plant

by George J. Drews

The Naturopath and Herald of Health, XVIII (1), 56. (1913)

Malva Crispa, L. Malvaceae

This mallow plant is well known in all the European countries. The French call it *Mauve frisee* and the Germans call it *Krausblaettrige Malve*. It is a large plant, with an erect, simple or slightly branched stem, four to six feet high, and leafy to the top. The leaves are large, round, light green in color, very elegantly curled and puckered at the edges. The seed may be sown in April in a seedbed, from which the young plants should be transplanted at any time before they are three inches high; or it may be sown into its permanent place. The plants should stand about two feet apart. In sowing mallow seed, do not cover it with more than one-eighth inch of heavy soil or one-quarter inch of light soil. After they are started, they require no particular attention. This plant has the power to digest and absorb from the soil a large quantity of basic elements and transform them into organic salts. The character of the organic salts in each variety of plants is different as the character of their growth, flavor and odor. The salts organized by the curled mallow are easily absorbed by any depleted system, and hence it makes a most valuable green food for people whose blood is not proper tone. The mallow salts can be more easily used by the liver and other secretory glands for reorganizing and solidifying undesirable elements in the blood than the organic salts of more common herbs. The mallow salts, however, are no less valuable to the kidneys for making undesirable elements in the blood eliminable.

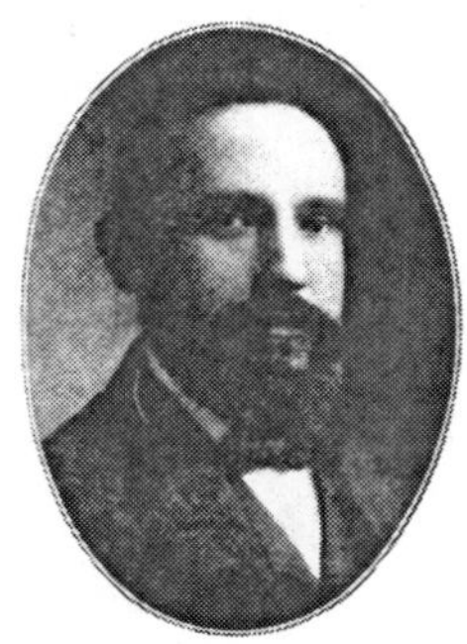

George Julius Drews

Considering the properties of the curled mallow for toning the blood and for promoting proper secretion and excretion of the glands deserves to be called *Hygeia Plant.* The leaves have a mild, pleasant flavor and can be used for aesthetic synede (salads) like any other esculent [vegetable, fit to be eaten] herb. The dried leaves are very valuable for therapeutic purposes, (drinks.) For the purpose of making a strong infusion, soak the leaves in cold water over night or for twenty-four hours. Most refreshing euposes* can be made of a mixture of dried mallow and other wholesome sweet or aroma dried herbs.

Every apyrotropher should have a trophery garden** regardless of size, for a small garden is better than none. One would be surprised how much a small trophery garden can produce when properly arranged and cared for.

Those who have only a very small garden space should have at least six more mallow plants.

The editor had six mallow plants in his trophery garden last summer and gave him much more pleasure to see the mallows grow in very poor soil. This year, the editor has imported from Europe enough mallow seed to supply all apyrotropher friends.

For fifteen one-cent stamps, he can send anyone a packet containing enough mallow seeds to start with a generous crop from greens during the summer for euposes next winter.

Please send your orders to George Drews, Al.D., 3220 Thomas St., Chicago, Illinois.

The mallow salts can be more easily used by the liver and other secretory glands for reorganizing and solidifying undesirable elements in the blood than the organic salts of more common herbs.

Considering the properties of the curled mallow for toning the blood and for promoting proper secretion and excretion of the glands deserves to be called Hygeia Plant. *The leaves have a mild, pleasant flavor and can be used for aesthetic synede (salads) like any other esculent herb.*

---

*An eupose was a drink composed of herbs and fruits and / or vegetables made by Apyrotrophers. The word, apyrotropy, meant unfired food. The apyrotrophy movement started with a book, *Unfired Food and Tropho-Therapy* by George J. Drews who initiated a raw vegan diet in 1912, long before the dietary trends that we find today. —*Ed.*

**A trophery garden included herbs and vegetables providing the basic ingredients for an apyrotroph. —*Ed.*

Curled Dock

by George J. Drews

The Naturopath and Herald of Health, XVIII (4), 266. (1913)

From the standpoint of diet, the apyrotrophers are the most economical people known, for they know how to use to best advantage every fruit, every wholesome wild and cultivated vegetable, the nuts and even the flowers of wholesome plants.

Nearly everywhere in the northern states, next to the dandelion, in the woods, in the meadows, in the waste fields, in the waste lots of cities, in the back yards, in the hedges and by the roadside grows the curled or yellow dock.

This dock comes to usefulness about the same time as the dandelion and like the dandelion, it is an excellent spring tonic food herb. It is, like spinach, rich in all the essential organic salts for toning the blood for aiding the kidneys and the other glands in eliminating from the blood and tissues accumulated impurities, wastes and irritants.

The leaves of this dock are from 6 inches to 12 inches long, tapering towards both ends and about one and one-half inches wide. The surface and the edges of the leaves are sometimes slightly crimped and this is the reason why it is called curled dock. The flavor of the leaves is acid at first taste, but the acidity quickly leaves when the leaf is properly masticated and then changes into a pleasant bread-like flavor.

Bitter dock looks like curled dock in every respect except that its leaves are twice as wide and has no acid flavor.

The curled dock plant can be forced to furnish tender leaves during summer and fall when prevented from running to seed. When you must go far to get curled dock, then gather enough for a few days and on arriving home place the leaves, stem end down, into a bucket containing about two or three inches of water and let it stand in a cool place.

There is nothing in dock roots that is superior tonic food that what the system can get from the leaves.

From the standpoint of diet, the apyrotrophers are the most economical people known, for they know how to use to best advantage every fruit, every wholesome wild and cultivated vegetable, the nuts and even the flowers of wholesome plants.

This dock. . . is, like spinach, rich in all the essential organic salts for toning the blood for aiding the kidneys and the other glands in eliminating from the blood and tissues accumulated impurities, wastes and irritants.

Dandelions

by George J. Drews

The Naturopath and Herald of Health, XVIII (4), 267-268. (1913)

Now is the time when the dandelion comes out from its winter retreat on the sunny side of the hills or any place exposed to the warm rays of the sun.

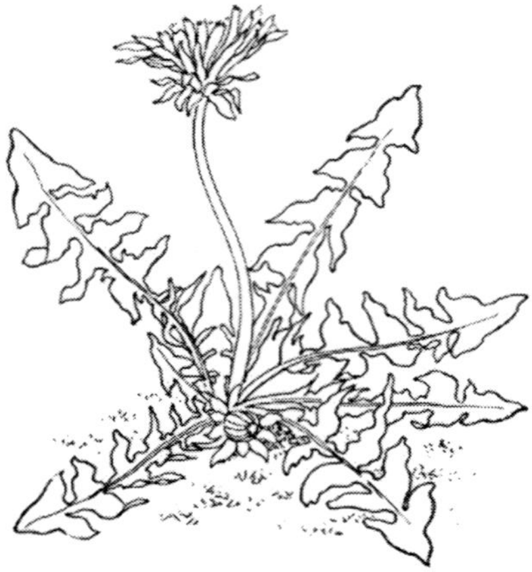

Dandelion
(*Taraxacum officinale*)

The early, young and tender leaves of this vegetable have only a trace of the bitter flavor which they develop later in the season. The particular bitter flavor which the dandelion possess is what makes it so desirable as a synede herb.*

All herbs that are bitter like the dandelion are known as stomach tonics because their bitter juice stimulates the stomach to normal activity and after it combines with the secretions of the stomach, it leaves a very pleasant after-taste.

It is the dandelion that gives cow's milk in spring the rich flavor which we miss later in the season.

Most people who have learned to like the dandelion for a spring vegetable, especially the Italians, are too greedy in gathering it in that they cut it too deep beneath the soil and thus gather too much of the root, which is not desirable for food and besides ruins the plant for the season. For the market it is necessary to cut the root deep enough to hold the leaves for their own use. For synedes will do better by simply pulling the leaves that are from four to six inches long. By doing this, you will not ruin the plant and besides, it saves you a lot of tedious work by not having so many small leaves to wash and pick over.

The dandelion is known to the world over as a spring tonic for which the roots, the leaves and the flowers are used; but the value of its tonic elements is mostly destroyed by cooking and concentration.

The best way to get *your money's worth* out of the dandelion for tonic purposes is to eat the leaves in the form of a synede (saltless salad).

---

*The Aprotrophs made synedes that were salads made with a variety of herbs, roots, and greens without salt. —*Ed.*

Most people who believe in concoctions, dope and witch broths have the idea that the tonic properties reside in the roots of this herb; but the truth is that the tonic elements are more highly developed in the leaves and the flowers.

Vilmorin, the best authority on vegetables, says, "People contented themselves with gathering dandelions in the meadows or fields until, as they became an important article of commerce in the Central Market of Paris, it occurred to some that it could be cultivated and improved by selection of seed from choice plants. Thus the plant was improved to a remarkable degree."

He describes the cultivated varieties as follows:

Large Green Montmagny Dandelion

This, now largely grown in the vicinity of Paris, is a more vigorous form of the common dandelion.

Thick Leaved, Or Cabbaging Dandelion

A very distinct variety, obtained by cultivation and surpassing the wild plant not so much in the size as in the very great number of its leaves, which form a regular tuft or clump, instead of a plain rosette. It yields a very abundant crop without taking up much ground.

Improved Very Early Dandelion

Increasing the breadth of the leaves of dandelions has resulted in fewer leaves being produced. The variety known as the Improved Broad-leaved Dandelion forms a simple rosette of very large and broad leaves, sometimes 20 inches across. The Improved Very Early is a sub variety of the Improved Broad-leaved variety.

Moss Leaved Dandelion

A distinct variety with dense and compact curled leaves and apparently permanent in its characteristics. The plant can be easily blanched, and in that condition affords a vegetable not unlike curled endive, but coming in in spring, when it is very difficult to have any endive fit for table use.

Improved Giant Erect Dandelion

A distinct variety which, instead of forming into a rosette like other dandelions, grows in erect, strong, and thickly-set tufts. The leaves are long and stout, toothed, and slightly brown.

During the last few years the demand for dandelions in Chicago has so increased that, last spring, it was found in every up-to-date grocery store.

The year before last, we sowed a bed of cultivated dandelions early in spring, which grew vigorously during that summer. In the fall, before the frost set in, we laid a foundation around this bed for glass covering; but we allowed the bed to undergo the winter until last February the first, when we covered it with glass. The dandelions started to grow at once so that by the first of April the leaves were 13 inches tall and as tender and sweet as the finest of lettuce. We do not know any other that we could have forced so early with so little expense and trouble.

Those who have not yet procured a copy of our book, *Unfired Food,* may wonder how we prepare a dandelion synede; but we will tell you how in the following lines.

Dandelion Synede

Take a cup loosely filled with chopped dandelion leaves and put them in one side of an oatmeal dish. Now spin a teaspoonful of honey over the chopped leaves and then drip over them a teaspoonful of lemon juice and one of olive oil. In the vacant side of the dish put four heaping table spoonsful of ground (or flaked) almonds or flaked unroasted Spanish peanuts. Now the synede is ready to be served and the one who eats it is to mix the ground nuts with the greens with his fork, little by little as he eats it. For those who are not acquainted with the apyrotropher diet, it is best to mix the synede completely before serving it.

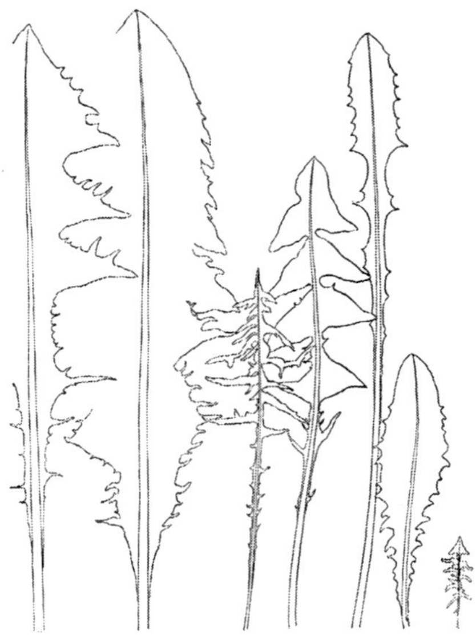

Variations of dandelion leaves

For the form of an aesthetic spring synede see *Unfired Food*, page 142.*

The dandelion flowers are composed of the essence of this plant. They are not as bitter as the leaves and slightly sweet if picked at sunrise, before the bees are out to gather the honey. They are not as tender as the leaves, giving pleasant resistance to the teeth, and being compact, they easily satisfy hunger without any other additional food.

---

*I have included this recipe for a spring synede in Herbal Formulas, p. 345. —*Ed.*

Between the fifteenth of April and the fifteenth of May when the dandelion flowers are most profusely produced, one can gather enough flowers for a mess in a few minutes.

If your blood is not in the most perfect tone, if you suffer from some form of alimentary trouble, if any disease troubles you, if you are convalescent, if you are about to become an apyrotropher or if you are already a confirmed apyrotropher, YOU CANNOT AFFORD TO MISS THE EATING OF A DANDELION SYNEDE OR TO EAT A MESS OF DANDELION FLOWERS.

We advise you to sow a bed of dandelions in drills 10 inches apart this spring for early green to be used next spring.* For economy of space you can sow a drill of curled cress between the dandelion drills. This curled cress will save you the need of picking the weeds out of this dandelion bed, but you must pull the cress for synedes before it gets two inches tall, to make room for the young dandelions.

During last November we went to Sault Ste. Marie, Michigan, to deliver a course of Trophotherapy, Trophoprofilactices and Eutrophy to a large class of chiropractic students of Dr. Robbins' chiropractic school, and while there we were much surprised to find so far north and so late in the year, plenty of large dandelion flowers for a daily mess in the Government Park and elsewhere.

All herbs that are bitter like the dandelion are known as stomach tonics because their bitter juice stimulates the stomach to normal activity and after it combines with the secretions of the stomach, it leaves a very pleasant after-taste.

The dandelion is known to the world over as a spring tonic for which the roots, the leaves and the flowers are used; but the value of its tonic elements is mostly destroyed by cooking and concentration.

The best way to get your money's worth out of the dandelion for tonic purposes is to eat the leaves in the form of a synede (saltless salad).

If your blood is not in the most perfect tone, if you suffer from some form of alimentary trouble, if any disease troubles you, if you are convalescent, if you about to become an apyrotropher or if you are already a confirmed apyrotropher, YOU CANNOT AFFORD TO MISS THE EATING OF A DANDELION SYNEDE OR TO EAT A MESS OF DANDELION FLOWERS.

---

*After reading this article several years ago, I transplanted some of the best dandelions found in my neighborhood and created a year round dandelion patch for my dandelion juices and salads. —*Ed.*

AUTUMN'S PEACE, AUTUMN'S BLISS

by Benedict Lust, N.D.

The Naturopath and Herald of Health, XVIII (10), 645-646. (1913)

Yes, Nature is now at rest, resting from the summer's storms which were mightier this time than ever before. She rests from the burning sun that threatened to singe the plants down to the very roots; from the streaming showers and destroying hailstorms and from lightening cleaving trees, and God's clear, quiet peace reigns smiling over all. Most plants' flowering time is past, but the seeds are coming to their own, and many a healing power, hitherto not heeded, has developed within them. The sun's warmth has dissolved the chemical ingredients and formed combinations whose qualities are welcome blessings to suffering mankind. But not alone the seeds contain such healing powers; *the roots* of many plants are likewise valuable.

Thus, now in September and October the root of the elecampane must be dug out, peeled, cut and dried. It smells of camphor, spicy, and when dried, of violets. The chemical ingredients of the plant are inulin, a bitter extract, a camphoric substance, etheric oil, rosin and acetic acid. The beautiful plant is nowadays much being used in gardens and parks, but there are only a very few people who know of the wonderful drugs for chest and stomach disturbances contained in its roots. They constitute a remedy for asthma, facilitate mucous expectoration, and clean the breast. As a tea it acts as a stomach strengthener.

Just as therapeutic is the root of the angelica plant. It has to be dug out late in fall and contains the same chemical ingredients as elecampane. It acts on sweat and urine furthering and strengthening on the heart, stomach and liver. It is used as tea or powder and is found on mountainous woods, on humid meadows and brooks.

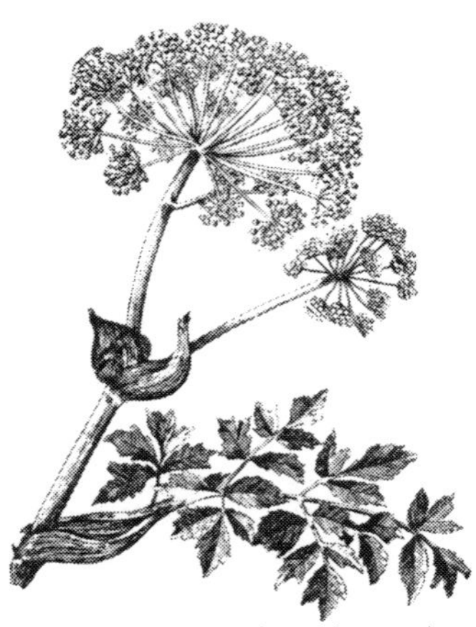

Angelica (*Angelica silvestris*)

In the autumn ripens also the seed of anise. It is good for colic, infantile cramps, chronic catarrhs of the stomach and intestines. Anise acts by warming and [relieving] gas. The seeds contain etheric oil, rosin, sugar and gum. The plant is being cultivated on fields and grows wild on dry meadows.

At this time of the year, the wormwood shrubs are being cut in the gardens and put in a dry place for the winter. Wormwood tea strengthens the stomach and is a splendid remedy for disordered bowels.

It is also advisable to collect the strawberry and blackberry leaves on dry, sunny woodland as long as they still smell spicy and before the autumnal dampness has changed their color into brown. They replace the Holland or Russian tea excellently, have no exciting effects and are much more aromatic in taste.

The barberry bush looks like red corals. The farmer does not like it near his field as it generates the spores of the blight. But we enjoy its pleasant appearance and know that the extremely sour berries refresh the thirsty wanderer. They contain malic acid and therefore give a good vinegar and are frequently used for cooling drinks.

There blooms in violet petals the wild marjoram. It is a splendid remedy for gripes and colic.

In October, the ripe acorns fall from the trees. They should be gathered, dried thoroughly on a warm hearth and then further dried. They are a fine substitute for coffee, for while the latter excites and consumes, they nourish and calm the worst diarrhoeas.

By the end of September the elder berries are ripe. They are gathered and thickened by boiling with sugar, for they make a mitigating and cooling drink for fever stricken patients.

There we see the burdock with its large leaves and carmine flowers whose capsules so easily stick to the clothing of passers-by. It contains in its root a strengthening oil furthering the growth of the hair. The tea made of it increases the sweat and urine. The tea is good for herpes and eruptions. The oil heals also abscesses and ulcers. Who suspects so many healing powers in the plant so much hated by the farmer?

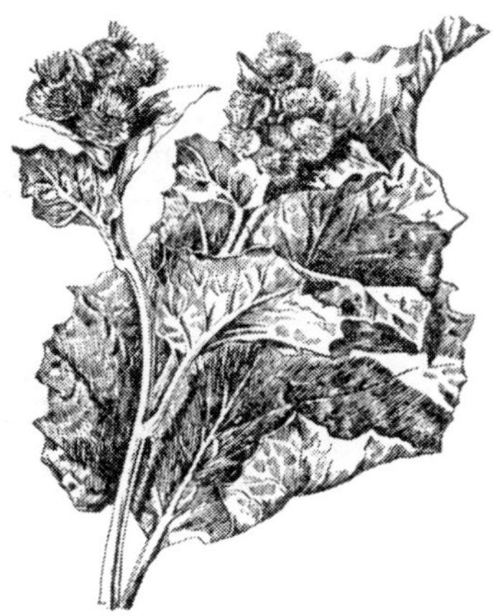

Burdock (*Arctium lappa*)

A remedy for the lungs is found in the Iceland moss which contains an easily dissoluble slime and a splendid remedy for dry cough. It furthermore possesses a bitter matter and is therefore to be recommended as a tea.

But let us not overlook the bristly juniper there in the woods, gladdening our eyes late in autumn and offering its berries for cure. Peculiar powers are ascribed to them—giving the weary new vigour of life, rest and alleviation to the sick, dropsical and paralytic, and protection from contaminating diseases and from the effects of damp and foggy weather in autumn to the healthy. The ripe berries contain oil, rosin and sugar and act softly stimulating on the digestion, on the mucous membranes, increasing the urination and skin exhalation. Juniper twigs, berries and also the aromatic wood are the best fumigatives in sick rooms.

Thus, the flora gives us until late in fall manifold remedies which we should not overlook. Let us enjoy to the fullest the pure air filling garden, fields and woods. Let us taste the fruits of the trees so wholesome to the health. But let us also be thankful that an omnipotent painter colors trees and flowers, so richly shading and brightly dyeing them! Alas, this quiet splendor and glorious peace last but a short while longer, for soon the storms of winter will be here.

But he who has strengthened body and soul in the enjoyment of Nature may calmly await the arrival of winter. And if little affliction should again trouble him, the knowledge of Nature and her hidden healing powers will now give him sufficient remedies to fight all evils of this kind.

Thus now in September and October the root of the elecampane must be dug out, peeled, cut and dried. It smells of camphor, spicy, and when dried, of violets. The chemical ingredients of the plant are inulin, a bitter extract, a camphoric substance, etheric oil, rosin and acetic acid.

Just as therapeutic is the root of the angelica plant. It has to be dug out late in fall and contains the same chemical ingredients as elecampane.

There blooms in violet petals the wild marjoram. It is a splendid remedy for gripes and colic.

[Burdock] contains in its root a strengthening oil furthering the growth of the hair. The tea made of it increases the sweat and urine. The tea is good for herpes and eruptions. The oil heals also abscesses and ulcers.

The ripe berries [of Juniper] contain oil, rosin and sugar and act softly stimulating on the digestion, on the mucous membranes, increasing the urination and skin exhalation.

1914

Licorice

George J. Drews

THE NATUROPATH AND HERALD OF HEALTH'S

Apyrtropher Section

DEVOTED TO

APYRTROPHY—the Science, Art and Practice of Living on the Moral Unfired Diet for the Perpetuation of Perfect Health and Cure of Disease.

It is also the organ of the Apyrtropher (*Unfired-fooder*) Society. Address all communications for this department to its editor.

GEORGE J. DREWS, M.D., D.C., 1910 North Harding Avenue, Chicago, Ill.

LICORICE

by George J. Drews

The Naturopath and Herald of Health, XVIX (12), 830-831. (1914)

Since the first publication of our book *Unfired Food* we have amply proven, over and over again that licorice is richer than any other edible root can be verified by chemical analysis.* That beet roots, beet leaves, Swiss chard and spinach are richer than any other succulent vegetable has already been determined by analysis.

Licorice, however, when dried and ground, is superior to the sugar beet in that it requires no boiling (denaturing) and refining to render it useful as a condiment food and then on account of the organic salts it contains, it is a tonic food beside.

The equivalent of organic salts that the licorice root contains can be roughly determined in the following way. Take three glasses full of water; put a teaspoonful of sugar into the first; into the second put a teaspoonful of sugar and a half teaspoon of table salt; and into the third put a teaspoonful of powdered licorice root and stir all briskly. Now taste each glass in order and you will find that the last two have about the same intensity. This experiment is not in the least intended to convey the idea that there is anything common in table salt and organic salt, nor in the con-

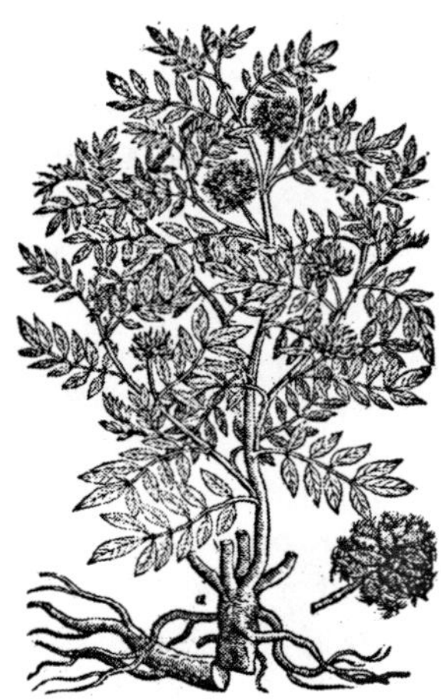

Licorice (*Glycyrrhiza glabra*)

This illustration is from John Gerard's *The herbal, or Generall historie of plantes* (1633).

*Drews published a complete article on licorice in *Unfired Food* found on page 296. —*Ed.*

tents of the last two glasses, except the resultant intensity, which is to convey a conception of the percentage of organic salts the root may contain. The full value of this experiment, however, cannot be understood until the experimenter has tasted the crystals of organic salt that form on the outside of a drying Swiss chard leaf stalk, for those crystals taste sweet instead of salty without containing an ingredient of sugar.

The value of licorice cannot be determined by the above experiment nor by a chemical analysis. Only the effect it has on the sick and the convalescent can determine its true value. We cannot quite say that the organic salt in licorice is an elixir of life, but it has proven itself a wonderful blood tonic to those whose blood is impoverished by denatured food and resulting disease. If the entire world had seen how some of our resident patients improved on using it and had read the letters we have telling of its results, we fear it would prove the extermination of the licorice plant.

For children of all ages, there is no more wholesome substitute for candy than a stick of licorice root. It gives all the pleasure that candy can give. It is sweeter than rubber or clothespins for teething, it gives plenty of exercise to the teeth for preserving tooth health, it is the finest cure for the tobacco chewing and smoking habit, and it can be eaten, not only with impunity, but with benefit in those diseases in which commercial sugar is forbidden.

The powdered licorice root is useful for drinks, vegetable salads and for some fruits. There is only one warning that must not be forgotten on account of the intense sweetness of the powdered root lest too much is used and the food becomes unbearably sweet.

To those who taste the powdered root for the first time on vegetables or fruits, it may taste bitter on first contact; but this introductory bitter taste soon gives way to an intensely sweet taste which at once becomes agreeable and pleasant, provided it is used sparingly. The powdered root cannot be recommended as a universal condiment, because some people will never learn to like it, nor does it combine well with all food; but still all may use it, in some way or other, as a **tonic food.**

The therapeutic use of licorice for lung troubles, coughs and colds is so old that its history cannot be traced. The present and customary habit of making licorice concoctions by boiling the licorice destroys more than half of its therapeutic value, for the boiling temperature so destroys the organic state of the salts that its usefulness as a tonic for the blood, nerves and glands is practically out of the question. The scientific world of today, however, would rather have us use the terms *activator* or *vitamins* when writing on the destructive power of fire on therapeutic food.

The several best ways for using licorice root for therapeutic and prophylactic purposes are the chewing of the root, the powdered root in drinks and on salads.

Of all the sweets that man may eat, licorice root is the most fortunate in that it does not favor fermentation in the stomach nor the intestines. There is only one unfortunate condition about licorice and that it does not form a habit. No one is able to eat too much of it because at the moment of satisfaction it forms an aversion as most of the undenatured foods do.

The following is a quotation from *Unfired Food*:

> LICORICE (*Glycyrrhiza glabra*)
>
> The licorice roots are most wholesome for the children as well as for the grown-ups. The dried or fresh roots are chewed to extract the sweet juice which is most rich in saline sugar. The pulp should be rejected when it ceases to taste sweet. These roots may be chewed with benefit by all whose blood requires to be toned with organic salts. The licorice sticks and licorice candy on the market is worse than useless because its organic sugar and organic salts have been rendered inorganic in the process of extraction and concentration. Dried licorice root ground or powdered is the most wholesome substitute for commercial sugar. It is so extremely sweet that it must be used in very minute and sparing quantities, otherwise the dish, so flavored, may become repulsively sweet; especially to those who are not accustomed to the licorice flavor. Therefore, powdered licorice root is best served like sugar to be used by each individual in drinks or soups, and on salads or brawn foods as desired.

The price of the root used to be about twenty-five cents per pound, but since the war it has been raised to fifty cents per pound. We are not interested in the licorice trade, but to those who need it for their health, we will be pleased to send by parcel post from four to twelve ounces at the above rate, provided the parcel postage is added to the price. Do not send for more.

We cannot quite say that the organic salt in licorice is an elixir of life, but it has proven itself a wonderful blood tonic to those whose blood is impoverished by denatured food and resulting disease.

The therapeutic use of licorice for lung troubles, coughs and colds is so old that its history cannot be traced.

Of all the sweets that man may eat, licorice root is the most fortunate in that it does not favor fermentation in the stomach nor the intestines. There is only one unfortunate condition about licorice and that it does not form a habit.

1915

Honey

Benedict Lust, N.D.

Plantain

George J. Drews

Yarrow

M. G. Young

HONEY

From Producer to Consumer

Honey is a purely vegetable product—a natural food, delicious strength giving and health giving.

The craving of the human system for sweets is perfectly natural and Honey is a perfectly *natural* sweet to supply this need.

I am a *specialist* in Honey selling directly to the consumer. My Honey is ripe, rich, thick, delicious, and *I fully warrant it's purity under all Pure Food Laws.*

Place Honey on the table every meal. Use it partly in place of nut butters or creamery butter. Costs only half as much and will take its place in part. Give it to children in place of candy.

I sell two colors and flavors—light and dark. The dark is preferable for flavoring.

Prices;—10 lb. pail $1.30 by express. 4 (10lb) pails $5.00 by freight. *Freight charges much less than express.*

Sample by mail and copy of "Honey as a Health Food". 10c.

ALBERT G. HANN, Pittstown, New Jersey

RAISE YOUR OWN REMEDIES.

We make a specialty of all kinds of seeds recommended as natural medicines. Write for our catalogue, ready February 1st.

We are headquarters for

"Silber-Eschen-Blätter-Tea,"

A sure cure for Rheumatism. By mail, prepaid, $1.00 per lb.
JIJ

Herrmann's Seed Store,

413 EAST 34TH STREET,

NEAR L. I. FERRY, **NEW YORK CITY**

Honey

by Benedict Lust, N.D.

The Naturopath and Herald of Health, XX (2), 120-121. (1915)

If the English, as is stated, eat less honey than almost any other nation, then the fact certainly provides food for reflection, for while refined sugar is entirely deficient in mineral matter, and therefore injurious to health, honey is one of the most wholesome forms of sugar, mildly laxative in its properties.

It is largely used in the East, for the preservation of fruit, and the making of cakes, sweetmeats, and other articles of food. To the ancients, who were almost unacquainted with sugar, honey formed an alimentary article of great importance thousands of years before the first sugar refinery was built.

Almost all pure honey, when exposed to light and cold, becomes more or less granular in consistency. Any liquid portion can be readily separated by straining though linen.

The mean composition of pure honey, according to Dr. Sieber, is as follows:

Moisture	19.98%
Grape Sugar (Dextrose)	34.71%
Laevulose [Fructose]	39.24%
Substances other than sugar	6.07%

Imported honey sold out of the comb is now usually extracted by a machine called a honey extractor. The combs are rapidly revolved and the centrifugal force throws out the honey into the cylinder. The combs can then be returned uninjured to the hive to be again refilled with honey; thus is brought about a great saving over the old method of melting the combs and straining the honey.

It is especially valuable as a restorative during prolonged muscular exertions, as it quickly affords a fresh supply of vital force. It is well known how serviceable is honey combined with other ingredients as a medicinal agent for throat conditions, etc., but as a regular article of food it is less appreciated, although it has a therapeutic value which it is difficult to overestimate. The harmful effects of over-indulgence in sweets by the young are well-known, but honey carries with it no such detrimental results. On the other hand, honey can be eaten freely both by children and adults, and will be found as economical as it is beneficial. With a good supply of honey, little or no butter need be used in fact, bread and butter, if replaced by honey thickly spread on the bread, will not only be much preferred by the little ones, but good results will usually follow. With delicate children and those with weak digestive organs, it will be found of great service; if substituted for cane sugar and sweets made therefrom, not only will their digestive apparatus be saved much work, but the honey will be easily assimilated, their bodies will be nourished, and much will be done to build up strong, bonny brains. The finest Jamaica honey can now be purchased at about half the price of butter, and unlike butter, the longer it is kept, the more pleasing it becomes. If children are given all the honey they desire at meal-times, it will do much to satisfy their natural longing for sweets, and if the one is substituted entirely for the other, nothing but good results can follow. The old man may crave for fat, the child wants the sweets, and honey provides it in a harmless and nourishing form, and the best of sweets for the sweet. With mashed bananas or strawberries, with or without cream, it is delicious. Honey can also be substituted for sugar in sweetening stewed fruits, fruit juices, and hot drinks. One or two tablespoonful of honey in a glass of hot water will make an ideal drink for children; this beverage is taken largely in Germany by adults, and many attribute their great age to this life-long use.

Quite apart from the high position honey occupies as a food, it possesses valuable medicinal qualities also. The Koran, in the chapter entitled "The Bee," remarks with reference to bees and their honey: "There proceedeth from their bellies a liquor of various colors, wherein is a medicine for men." Before sugars, such as cane and beet, can be digested in the human stomach, they must be converted by the digestive organs into grape sugar; very often the overtaxed stomach fails to properly perform this operation, when extra work is thrown on the kidneys with baneful results, but in honey we have the grape sugar already prepared, which renders it more easy to digest and assimilate than perhaps any other form of sugar. Many now troubled by indigestion, dyspepsia and loss of flesh, who have sought but never found relief in medicines, would find a wonderful benefit accrue by giving up the use of drugs entirely, and by living on brown bread, "Placobred", or other health biscuits, together with a liberal supply of honey. Honey is said to be the only food that leaves no residue when taken into the stomach, being entirely absorbed into the system by the action of the blood, and is not digested by any action of the stomach. The medicinal value of honey appears to have been better understood in olden times than at present. In recipes of the Saxon and later periods it is a common ingredient.

On the other hand, it should not be looked upon as a quack medicine to give temporary relief, but as a health food of great value, and should be taken regularly as such, in place of foods which too many experience as harmful. The daily use of honey will tend to bring about a healthy condition of the bowels, and thus enable them to properly perform their functions, and so prevent many of the ills arising therefrom. For coughs, colds,

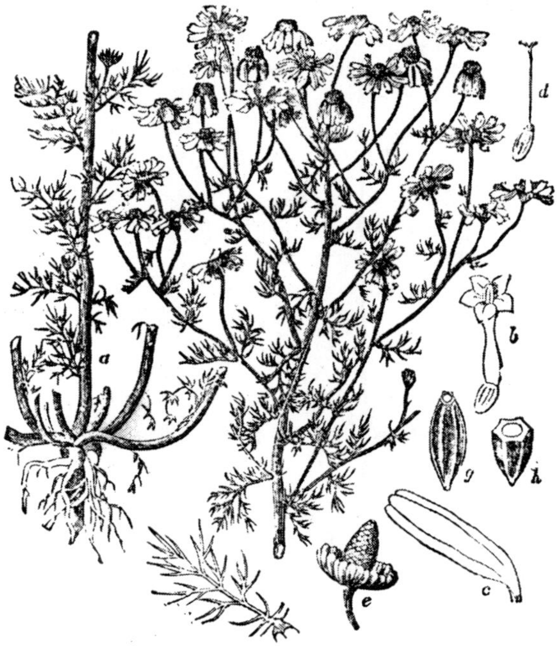

Chamomile (*Matricaria chamomilla*)

a. Upper and lower part of the plant, b. central yellow flower, c. outer white flower, d. pistil magnified, e. calyx and bottom of the flower, f. leaf, g. fruit, h. cross-section of the fruit.

and sore throats, honey and lemon juice mixed together in equal quantities will be found a remedy as useful as it is old. Old people, who suffer with a tickling sensation at the bottom of the throat will find great relief in the following. Simmer together for several hours 8 oz. of honey and 2 oz. chopped onion, and strain; take a teaspoonful at a time as desired. The following is a remedy for colds on the chest, for use just before going to bed. Boil a quart of water, stir in 2 oz. honey and ¼ oz. of chamomile flowers, quickly remove the vessel to a table, cover the patient's head and the vessel with a rain-proof or similar cloth, let the patient inhale the vapor till cold, stirring occasionally. If the desired results are not brought about by the first treatment, repeat once or more often. A splendid candy for colds, whooping coughs, etc., can be made as follows: Boil a strong solution of horehound leaves in soft water, strain through muslin, add as much honey as desired, boil until all the water evaporates, pour into shallow vessel and allow to set. The eating of honey while otherwise fasting is said not only to provide a remedy, but a cure for tape worms. Honey will also be found useful for children suffering with indigestion and sickness. For frost bites on ears, fingers, etc., wrap up in honey, when the swelling will be quickly reduced and no ill effects follow. For inflamed and sore eyes, a drop or two of liquid honey put in the eyes several times a day had been known to bring about wonderful results, when all else has failed. Equal parts of honey and cream mixed together, rubbed on the affected parts is said to be a good thing for freckles. Honey spread on a cloth and applied to the affected parts in cases of erysipelas will usually relieve the pain immediately, and if the application is renewed about every four hours, convalescence should follow in a very few days.

[Honey] is especially valuable as a restorative during prolonged muscular exertions, as it quickly affords a fresh supply of vital force.

With delicate children and those with weak digestive organs, it will be found of great service; if substituted for cane sugar and sweets made therefrom, not only will their digestive apparatus be saved much work, but the honey will be easily assimilated, their bodies will be nourished, and much will be done to build up strong, bonny brains.

The daily use of honey will tend to bring about a healthy condition of the bowels, and thus enable them to properly perform their functions, and so prevent many of the ills arising therefrom.

For coughs, colds, and sore throats, honey and lemon juice mixed together in equal quantities will be found a remedy as useful as it is old.

The following is a remedy for colds on the chest, for use just before going to bed. Boil a quart of water, stir in 2 oz. honey and ¼ oz. of chamomile flowers, quickly remove the vessel to a table, cover the patient's head and the vessel with a rainproof or similar cloth, let the patient inhale the vapor till cold, stirring occasionally.

The eating of honey while otherwise fasting is said not only to provide a remedy, but a cure for tape worms.

For frost bites on ears, fingers, etc., wrap up in honey, when the swelling will be quickly reduced and no ill effects follow.

Plantain

by George J. Drews

The Naturopath and Herald of Health, XX (9), 580-581. (1915)

It seems that most people do not appreciate the useful plants that grow wild around them without care and attention; but they may take fancy to a wild plant of some distant place country and try to grow it in their home field, garden or in their house, often in spite of the unfavorable climate that may be at their home for that plant.

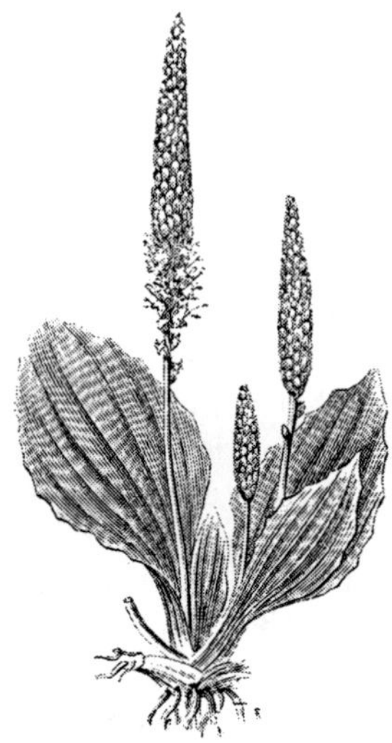

Broad leaf plantain
(Plantago major)

The common sweet clover used to be despised because it could be found wherever man had stepped or somehow turned the soil. This same sweet clover now, however, is cultivated and dried for both animal and human food. In this same way, many plants are carelessly stepped upon until someone proved them extremely useful.

The broad leaved plantain, which grows everywhere man has often placed his foot, tries to cover his path with a carpet of its broad green leaves.

The macerated leaves of this plant are known to have drawing and healing properties in poultices for fresh and chronic wounds. The infusion of the dried leaves tones the blood and is used medicinally for nervousness, bladder trouble and leucorrhoea.

Some people have the idea that all medicinally used plants or herbs must be poisonous when used in health. This is not always true; for there are many of these plants that are wholesome for food, having no unpleasant flavor nor any medicinal effect in health. The following axiom is to the point here. "All vegetable-herbs, roots, fruits and even cereals and nuts have medicinal properties in their uncooked and unsalted state when properly selected and used for that purpose; but the medicinal properties manifest **only** in and during the disease for which they are specifics."

The above axiom also holds well with the plantains of which there are a number of varieties. The writer has experimented with the broad leaved plantain, as that is the most common in Chicago.

This spring we rooted up the plantains in the lawn, because they make [the lawn] look unkempt. While we were doing this, the thought came to us that we should cultivate some of these plants for experience. We chose to plant ten plants in a row ten inches apart. Three of these plants we plant as carefully as we would any other flower or vegetable plant. The fourth plant we put in with the roots up and the heart down and only slightly covered the roots. The fifth plant we put in three inches deep with the root end up after we had cut off all the roots and leaves. The sixth plant we treated the same as the fifth, but put it in six inches deep. The seventh plant we simply carelessly forced down two inches and covered it in the same way. From the eighth plant we again cut the roots and leaves and put it in, heart up, four inches deep. From the ninth plant, we only cut the leaves and put it in six inches deep. The tenth plant we put in eight inches deep with roots and leaves as it was pulled from the lawn. After four weeks these plants all looked alike. Although, it took the deepest one a week to come to the surface; but after that it took no exception to the other plants. In five weeks from planting some of the leaves were fourteen inches tall, crisp and tender, with only a deliciously mild plantain flavor; while the largest leaves of unkempt plants in the lawn (left there for contrast) were only eleven inches tall and four and one half inches wide and were hard, leathery and strong in flavor. We forgot to say that the largest leaves of the cultivated plants were nearly six inches wide.

Now we gave these plants no more attention than we give to other vegetables, pulling the weeds and sprinkling when the soil becomes too dry. The average leaves of the uncultivated plantain are seven inches long and three inches wide and lay as close to the ground as other vegetation around them permits. The leaves in footpaths more often are dwarfed and grow nearly as wide as they are long, measuring about two and a half inches.

Six or ten cultivated plants produce an abundance of tender leaves for a family of three from spring until frost. For a general diet, a plantain synede (salad) may be enjoyed every third day. Such a plantain synede may be composed of chopped plantain leaves and ground raw peanuts (or other nuts) dressed with honey if desired sweet; though some people prefer the plantain leaves as an admixture to other synede herbs for that particular flavor they impart. Those who wish to prepare a larger variety of plantain synedes may be referred to our book *Unfired Food*.

It is very important to remember when cultivating plantains in a vegetable garden to be sure and pull all the seed stalks while young, for in case they get ripe and the seed is spread it produces a hundred times more work the next year than it takes to carefully pull the seed stalks.

It seems that most people do not appreciate the useful plants that grow wild around them without care and attention; but they may take fancy to a wild plant of some distant place country and try to grow it in their home field, garden or in their house, often in spite of the unfavorable climate that may be at their home for that plant.

The macerated leaves of this plant are known to have drawing and healing properties in poultices for fresh and chronic wounds.

All vegetable-herbs, roots, fruits and even cereals and nuts have medicinal properties in their uncooked and unsalted state when properly selected and used for that purpose; but the medicinal properties manifest only in and during the disease for which they are specifics.

Phytotherapy Department

(The American Herb Doctor)

Address all communications for this department to its editor

Prof. M. G. YOUNG, 4156 Arcade Building, Seattle, Wash.

Yarrow

by M. G. Young

The Naturopath and Herald of Health, XX (12), 775-776. (1915)

For reasons that I am not able to give, there seems to be an idea among the people that any herb which has real medical qualities of value does not grow here. They seem to think that the more remote and difficult to obtain a plant is, the better it is. Also, the same kind of reasoning is used in regard to any other remedy. If the medicine comes with a Latin name or some obsolete conglomeration of letters which they can't understand, then it is *all right*, and they desire to try it at once.

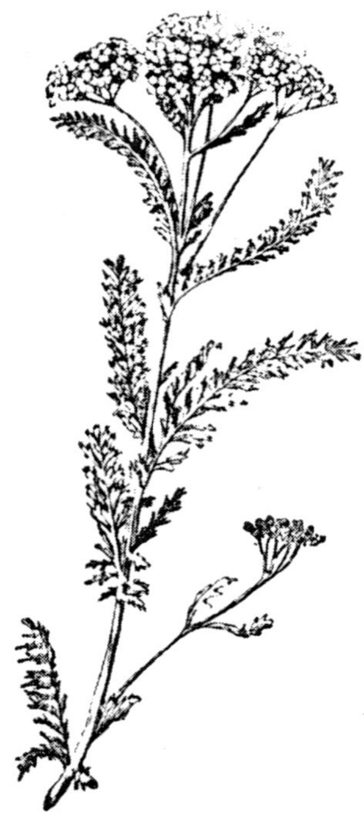

Milfoil or Yarrow
(*Achillea millefolium*)

But there are many valuable herbs which you see every day and perhaps are walking over them, which contain the most desirable medical qualities, and in many instances would heal the disease of the one who is treading them down. But, alas, this knowledge has been lost years ago. The good old fathers and mothers knew and praised these God-given, healing plants. It is the avowed purpose of the editor of this department to restore this lost art to suffering humanity. Although I am a very busy man, I feel keenly a conviction of duty upon me; and hence I have added this much more to my daily duties.

Yarrow is one of the most common and yet one of the most valuable herbs of America. It grows here in great abundance. Yarrow, milfoil, and wild tansy are a few of the common names by which it is known. Its Latin name is *Achillea millefolium*.

Description

It is common in Europe and North America, has a hairy stem, branched at top, bearing the large corymbs or clusters of white flower heads. Each is composed of five pistillate ray-florets and greenish white perfect disk florets, and leaves lanceolate thrice pinnatifid, with linear divisions. The herb's odor is chamomile-like and its taste is aromatic, bitter and astringent.

This is the regular botanic description of this herb. I will now give you a somewhat plainer description. It grows from 12 to 30 inches in height, is perennial and grows continually from the same root. It has leaves somewhat resembling carrots and flowers from June until October. It may be found growing in waste places, old fields, and hedgerows. The entire plant, including the root, may be used as medicine. It possesses the following medical qualities. It is aromatic, having a rather strong aroma or smell. It is bitter and is therefore a tonic to the liver and kidneys. It is also an astringent in mild degree. Its qualities are numerous. The next I will mention is its diaphoretic effect; that is, having the effect to increase perspiration. It also is a valuable stimulant. The medical qualities of yarrow can be extracted by steeping in water, soaking in alcohol, or by chewing it and swallowing the saliva. This last method was employed by those true sons of Nature, the *American Indians*.

If the astringent qualities of this plant are desired, it should be boiled.

I will now direct you as to the proper method of gathering and preparing yarrow for medical use. It should be gathered when in full bloom. Either dig or pull up the plant root, and all care should be used not to gather that which is dusty or otherwise damaged. The dirt should be shaken from the roots, but do not wash them, as they yield their medical qualities so readily to water; you will damage by washing them. They should be spread out thin on paper in a clean, dry place, where the sun will not shine upon them until they are thoroughly dry. The roots may then be cut off and placed in a sack by themselves. The remainder of the plant should be broken up and put away in a dry place in large paper sacks and tied tightly.

You now have a remedy which experience will teach you, is a most valuable asset in the treatment and cure of a large number of human ills. It is not a cure-all, but you will become enthusiastic about its virtues if you put it to the test. An amusing story is told by Dr. A. I. Coffin of England, of a venerable old minister of the *Society of Friends*, who had studied medical botany. When asked: "What would cure a cold?", he answered, "Take a pint of yarrow tea, made strong, on going to bed, and put a hot brick to thy feet wrapped in cloth wet with vinegar, and thou wilt surely be well in the morning." The old gentleman was again asked, "What he would recommend for rheumatism?" The answer was: "Take a pint of yarrow tea made hot on going to thy bed, with a hot brick to thy feet wrapped as before, and thou wilt soon be well." And again he was asked: "What would expel worms from children?" He answered as before: "Give them a strong tea of yarrow and a warm brick to the feet and they will be cured speedily." A number of other questions were also asked, and his answer was invariably given with great patience and earnestness: "Take a pint of hot yarrow tea, etc." Chimerical, as the old friend's advice may appear to many, its correctness may be proven in a large degree in your own experience. Dr. Coffin also adds that it is his opinion, that if yarrow was the only medicine sold at the drug store, there would be far less suffering and distress among the people. Many forms of disease owe their origin to what is termed a cold. It will be seen, therefore, that when the skin is stopped up and generally obstructed that the means which would clear it out by sweating and promoting the action of the kidneys, would be a most desirable one. Such, indeed, is the fact with yarrow. It will aid in equalizing the circulation by inducing a determination of the blood to the surface, and promotes a free discharge of urine.

A strong tea made by boiling the roots and tops of yarrow is a good wash for old sores; such as scaled head, chapped hands, dandruff and scurvy. It will really stop the falling of the hair and renders it soft and glossy. It is one of the ingredients in my herbal hair tonic. A very desirable ointment can be made from the green flowers and leaves with equal parts of ground ivy and red raspberry leaves, also green, and the green bark of dogwood (sometimes called green ozier). Bruise them well, place in kettle and add sufficient Vaseline to cover the herbs. Let it simmer over a slow fire so as not to make the Vaseline too hot (and thus burn the herbs) for two or three hours. Then strain through a piece of cloth and box for use. You have now one of the best ointments for scurvy, old sores and cracked hands. If you wish it still more active, which is sometimes necessary in sores of long standing, add to each pound of Vaseline two teaspoonfuls of best cayenne pepper.

In fever cases, yarrow made by steeping may be drank freely. I have also found it good for cramps, colic, and pains in the bowels. Should you be troubled with passing bloody urine, you will find a pint or two of the tea, drank cold, a sovereign remedy.

If you boil yarrow in white wine, it is good to relieve the flux or bloody discharge from the bowels. The Indians used to chew the roots for tooth ache. A strong tea made by boiling and drank frequently will relieve the inability to hold water.

I hope now, good reader, you will have become acquainted with this valuable herb and its medical uses. And that you will ever hold it in respect and not class it as a mere weed and pest.

For reasons that I am not able to give, there seems to be an idea among the people that any herb which has real medical qualities of value does not grow here.

But there are many valuable herbs which you see every day and perhaps are walking over them, which contain the most desirable medical qualities, and in many instances would heal the disease of the one who is treading them down.

"What would cure a cold?", he answered, "Take a pint of yarrow tea, made strong, on going to bed, and put a hot brick to thy feet wrapped in cloth wet with vinegar, and thou wilt surely be well in the morning."

A strong tea made by boiling the roots and tops of yarrow is a good wash for old sores; such as scaled head, chapped hands, dandruff and scurvy. It will really stop the falling of the hair and renders it soft and glossy.

A very desirable ointment can be made from the green flowers and leaves with equal parts of ground ivy and red raspberry leaves, also green, and the green bark of dogwood.

Should you be troubled with passing bloody urine you will find a pint or two of the tea, drank cold, a sovereign remedy.

1916

Garlic Juice And Medicine

Benedict Lust, N.D.

Sage

M. G. Young

Sassafras, Laurus Sassafras

M. G. Young

Comparative Therapeutics

W. Wallace Fritz, M.D., D.D.S., N.D., D.O., D.C.

Cascada Sagrada

M. G. Young

Impure Blood

M. G. Young

Dandelion

M. G. Young

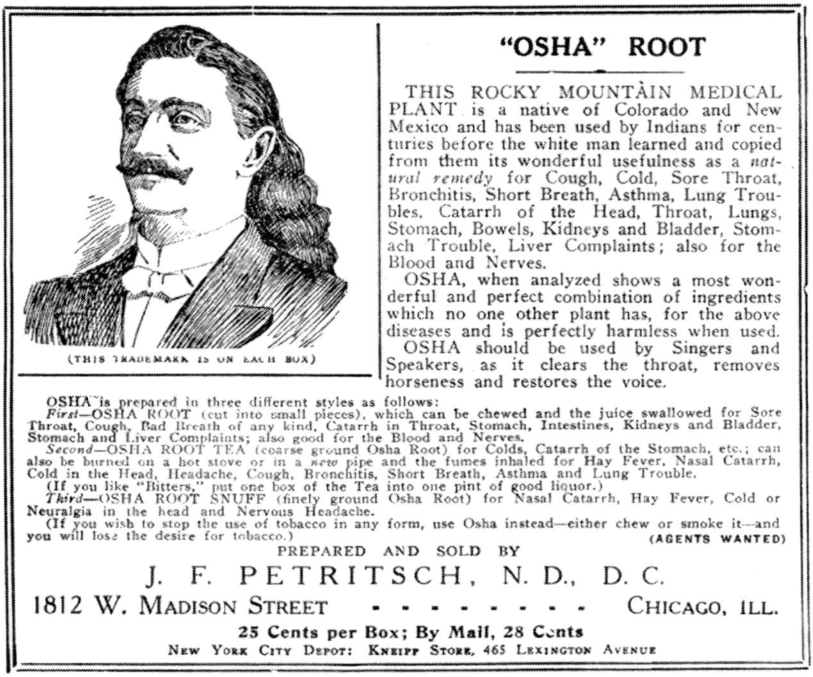

Osha is a native plant of America and this ad is a departure from the reliance upon European and Kneippian herbal products.

GARLIC JUICE AND MEDICINE

by Benedict Lust, N.D.

Herald of Health and Naturopath, XXI (1), 11. (1916)

An army surgeon in the war zone *rediscovered* that garlic juice diluted in distilled water is almost a cure-all when applied to infected wounds, stopping infection and healing quickly. The *discovery* was made by an army surgeon observing an old French peasant woman who was using it so successfully to dress soldier's wounds, and he not only adopted it with proper credit to the unlettered old lady, but he spread the news throughout the battle fields of Europe. Now common garlic and brown sugar have superseded drugs and chemicals with high-sounding names.

How different the outcome of this rediscovery would likely have been had it occurred in these civilized United States. In the first place, the old lady would probably have been arrested and sent to jail as a *quack* and impostor, as it would be impossible for such a homely remedy originating outside the pale of the American Medical Association to be of merit and worthy of recognition by that august body which we are solicited to look up to.

Should a state of war have existed here as there, no doubt this benevolent woman would have been court-martialed and shot as a menace to the *regular* profession, and a dangerous woman to run at large. So, it is indeed fortunate that this truly wonderful rediscovery occurred in war-torn Europe, where it received the instantaneous acceptance of the whole medical fraternity for the real benefit of the greatest number.

The discovery *was made by an army surgeon observing an old French peasant woman who was using it so successfully to dress soldier's wounds, and he not only adopted it with proper credit to the unlettered old lady, but he spread the news throughout the battle fields of Europe.*

Phytotherapy Department

(The American Herb Doctor)

Address all communications for this department to its editor
Prof. M. G. YOUNG, 4156 Arcade Building, Seattle, Wash.

Sage

by M. G. Young

Herald of Health and Naturopath, XXI (1), 50. (1916)

I have chosen for this issue of the *Herald of Health* one of the oldest, if not the very oldest herb that has a place in medical history. For thousands of years humanity has known the helpful qualities of sage. It has been used for many centuries by the inhabitants of Europe and the people of America.

A few hundred years ago it was used very extensively in curing the sick, but in recent years it has, like many other valuable plants, gone into disuse. The reason, I suppose, is the same for its neglect, as it is with many other plants, because it was known, and commonly known, and to be of little or no value.

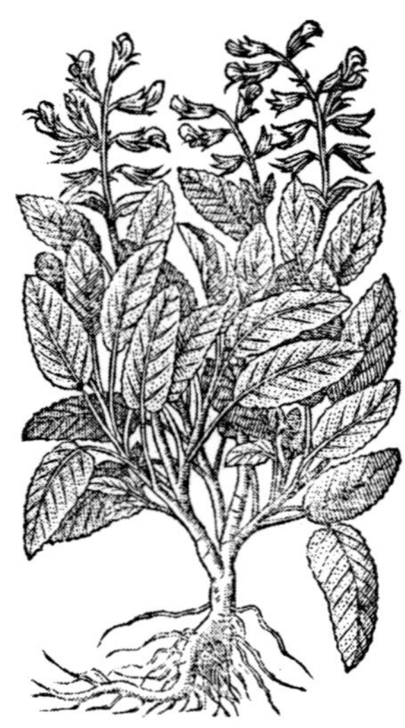

Sage (*Salvia officinalis*)
This illustration is from John Gerard's *The herbal, or Generall historie of plantes* (1633).

It is a fact that in the dooryards of the majority of people are medicines that would cure their ills if they only knew what they were and what their medicinal qualities were. It is my object to reinstate their valuable God-given remedies to that degree of appreciation in the minds of the people which they once held. The name sage is derived from the Latin word *Salvia*, which means safe.

It was regarded as it truly is, absolutely harmless. Its healing properties are most in its volatile oil. It grows wild in South Europe and is cultivated in America. It is so common and so well known that it will be unnecessary to give it any further botanic description.

It has a penetrating, aromatic smell, and a bitterish and somewhat astringent taste. It contains much essential oil. Its medicinal qualities are obtained by infusing or steeping. They are tonic, carminative and astringent. It also possesses diuretic and sudorific qualities. In common language I would say, it will tone the system and is soothing and somewhat astringent or binding, has the ability to cause sweating, and acts nicely upon the kidneys. It is very grateful to the nerves and might therefore be called a nervine.

I employ this valuable herb in the manufacture of several of my medicines. It is the ingredient I most depend upon in my hair tonic. I also use it in preparing a medicine for washing catarrhal ulceration, internally or externally. I also use it in my vermifuge. There is not anything I know of more grateful to a raw, irritated, inflamed condition of the stomach than a mild cup of sage tea. It is very pleasant to the taste if it is not made too strong and a little sugar is added to it.

It is a thousand times better to drink a cup of sage tea than the very best China or Ceylon tea. I have used it with good results as a wash for sore eyes. Those who are troubled with a coated tongue and a bad or unpleasant taste in the mouth in the morning would do well to take a cup of mild sweetened sage tea before eating. It may be relied upon in all cases of night sweats if a strong tea of it is made by steeping and then allowed to become cold and a cup of it drank on retiring. It should never be drunk warm if you desire to stop night sweats.

A tea made of sage and sweetened well with honey is excellent for sore mouths in children. I would advise all my readers to cultivate this valuable herb and as soon as it blossoms begin picking the leaves. Pick off all of the mature leaves and spread them on clean unprinted paper and dry them in the shade. In about four weeks from the first picking you may pick another crop, and so continue until frost comes in the winter. As soon as the leaves are dry, they should be put in clean paper sacks and tied up, or may be put in glass jar or tin boxes, but should be covered tightly.

Five or six leaves are sufficient to make a cup of pleasant tea. There is not anything more grateful to the stomach and bowels in the case of diarrhea or dysentery. Also, during the treatment of a fever case you would do well to give frequently a cup of sage tea. It would be best, however, in this case not to sweeten it. The wild sage that grows on the mountains in the eastern portion of this State and also all over the country to the eastern foot hills of the Rockies is equally valuable as medicine. A strong infusion of it will be found to be a very good wash for those who have diseased scalps and are suffering the loss of hair.

The name sage is derived from the Latin word Salvia, which means safe.

[Sage teas] are tonic, carminative and astringent. It also possesses diuretic and sudorific qualities. In common language I would say, it will tone the system and is soothing and somewhat astringent or binding, has the ability to cause sweating, and acts nicely upon the kidneys.

I also use it in preparing a medicine for washing catarrhal ulceration, internally or externally. I also use it in my vermifuge.

Those who are troubled with a coated tongue and a bad or unpleasant taste in the mouth in the morning would do well to take a cup of mild sweetened sage tea before eating.

[Sage] may be relied upon in all cases of night sweats if a strong tea of it is made by steeping and then allowed to become cold and a cup of it drank on retiring. It should never be drunk warm if you desire to stop night sweats.

Five or six leaves are sufficient to make a cup of pleasant tea. There is not anything more grateful to the stomach and bowels in the case of diarrhea or dysentery.

Phytotherapy Department

(The American Herb Doctor)
Address all communications for this department to its editor
Prof. M. G. YOUNG, 4156 Arcade Building, Seattle, Wash.

Sassafras, Laurus Sassafras

by M. G. Young

Herald of Health and Naturopath, XXI (4), 261. (1916)

I have selected this medical tree for the subject to be explained in this issue of *The Naturopath*, because those who remember anything they ever knew about herbs will doubtless recognize it as one of the spring medicines which was once very popular among those who used herb medicines.

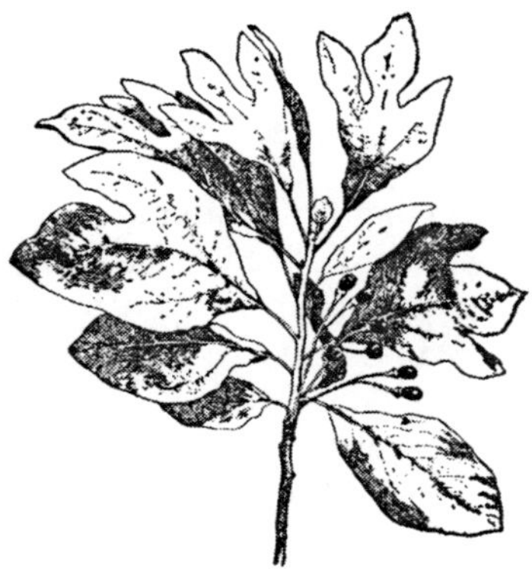

Leaves from the Sassafras (*Sassafras officinale*)

Sassafras is so well known where it grows that a description of it is unnecessary. I will therefore proceed to the notice of its properties and uses.

Sassafras is a rather warm, aromatic stimulant, alterative, diaphoretic, and diuretic. The bark of the root is the principal part used. It is an aromatic stimulant, yielding most of its properties to water, but is almost worthless if boiled. When steeped, the warm infusion is a very good stimulating, sweat-producing nervine. It is very useful in colds and recent obstructions of the menses, and is a very popular drink in skin conditions. Years ago, many people used it as a spring medicine by drinking it with sugar at the table as tea or coffee is drunk. But this custom if followed for long [duration] causes a great general weakening of the whole body.

One week is as long as it should be used at one time. Some years ago, I was called to see a family who were strangely afflicted with weakness and although they experienced no pain or real loss of strength, there was a general weak, tired feeling. At once, I asked them if they had not been drinking sassafras tea. Yes, they had been drinking it for a month or longer, because they liked it very much. I explained to them the nature of the bark and they were soon feeling as strong as ever.

This bark is of great value when combined with other suitable vegetable medicines in the treatment of syphilis, scrofula, rheumatism, and skin diseases. But in no case should it be boiled. When used alone, its most desirable qualities are its influences upon the capillary circulation of the blood and upon the absorbent organs.

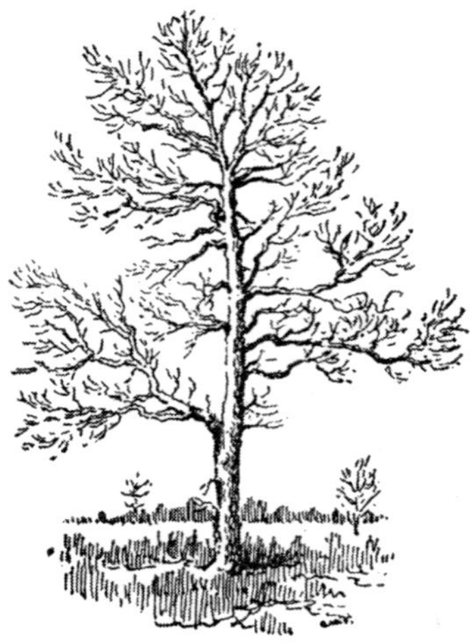
Sassafras tree

The powdered bark is of great value in cases of bruises, congested swellings and old sores. It should be mixed with or sprinkled over the surface of poultices for the above use.

When mixed with ground mullein and boiling water poured upon it, it is a superior application for swollen face, chronic abscesses or any condition where the flesh is swollen and congested. In such cases, it relieves the pain and reduces the swelling quickly, and may be used in local dropsies.

The oil of sassafras is among the very best of the nervine stimulants and relaxants. It is very valuable in almost all liniments for rheumatism, deep congestions and inflammations, abdominal and pelvic swellings, dropsies, sprains, bruises, etc. It may be used internally in doses from 2 to 4 drops on sugar for painful menses, but is not as good as the infusion of the bark for this ailment.

The young branches of this tree have a large pith which is very mucilaginous. If placed in cold water for a short time it yields a very large amount of mucilage, which is very agreeable to irritated conditions of the stomach and bowels, and excellent for highly inflamed conditions of the eyes.

I make use of the bark, oil and pith in my remedies and value it very highly as a remedy when used as before described. This is the season of the year to gather the bark. It should be scraped free of all dirt or washed quickly and dried in a cool, dry place, then put into paper bags and tied up to exclude the air. The pith should be gathered in midsummer and carefully dried free from dust. Be sure to provide yourself with a generous quantity of both bark and pith if it grows where you live.

Sassafras is a rather warm, aromatic stimulant, alterative, diaphoretic, and diuretic. The bark of the root is the principal part used. It is an aromatic stimulant, yielding most of its properties to water, but is almost worthless if boiled. When steeped, the warm infusion is a very good stimulating, sweat-producing nervine.

This bark is of great value when combined with other suitable vegetable medicines in the treatment of syphilis, scrofula, rheumatism, and skin diseases. But in no case should it be boiled.

The powdered bark is of great value in cases of bruises, congested swellings and old sores. It should be mixed with or sprinkled over the surface of poultices for the above use.

When mixed with ground mullein and boiling water poured upon it, it is a superior application for swollen face, chronic abscesses or any condition where the flesh is swollen and congested.

The oil of sassafras is among the very best of the nervine stimulants and relaxants.

The young branches of this tree have a large pith which is very mucilaginous. If placed in cold water for a short time it yields a very large amount of mucilage, which is very agreeable to irritated conditions of the stomach and bowels, and excellent for highly inflamed conditions of the eyes.

Neuropathy Department

Address all communications for this department to its editor

W. WALLACE FRITZ, M.D., D.D.S., N.D., 1600 Summer St., Philadelphia, Pa.

Professor of Neuropathy and Dean in the American College of Neuropathy, and President of the National Association of Drugless Physicians

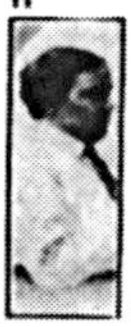

ASSOCIATE EDITOR:

SARAH E. GROVES, N.D.

Professor of Physiology in the Am. College of Neuropathy and Secretary of the National Association of Drugless Physicians

1113 Spruce St., Phila., Pa.

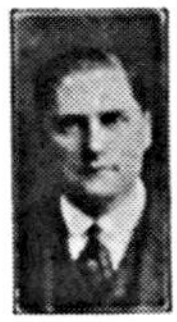

ASSOCIATE EDITOR:

THOMAS M. JACKSON, D.D., N.D.

Professor of Anatomy in the American College of Neuropathy

1533 Diamond St., Phila., Pa.

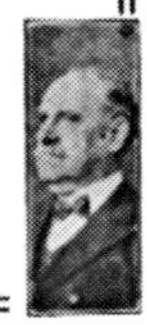

COMPARATIVE THERAPEUTICS

by W. Wallace Fritz, M.D., D.D.S., N.D., D.O., D.C.

Herald of Health and Naturopath, XXI (5), 314-316. (1916)

Lecture delivered to the classes of the American College of Neuropathy

Today I will invite your attention to the subject of quinine. Quinine is a very light, snow-white, fragile crystalline, of a very bitter, persisting taste, soluble in sixteen hundred parts of water, and six parts of alcohol, at a temperature of 59°F/15° C. It is hardly necessary for me to enter into discussion of where this drug comes from, as you all know from your lectures on Materia Medica that quinine is derived from the cinchona tree. The cinchona tree belongs to the natural order of *Rubiaceae*, and is a native of the Eastern Andes, but has been largely planted in India, Ceylon, Java and Burma, with the result of improving the quinine yielding value of many species of cultivation. In late years, the test of appearance has given way to that of assay in the changing of various barks of commerce; and, only those are official which yield three per cent of total alkaloids of which at least two percent must be quinine. From the cinchona tree there are a number of preparations made, but of the number of preparations made, the sulphate of quinine is probably used more than any other preparation. It is not my object to enter into discussion upon the Materia Medica of the drug, but to take up its physiological action so that we can understand the comparative therapy between medicine and neuropathy. Quinine is known as astringent and bitter, and contains tonic acids. It is supposed to act as a stomach tonic, promoting the appetite, increasing the flow of gastric juices, and aiding the digestive powers. If quinine is long continued, it will produce gastric catarrh, and the digestion becomes painful and labored. The astringent action will cause constipation. The alkaloids are distinctive to the minute organisms in the presence of which fermentive changes take place. When quinine is added to milk, it will prevent decomposition, acting as a preservative. Sulphate of quinine is the most active of the alkaloids and is not equally destructive to all minute organisms; some, it merely inhibits and others it kills. The bacteria of septic fluids resist its tonic action to a great extent and are only inhibited by the largest quantities. The alkaloids are readily soluble in gastric juices; in escaping from the action of the gastric juices, it will pass out unabsorbed into the intestinal tract. The alkaline reaction of the intestinal juices will cause precipitation of the quinine which will form insoluble combinations with the bile acids, and will not be absorbed. It is supposed that, when quinine leaves the stomach, it is diffused into the blood with facility. In the blood this alkaloid is probably held in solution by the carbonic acid as there are no changes discernable in the blood.

Quinine acts in a definite manner on certain constituents of the blood. On the hemoglobin, it impairs the power to destroy active oxygen or ozone into which the ordinary oxygen is converted. In conclusion, we find that quinine lessens the oxidizing functions of the blood. Quinine inhibits or lessens the activity of the white blood corpuscles, and indeed destroys them or arrests the ameboid movement as one part to four thousand, and is called a protoplasmic poison outside the body. Quinine also has the power to arrest the migration of the white blood corpuscles from the capillaries, interfering with the process of diapedesis, although it has been stated by some authors, that no amount short of a fatal dose can affect the movement of the white blood corpuscles in warm blooded animals. Quinine affects the rate of the movement of the heart, depending upon the size of the dose. Some authors claim that artificial hyperemia is the result of medicinal doses on the brain. It also acts on the cardiac motor ganglion, and causes the feebleness of the heart's movements and a general lowering of the vascular tension. Besides these effects, it unquestionably depresses the vasomotor system after a short preliminary stimulation. In small doses quinine produces a stimulating effect on the cerebrum, increasing the mental activity, and even accelerating and producing slight hyperemia. In full doses quinine accumulates in the brain producing a sense of fullness in the head, causing a constriction of the forehead (tinnitus aurium), more or less giddiness. Even decided vertigo, dullness of hearing and deafness have been permanent. It has also caused atrophy of the optic nerve and subnormal acuteness of vision (amblyopia). In fatal doses the symptoms presented are intense headache, constrictions of the forehead, dimness of vision, or complete blindness, deafness, delirium or coma, dilated pupils, weak, fluttering pulse, irregular and shallow respiration, convulsions, collapse, and death. It has been proven that quinine lessens the activity of the spinal cord, depresses the functions of the sympathetic nervous system, causing contraction of the uterus and causes an eruption to appear on the skin. It diminishes the excretion of the urea, uric acids, creatinin, phosphoric and sulphuric acids, and is supposed to reduce enlargement of the spleen. Quinine is excreted out of the blood into the urine chiefly, but also by the sweat glands, saliva, milk, and pathological exudations.

Now, I have placed before you the physiological action of this alkaloid of the cinchona tree, "quinine sulphate". You must bear in mind the action of this drug, so that you may be able to understand how it acts upon the human body, and what beneficial effects it may, if any, produce. It is for us now to analyze and understand the neuropathic treatment. By means of our neuropathic treatment we are able to get better results than those produced by this drug. As I have stated to you that quinine given in small doses stimulates the activity of the brain producing slight hyperemia, it is not necessary then, in cases where you wish to produce an active condition of the brain or assimilation of any part of the body, to administer a drug, for with our neuropathic treatment we immediately begin to increase the activity of the passive condition of the body by regulating the blood supply to the involved areas through the nerve mechanisms, producing a relaxation of the pathological area by controlling the vasomotor system.

Our Creator has placed in our bodies two grand nervous systems, the cerebral spinal [autonomic] and sympathetic. The cerebral spinal brings us in closer relation to several parts of the world at the same time, and through it we have our willpower, our thinking faculties, etc. The sympathetic nervous system controls the growth and development of the body. These two nervous systems work together hand in hand, the cerebral spinal acting as a medium of which it increases or depresses the activity of the sympathetic. There is no part of the body to which these two nervous systems do not pass. Every minute cell of the body is controlled in this manner. Therefore, when you wish to increase the activity of any part of the body, you take up the sentinels and pass the message to the nerve center controlling that part. The mode of administering to the sentinels is either stimulating or sedative action. Therefore, in producing the activity to the brain as in this particular case of administering quinine, you would decrease the activity of the nerve cells. In case of chills and lymph stasis, you would decrease the messages to the nerve centers and empty out the waste from the tissue that is involved.

Administering quinine interferes with the normal function of the white corpuscle which is the phagocytes (the warriors of the body), therefore, producing a harmful effect to these organisms which are the best friends that the body has. With Neuropathy, we do not depress the phagocytes or interfere with their normal function, but we increase the phagocytes, and by increasing the phagocytes, they devour the bacteria that is doing harm to cell life. Remember one point: that no disease can enter the body of any individual who has proper circulation and nerve tone. Disease only enters the body when there is a lack of nerve force to the part affected. If you keep the circulation normal and the nerves normal which control the circulation, the phagocytes of the body will do the rest as they will destroy and devour the enemy as it enters the body. Instead of decreasing the activity of the spinal cord which quinine does, we keep the spinal cord in a normal condition by regulating the blood pressure to it and to the brain through the nerve mechanisms, keeping up the normal compensation of blood throughout the body. You know from your lecture upon Neuropathy and Neurology how this is done.

As I do not wish to encroach upon this subject, therefore, I leave this subject with you, that you may understand, where diseases are involving the body, it is useless to prescribe this alkaloid from the cinchona tree, as recommended by the medical fraternity. When the Almighty created our bodies, He placed within them the different organs to produce the proper secretions to keep the body in health by continually secreting its own antitoxins, to preserve and keep it as the Creator wished us to have. It is not necessary, then, for us to place into the body any foreign substance, as it cannot, of itself, produce any cure.

People have strayed so far from Nature that the road back is totally obliterated. Getting back is to undo the work of the fathers, the grandfathers and a lot besides.

Quinine is known as astringent and bitter, and contains tonic acids. It is supposed to act as a stomach tonic, promoting the appetite, increasing the flow of gastric juices, and aiding the digestive powers.

Remember one point: that no disease can enter the body of any individual who has proper circulation and nerve tone.

Phytotherapy Department
(The American Herb Doctor)
Address all communications for this department to its editor
Prof. M. G. YOUNG, 4156 Arcade Building, Seattle, Wash.

CASCARA SAGRADA

by M. G. Young

Herald of Health and Naturopath, XXI (5), 335-336. (1916)

I have chosen this medicinal herb or tree as the subject of this issue of the *Herald of Health* because it is one which many people are using in their effort to help themselves in a medical way.

This medical agent is like many others, poorly understood even by those who employ it. It is my purpose to so treat this subject that those who read what I say will be able to get the virtues of this medicine which should be obtained from it and that in an intelligent way. There are very few people who are employing it properly at this time. Many are injuring themselves with it because of not knowing how to use it.

I will first give its botanical description. Botanists call it *Rhamnus purshiana,* the common name is chitten bark. It is described as attaining a height of from 10 to 20 feet, but I have seen it in the State of Washington much taller. The leaf is ovoid and from three to five inches in length and rather narrow serrate except at the base. Flowers are small and white appearing after the leaves have matured. The fruit is a plain, round, black berry, is about ¼ inch in diameter and contains three seeds. This species differs from other species of *Rhamnus* in that it is a larger tree and bears a larger fruit.

Source: Several allied species grow in the *Cascara* districts of California and seem to contribute largely to the stock of *Cascara sagrada.* The official species grow abundantly in Northern California and throughout the States of Oregon and Washington. If the bark is actually collected in Northern California, it is presumptive evidence that it is the genuine *Cascara sagrada.* The likelihood of its adulteration increases as the source of its collection extends southward, and if collected in the central or southern parts of California, it may be looked upon with suspicion.

DESCRIPTION OF DRUG

It generally appears in curved pieces or quills, from 1/16 to 1/8 inch thick. The outer surface is brown or brownish gray, sometimes mottled or figured and is occasionally marked with corky warts; inner surface smooth and yellowish, turning brown or nearly black on exposure; fracture short, of the inner layer somewhat fibrous. A cross-section shows numerous thin, almost straight, broadening medullary rays which run on the average about three-fourths of the distance across the bark.

What It Contains

Volatile oil, malic, and oxalic acids, a neutral crystalline substance, a red resin, a yellow resin, and a brown resin. The resins are turned a vivid purple red by caustic potash. The fresh bark is active as a purgative, causing much gripping. By keeping and properly curing, however, this gripping principle is destroyed, and the bark becomes more accurate in action and less likely to cause this discomfort and is less injurious to the intestines. There is a very erroneous notion among the people that the more physical effect they notice from the taking of a remedy, the better it is for them.

They seem to go under the idea that used to prevail with the Indian who said, "No smart 'em, no cure 'em." It is due to this fact that many almost incurable cases are found, who have been endeavoring to cure themselves by carrying out the above principle.

I have said a number of times that physic was injurious, and have discouraged the use of cathartics and I must still adhere to this doctrine. I am positive no material can be used to physic out the contents of the bowels which does not do as much damage as it does good.

Thousands of people are incurring this damage daily. All physic or cathartics are irritating to the lining of the bowels, hence weakening. Each dose of physic taken makes it necessary to take another, provided there is nothing done to remove the cause of the constipated condition. The average person who receives a medicine which causes a decided action on the bowels is likely to praise it, whereas they really should discard it. If the medicine taken is such as superinduces the flow of bile, so that the bowels discharge a yellow feces, they have the proper remedy. The bile is naturally physic and is the only one which should ever cause action of the bowels.

Cascara taken alone is a drastic physic, especially when it has not been properly cured and is not three years old. It is a valuable tonic to the liver and stomach when compounded with other tonic and aromatics and carminatives (by this I mean medicine which aid nature in the relief of flatulency). I never employ cascara singly. It is one of the ingredients of my celebrated remedy for constipation called *Herbal Laxative*.

Therefore, those who desire to use the *Cascara* should peel it in the spring of the year, before the leaves start, and should cure it under cover so that it will not get wet when drying. When thoroughly dry, it should be put away in tight boxes, or barrels or paper sacks and kept where it will not draw moisture or it will mildew or mold. When it is aged, it may then be made into infusion or syrup with an equal quantity of Oregon grape root, licorice root, dandelion root, burdock root, and lady slipper root. This may be boiled to a moderately strong tea. Then sweeten with loaf sugar and you will have a very desirable medicine for the bowels because of its aid to the liver, stomach, and nervous system.

The dose may be as indicated by your experience in its use.

The official species grow abundantly in Northern California and throughout the States of Oregon and Washington.

The fresh bark is active as a purgative, causing much gripping. By keeping and properly curing, however, this gripping principle is destroyed, and the bark becomes more accurate in action and less likely to cause this discomfort and is less injurious to the intestines.

I am positive no material can be used to physic out the contents of the bowels which does not do as much damage as it does good.

Cascara taken alone is a drastic physic, especially when it has not been properly cured and is not three years old. It is a valuable tonic to the liver and stomach when compounded with other tonic and aromatics and carminatives.

When it is aged, it may then be made into infusion or syrup with an equal quantity of Oregon grape root, licorice root, dandelion root, burdock root, and lady slipper root. This may be boiled to a moderately strong tea.

Phytotherapy Department

(The American Herb Doctor)

Address all communications for this department to its editor

Prof. M. G. YOUNG, 4156 Arcade Building, Seattle, Wash.

Impure Blood

by Prof. M. G. Young

Herald of Health and Naturopath, XXI (6), 398-402. (1916)

Ever since the editor of this department made his first visit to you through these columns, you will remember his advice and remedies have been appropriate to the season, and we trust his timely help has saved you much suffering and mental anguish, perhaps also saving many precious lives. Well, here he is again, this time, as before, to correct common errors and by his advice enable you and yours to walk in Nature's ordained path, that of safety, health and happiness. It becomes all good, honest, well informed doctors to arrest the attention of the unwary, and make them [aware of] the imminent dangers incident to the springtime.

But alas! To our surprise only silence reigns as one listens for advice, warning or counsel from the doctors who are now holding the reins of professional medicine. They are undisturbed, and yet wistfully waiting for the harvest which must inevitably come because of ignorance among the people of the unalterable laws of Nature.

Well, now as before, in the work of the *Herald of Health*, we want to begin in a plain, rational way to disclose to your minds the facts or exact conditions existing in the bodies of all, which are peculiar to springtime. Throughout all temperate zones the varying temperatures of the different seasons of the year produce very pronounced changes in all life, both animal and vegetable. These are facts moderately well understood by man as they apply to the vegetable world, but they are not clearly enough known about the human body to be thoroughly practical.

The bodies of all things that live are made up of the supply matter called food, and no product of food matter can be of better quality than that which was contained in the material upon which that body subsisted. I wish to apply this truth to the subject which we are now reasoning upon, the impurities of the human body at this season of the year.

What Is Meant By "Impure Blood"

"Impure Blood" is a phrase which is very common among the people and it is used also by those of the medical profession who are careless in their words while conversing with the laity. As a matter of fact, this expression would convey the idea that there is pure blood and impure blood. On this subject we find to be correct, as it is on many other supposed scientific subjects. The *Bible* asserts that the blood is the life, or that in the blood resides that spirit force called vital or life force. This fact precludes the statement that the blood is impure as life is a pure and unmixed principle. The moment the life principle leaves a corpuscle of blood, it becomes impure, and as long as the spirit of life remains in the body of the matter called blood, that matter remains pure. The blood is alive no longer than the spirit of life remains in it. Hence, the only absolutely pure principle in the body is the blood. But when we consider impurities of the body, which the live, pure blood must handle in order to clean the body, then we have the right idea.

Now observe that this work of cleansing the body of impurity constitutes a large part of the work done by the blood, and you will see of what importance it is to aid these live servants of Nature to perform their work. Especially is this help needed at this season of the year.

I will now direct your attention to the experience of the housekeeper. During the winter months, she is as diligent in her housework as she is at other seasons of the year, and does all she can to keep her house clean and healthful, but when the warmer days of spring come, she finds there is pressing need of a general house renovating and she finds it necessary to make a thorough campaign of overhauling and cleansing her house. This task is a big, heavy one. She feels the need of help and should have it right along until everything about the house shows it has been renovated and is clean and in order.

Some of the reasons of this general accumulation of filth are these: the cold, unpleasant weather has required her attention to keep up the heat temperature. There was a large accumulation of ashes and dust from the extra firing. There was less opportunity to open the outlets of the house, the doors and windows.

The cold winter temperature outside the house was very unfavorable to any other work than that which could be performed inside the house, and hence, much of the activities of the good lady were performed indoors, which could have been and generally are performed out of doors during the warmer weather. Consequently, there was very naturally a larger accumulation of wastes and filth throughout the entire house than there would have been in warm weather.

The walls, she observes, have become polluted. The cellar, the living rooms, yes, even the garret have come in for their share of this accumulation.

If this material is not removed effectively, it will soon begin the process of decay due to the rise of temperature. The effete smell will be noticeable. Therefore, all those who are inhabitants of this residence must suffer in a greater or less degree.

Now, my dear reader, you will please turn this illustration and apply it to your own body. Allow the good housewife to represent the life force, which is the faithful guardian of your entire body. This force has built and kept your body every moment of the time from its conception until the present moment. It has faithfully ministered to its every necessity, has diligently made the best of everything, and has frequently been compelled to do its cleansing without any intelligent assistance on your part, until perhaps at present your body needs a very thorough renovating, which should extend from top to bottom.

It would be quite unwise to presume that the good housewife, who is so zealous about cleaning her house, would herself be unclean. The facts are that the blood, like the housewife, is itself clean and energetically bent on a complete cleansing of its house—the human body.

In the human body the accumulation of wastes occur very rapidly during the winter months, owing to the fact that a larger amount of food is required to keep up the system in winter than in the milder temperature. Also, the foods eaten during the winter are condensed and of a drier character which render them harder for the life force to liquefy and carry out of the system.

If you will observe the lower animals, both wild and domestic, you will see the same thing is true in their lives, and guided by that grand endowment which we call instinct, they seek so eagerly the first sprouts of herbage that Nature sends forth in springtime.

If you observe their habits and watch the results of their obedience to instinct, you will soon see how nicely they meet the demands of Nature. The young, juicy herbage causes a mild, agreeable, thorough fluxing of their bodies. They soon have a completely changed appearance and become playful. They are cleansed not only inside, but outside. You will see the shedding of the old winter coat of hair and find it replaced with a bright, new, clean dress for springtime, of the best quality and latest style.

Why should not man, "God's masterpiece", have a similar transformation? Ah! Man! Poor Man! What a wise ignoramus! He has lost his instinct and will not reason on this vital question.

If I were to commercialize on this question and show men how by receiving and acting upon these suggestions their wealth would increase tenfold, what a sale this magazine would have!

It is indeed unfortunate that this is the case. If a man is not afraid he is going to die, he has little or no concern for this direction. It is the likelihood of death that arouses his sluggish mind on the subject of health.

"All men think all men mortal but themselves." This truism might be modified very appropriately by saying all men think all men should obey the laws of Nature but themselves. There are those who will read this article this spring and quite agree with me in all I say, and will yet so lightly regard the matter that the months will slip by and along next summer or autumn will notice that they are feeling *bad* and will notice that there is a hot feeling all over their body, that the heart beats rapidly, that they have lost their appetite, that their tongue is coated over with a white fur and that there is a bright, fiery red edge around the tongue. They will feel sleepy, have soreness all over the body, and a sickening dull headache. They will finally call a doctor, who will look grave and say he is afraid the patient has typhoid fever, but he can tell definitely when he calls again.

There he is, in for a long sick spell and may justly have doubts as to the final outcome. He will then have to close his eyes to every business interest and perhaps soon lose consciousness in delirium and be doped with poisonous drugs to *keep his fever down*, as the doctor says. (What a fool act this really is.) It is this *keeping the fever down act* that has dug many a grave in the bosom of this beautiful earth for the poor, typhoid patient.

This typhoid condition is one of supreme filth all through the body; it is the result of months of accumulation of body wastes, which should have been discharged long ago, but have remained and decayed in the body. Now, as the condition has continued until the clean life force can endure it no longer, this guardian of the body must either move out, or undertake its renovation.

This renovating effort is just what we call fever. Fever is only an act of Nature, and Nature is never in error; she never makes mistakes, and this fever is simply her effort. Then, why should the doctor give the death dealing drug to stop this intelligent effort of Nature? You can easily see that such medicine only hinders the work of Nature and makes her task harder by the subduing of her strength with poison drugs. But the fool will point with pride to the lowered pulse and temperature and vainly think he has achieved something desirable by his drugging, even though he has not reduced the amount of filth in the patient's body one atom.

He has the idea that this fever is a *thing*, at least he is sure it is a germ; and these animal germs are burning up and eating the patient. He therefore feels duty bound to kill the germ, and hence he supposes he has done the right thing, when he has lowered the temperature and pulse of the patient. But alas, what nonsense!

The poor vital force must now cure by cleansing the body in spite of what the wise medical man has done. So, by the time the fever has had its run, as they call it, which will be several weeks, if there is plenty of this meddling with drugs, the patient has either died of his own filth or has become cleansed of it by the vital force, independent of all that has been done by the doctor and nurse.

Well, if he lives through it, and has a successful recovery from convalescence, he finds his bank account has shrunk a great deal, or his unpaid bills are a handsome pile. Then all his former business and plans must be reconstructed and he must charge it all to *bad luck*. Poor fellow; how he is to be pitied. If he had only given attention to the supreme thing in this world, which is his bodily health, and have cleansed his body as did the bear and cow, he would have cleaned out the filth which necessitated Nature suspending all her other work for this supreme effort of house cleaning. Now, let us further consider what the real loss has been, and what damage has come as a consequence of the neglect of spring cleaning.

His own time, two or three months, has been really lost. His own vital energy has sustained a great damage. He will never again be as strong in constitution as before. It is true, however, he may feel better and look better than he did before the effort called fever occurred, because his entire system has been cleansed of the obstructing accumulations but he will not be as rugged and able to ward off intrusions upon Nature as he would have been had he not become polluted and had to have the fever method of cleansing. He will be often reminded of the fact that he once had typhoid.

When you read of some form of disease where the name ends with the letters *i-t-i-s*, you may know this ending means the inflammation of the organ mentioned in the first part of the word. Therefore, when you read of *meningitis* it means inflammation of the meninges, which means the membrane but specifically means the membrane covering the brain. There will be many cases of this disease this spring throughout the country because the patient has not cleansed the filth from his body when the spring or warmer weather came on. The inflammation is caused by the fluids of a vile character which have been carried to the brain (by the blood) and caused this membrane to be obstructed; hence the inflammation. No case of this kind would ever occur when the orders of instinct were obeyed and Nature was cleansed. Again, there will be boils, pimples, abscesses, quinsy, tonsillitis, constipation, gall stones, and other liver complaints which will take your time, cause you pain and anguish, cost you money and perhaps cost a funeral expense; all because of neglect of this very important house cleaning this spring.

There was a time when people all through the country knew pretty well the necessity of this cleansing and also knew what to use to affect it; but now this knowledge has been lost. Why? MONEY! An undue demand for it and an all absorbing love for it have made the rank and file of the people forego everything which was not in the direct line of acquiring it.

The doctors have been smart enough to let all such knowledge die out among the people. They have laughed at it and called it *old fogyism* and superstition and have succeeded in shaming the people out of it and have given nothing they could understand in its place. The doctor is now in almost undisputed control of the lives of the people and mark me, the time is not far distant when he will raise the heel of the despot and compel the people to obey and submit to his dictates. Just wait until a few more are elected to the legislatures of the States and to the Congress of the United States and we will have a set of laws which will compel your surrender of choice of means and medicine and doctors. It has already begun in our public schools.

Every month a medical man is forcing his services on your children under the pretext of protection of their health. He meddles himself into opening their mouths and examining their eyes. Did you ever hear of one of these chaps telling the children the cause of their ailments? Never! Not a word of it. He simply writes a note on his card to the parents and in forceful language, such as "You must" or "You should at once" have these tonsils removed, "these adenoids must be cut out," or "this child must have glasses". If you don't attend to this, the child will be suspended or reported to the Health Board. Whew! Just think of being reported to such an august body as this Health Board. M.! you'll have to obey and take your medicine.

Now, if you can read this handwriting on the wall you can foresee what is stealthily coming upon the people. You talk, think and read much these days about the sugar trust, steel trust, oil trust, and other combinations which exist to the hindrance of commercial interests, but, my reader, they pale in small magnitude with the doctor's trust. "He already holds it over all of us."

Medical freedom is as much your common right as religious freedom. It is your inalienable right; you will soon have to fight for it or lose it. May God help us when we will be compelled to submit to the dictum of the doctors who refuse to teach us anything about health or disease as it relates to its cause or prevention and then dope us with their rotten serums and poison drugs and cut us up with their ever bloody knife.

Well, we will not cease our efforts to plant in your mind the truth on these lines. We want you to know, yes, to know practically how to prevent disease and how to cure it in the only true way—Nature's way—with the use of Nature's means, which are always harmless. How I wish everyone knew that Nature ONLY cures disease, and she produces each year from the soil, every remedial means she can use or need to accomplish it, THE REMEDY FOR *IMPURE BLOOD*.

We will now tell you what herbs to use to aid Nature in cleansing your blood, or rather to aid the blood to get rid of the body filth which hinders its work. We will need a bitter principle to aid in the cleansing of the liver. Select dandelion root, culver's root, or yellow parilla. Either of the above. Then, we want a decided stimulant select, cayenne pepper, prickly ash bark, ginger, either of these. Then, we want a laxative for the bowels. Mandrake root, cascara bark, licorice root, senna leaves; either of these. Then, we want a remedy to aid the blood to cleanse the mucous membranes: blue flag root, sassafras bark, stillingia, tag alder bark, sarsaparilla; either of the last named may also be used in combination with the others. Then, add if obtainable a good handful of hemlock boughs, using of the other about two ounces of each. Boil this quantity in three quarts of water down to three pints, strain and add two pounds of cut loaf sugar; when this is dissolved, add about six ounces of alcohol to prevent it from souring. Dose, one-half a wine glass before each meal.

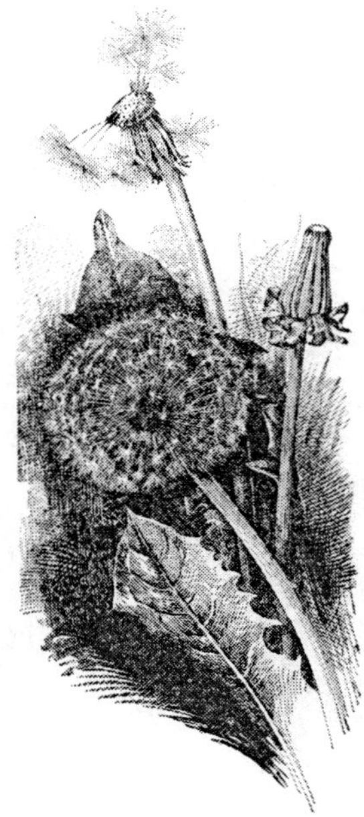

Dandelion
(*Taraxacum officinale*)

We have here mentioned those herbs which we suppose can be obtained very easily in almost any part of the country. We would advise that every family obtain the young vegetable sprouts as soon as they begin to grow this spring and cook and eat them freely. Dandelion and nettle sprouts, watercress, mustard, narrow and sour dock, poke sprouts, lambs quarter, turnip and beet tops; each of the above, singly or in combination, are good for food. Fresh or dried fruit should be used freely. Avoid cheese, dry beans, potatoes, white bread, and similar dry foods. Watercress and young dandelions may be served without cooking as lettuce is served. Let those who desire to assist Nature in its work of cleansing, abstain from tea and coffee. Water alone should be the drink.

Be it remembered that your blood is always clean, but that the other fluids of the body may be very unclean. Aid the blood in its work of cleaning house this spring and see how you will prosper in health and strength of both mind and body. Don't put it off in either your own case or that of your family.

"All men think all men mortal but themselves." This truism might be modified very appropriately by saying all men think all men should obey the laws of Nature but themselves.

This typhoid condition is one of supreme filth all through the body; it is the result of months of accumulation of body wastes, which should have been discharged long ago, but have remained and decayed in the body.

Fever is only an act of Nature, and Nature is never in error; she never makes mistakes, and this fever is simply her effort. Then, why should the doctor give the death dealing drug to stop this intelligent effort of Nature?

There will be many cases of this disease this spring throughout the country because the patient has not cleansed the filth from his body when the spring or warmer weather came on.

There was a time when people all through the country knew pretty well the necessity of this cleansing and also knew what to use to effect it; but now this knowledge has been lost.

The doctor is now in almost undisputed control of the lives of the people and mark me, the time is not far distant when he will raise the heel of the despot and compel the people to obey and submit to his dictates. Just wait until a few more are elected to the legislatures of the States and to the Congress of the United States and we will have a set of laws which will compel your surrender of choice of means and medicine and doctors. It has already begun in our public schools.

We will need a bitter principle to aid in the cleansing of the liver. Select dandelion root, culver's root, or yellow parilla. Either of the above. Then, we want a decided stimulant select, cayenne pepper, prickly ash bark, ginger, either of these. Then, we want a laxative for the bowels. Mandrake root, cascara bark, licorice root, senna leaves; either of these. Then, we want a remedy to aid the blood to cleanse the mucous membranes: blue flag root, sassafras bark, stillingia, tag alder bark, sarsaparilla; either of the last named may also be used in combination with the others.

Phytotherapy Department

(The American Herb Doctor)

Address all communications for this department to its editor
Prof. M. G. YOUNG, 4156 Arcade Building, Seattle, Wash.

Dandelion

by M. G. Young

Herald of Health and Naturopath, XXI (7), 461-462. (1916)

In each issue of this magazine I have written in such a way and upon such subjects as would be properly adaptable both to the season and the needs of my readers. I have chosen for this magazine this very common herb which will need no explanation or description, as it is found everywhere. But when I come to tell you of its many, many uses and of its true value, you will no doubt feel ashamed that you have walked over it and trodden it down so many times. Especially will this be true when you have tried it out for the troubles for which I recommend it.

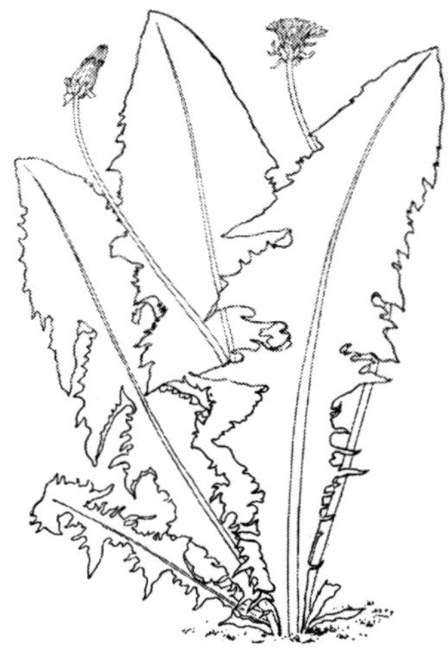

Large leaved form of dandelion.

Its Latin name is *Leontodon taraxacum [Taraxacum officinalis]*. Its medical properties are:

Diuretic—increasing the flow of urine.

Diaphoretic—promoting perspiration or sweating.

Aperient—promoting and aiding the action of the bowels in a mild way.

Anti-spasmodic and Expectorant—relieving spasm or periodic occurrences of spells and causing the secretions of the breathing organs to empty or come up easily and plentifully.

Tonic—prompting the action and secretions of the digestive organs.

Alterative—that which changes the system, by causing it to cleanse or empty its morbid or unusable material.

Now you will no doubt begin to think this herb is a *cure all*, but I can say I know of no other herb which is of more value to the human family. I would be glad to write a volume on this one herb and I don't think I would then feel I had done it justice.

In a case of dropsy, by adding common garden parsley to the dandelion roots and tops, say 2 parts of dandelion to 1 part parsley, and boiling them 20 minutes, straining the tea and drinking a wine glassful or more every 2 hours, you will be greatly relieved. Be sure to use plenty of the herbs so as to have it good and strong.

To use it for sweating and general benefit to the whole body at the same time, add to 2 parts of the dandelion, 1 part each of pleurisy root (*Asclepias tuberosa*), and 1 part boneset (sometimes called through wort; Latin, *Eupatorium perfoliatum*), boil this 15 minutes, strain and keep warm, give to patient a cupful every 15 to 20 minutes—give it hot. This will be found very sure and certain cure for colds, when accompanied by biliousness. Try it.

There is perhaps no single agent of greater value to the constipated patient, whose trouble generally arises from a torpid liver, than this same dandelion. To make it more effective, add 1 part blue flag root and 1 part culvers root to 2 parts whole herb and root of dandelion. Boil 30 minutes; take a cupful 2 to 3 times daily, if you find it necessary.

In lung diseases, I have found dandelion a most valuable remedy. I will venture this prediction: If any one article will cure consumption, it is dandelion, even confirmed consumption, I believe, can be better treated with it than with anything else.

Don't be afraid of using too much, or too strong. Boil all of it and use it as much as you choose. Sugar may be used in it, but don't make a thick syrup. Just take it as you would any article of food or drink, and persevere and you will soon see results, which will gratify you.

In asthma or bronchitis or catarrh, you will find it a very good help. Just go out and dig it up, wash it off and crush or bruise it well and put on water enough to boil out the juice and strength, then drink it often, say just like water, and if you find it acts too strong, lessen your dose or strength of it.

Say, I am telling the truth about this herb, if you are a sufferer, don't delay, use it and write me about your case and I will gladly help you.

The bitter principle of dandelion renders it one of the best remedies where a general strengthening is needed, and where there is general debility. Hence, the dyspeptic and especially the nervous patient can get very good results from it. By all means persevere in its use no matter what you may be taking beside it. Crush the roots and tops, dug at any season of the year, and boil the strength out and use it as often as you feel it is needed, always before meals.

As an alterative, it is very valuable, but is not rapid. Those who desire its benefit should continue its use, prepared as above, for months, but, be well assured there will be no failure. It will change the entire system in a very radical way and will completely change the liver, if kept up for months.

I will now direct you about collecting it for medicine. It may be gathered at any time of the year, but must be washed clean and then dried. It is best to separate the tops and root, then crush or rather slice the roots up rather thin and dry both in a clean, dry, shady place (not in the sun), then put them into sacks of paper and keep them in the driest place you have. If you will parch the common field peas, as you would coffee, and cut up fine these dry roots of dandelion and parch them also, then grind each separately, then take a teaspoonful of the ground dandelion, and a sufficient quantity of the ground peas to make a pea coffee. You will have one of the best substitutes for Mocha and Java coffee you ever used. You can scarcely tell the difference by taste or aroma.

You will also find that the green tops of dandelion will make excellent greens. They should not be cooked with meat, and should be used with any other kind of greens, such as spinach, turnip tops, mustard, or young sprouts of the common nettle. Season with butter, salt and pepper. Serve with vinegar or lemon juice.

By gathering the blossoms of dandelion, crushing them and properly treating them a very good and wholesome wine can be made.

Now, don't despise the dandelion, even though it grows in your lawn. I use it in many of my best remedies and will gladly answer all inquiries concerning it.

*To use it for sweating and general benefit to the whole body at the same time, add to 2 parts of the dandelion, 1 part each of pleurisy root (*Asclepias tuberosa*), and 1 part boneset (sometimes called through wort; Latin,* Eupatorium perfoliatum*), boil this 15 minutes, strain and keep warm, give to patient a cupful every 15 to 20 minutes—give it hot.*

There is perhaps no single agent of greater value to the constipated patient, whose trouble generally arises from a torpid liver, than this same dandelion.

In lung diseases, I have found dandelion a most valuable remedy.

1917

Mayweed

Elder

M. G. Young

Mayweed

by M. G. Young

Herald of Health and Naturopath, XXII (2), 97. (1917)

Mayweed is the common name for this herb. I have selected it because of its value and at this time of the year it may be gathered by those who desire its use. It has an annual, twisted, tapering, fibrous root with one or more stems, erect, branched, bushy, leafy, angular, furrowed, nearly smooth and solid, from one to two feet high. It may not be necessary to further describe this plant as it is commonly called dog fennel or mayweed and grows in all parts of the country. Its history is as follows; Mayweed is indigenous to Europe and is very common throughout the United States, where it is known by the following names: wild chamomile and dog fennel. It may be sought throughout in all waste places and hard, dry soil, especially along the roadside. Its flowers are white, and appear from June until September. Every part of the plant is acrid and fetid, according to Linnaeus; it is grateful to toads, and drives away fleas. For this purpose, it should be placed in the clothing which is to be worn so that its aromatic effect may become fused through the clothing, and it is also very annoying to fleas. If a portion of this herb is crushed and left exposed in a room the flies will soon disappear. The whole plant is useful as a medicine. Its taste is bitter and pungent. Water or alcohol extracts its properties. It has been found to contain oxalic, valenianic, and tannic acid, but Nature has so thoroughly and nicely distributed these qualities that they are of benefit and produce no injurious effect. It has coloring matter, albumen, and other qualities, such as volatile and various salts.

Its chief medical quality is tonic. In large doses, it is emetic and is an excellent article when used as an anti-spasmodic. It is also an emmenagogue and an excellent cuticle irritant or epispastic. The cold infusion or extract may be used as a tonic and [anti-] spasmodic. In all cases, this will be found an excellent article and may be taken freely, cold, for the above named troubles. A strong tea of it is excellent for sick headaches when taken at the time of the headache. It is also good for convalescence from fevers. A warm injection is useful as an enema and sweat producer. It is useful in suppressed menses. The bruised plant, when fresh, will cause a separation of the effete matter in sores when applied to such conditions and will cause them to heal rapidly.

A very powerful skin irritant may be made in the following manner. Take the fresh plant of mayweed and smart weed, equal parts, and bruise them together and moisten them with a small quantity of spirits of turpentine. This will be found an excellent application where severe skin irritation is suffered from. It would be excellent in all cases of neuralgia and as an external application for sciatica or any rheumatic pain. The dose of the infusion of mayweed is from one to four fluid ounces as often as may be required.

This herb should be gathered when in bloom and dried in the shade. Dust off the dirt from the roots. After it is dried, store it in paper sacks and keep in a dry place. All that I have said regarding its virtues will be found equally valuable when the dried herb has been properly prepared and used. I would suggest however, that the dry herb should be used in one-third larger quantities.

My friends, I have now told you of another very valuable herb which has been walked over, hated and despised by the very people who have needed its virtues, and because of their neglect of it have lost their money to the surgeon, the doctor and the undertaker. My God, when will the time ever come when the people will wake to the realization that the great and good God apprehended all of the necessities and fully supplied them in the vegetable kingdom? Oh, the ignorance of this wise being called man, but alas, the designing parties have succeeded in enlightening our minds and have led us to believe in error and superstition, having substituted ways and means which are remunerative to them in dollars and cents, and yet surely destructive of human life, health, strength and happiness.

May God help this article to fall under the eyes of many who need the virtues this plant contains. Dear reader, do you believe me conscientious and honest in this wish? I am doing everything I can or know to do to spread this valuable knowledge throughout the earth. Have you a duty in this direction? If so, evidence it by lending me all the aid you can.

Its chief medical quality is tonic. In large doses it is emetic and is an excellent article when used as an anti-spasmodic. It is also an emmenagogue and an excellent cuticle irritant or epispastic.

A strong tea of it is excellent for sick headaches when taken at the time of the headache. It is also good for convalescence from fevers. A warm injection is useful as an enema and sweat producer. It is useful in suppressed menses.

It would be excellent in all cases of neuralgia and as an external application for sciatica or any rheumatic pain.

My God, when will the time ever come when the people will wake to the realization that the great and good God apprehended all of the necessities and fully supplied them in the vegetable kingdom?

Phytotherapy Department

(The American Herb Doctor)

Address all communications for this department to its editor

Prof. M. G. YOUNG, 4156 Arcade Building, Seattle, Wash.

Elder

by M. G. Young

Herald of Health and Naturopath, XXII (3), 169-170. (1917)

Sambucus canadensis or common elder is an indigenous shrub growing in all parts of the United States in low, damp ground, thickets and waste places, flowering in June and July, and maturing its berries in September and October. This is such a well-known native plant that it is hardly necessary to give her the usual botanic description. The official parts are the flowers, the berries, and the inner bark. The odor of the flowers is characteristic and heavy, quite powerful when fresh, but faint when dry. They are slightly aromatic and bitterish, and impart their virtues to hot water. Boiling dissipates a volatile oil, which may be obtained by distillation with water; when cold it has the consistency of butter. Ammonia is present in water which has been distilled from the flowers.

Elder flowers contain volatile oil, acrid resin, tannic acid, malate of potassium and lime, mineral salts, a trace of sulphur, etc. The berries have little or no odor and acid-saccharine taste, and yield by expression a purple juice, called elder-rob, which gives a dark lilac color with alkalies and a scarlet with acids; acetate of lead added to the juice causes a blue deposit of its coloring substances. It contains malic acid, a little citric acid, sugar, and coloring matter. The inner bark is whitish with a green tint, odorless, of a saccharine taste, but subsequently bitterish, with some acrimony and imparts its properties to alcohol or water.

The properties and uses of the flowers are as a diaphoretic and gentle stimulant; in cold infusions they are diuretic, alterative, and cooling, and may be used in all diseases requiring such action, as in hepatic (liver) derangements of children, erysipelas and erysipelatous diseases, etc. In infusion with maiden hair [*Adiantum capillusveneris L.*] and beech drops [*Orobanche virginiana*], they will be found very valuable in all erysipelatous diseases. The expressed juice of the berries, evaporated to the consistency of a syrup is a valuable aperient and alterative; one ounce of it will purge. An infusion of the young leaf buds are likewise purgative and sometimes act with violence. The flowers and expressed juice of the

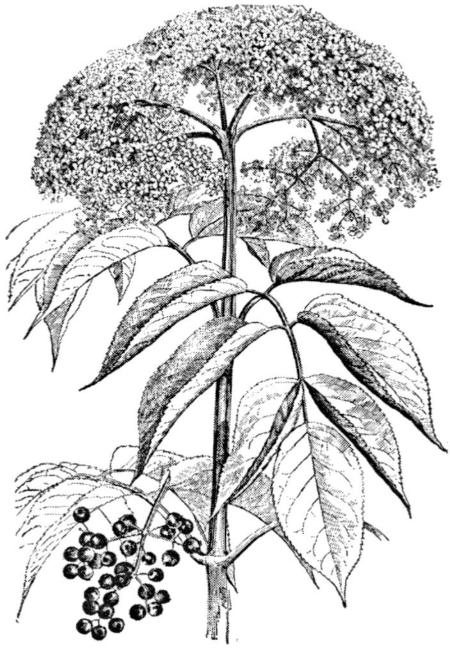

Elder (*Sambucus canadensis*)

berries are beneficially employed in scrofula, cutaneous diseases, syphilis, rheumatism, etc.

The inner green bark is cathartic. An infusion of it in wine or in the expressed juice will purge moderately, in doses from one half to a fluid ounce. Large doses produce vomiting; in small doses it proves an efficacious deobstruent promoting all the fluid secretion, and is very useful in dropsy, especially that following scarlet fever, and other febrile diseases as well as in many chronic diseases. Beaten up with lard, cream, or Vaseline, it forms an excellent discutient [dispersing agent] ointment which is of much value in burns, scalds, and some cutaneous diseases. The juice of the root in half ounce doses daily acts as a hydrogogue cathartic and diuretic and will be found valuable in all dropsical affections. It is also useful in epilepsy. Take the bark from branches one or two years old, scraping off the gray outer bark and steeping two ounces of it in five ounces of cold or hot water for 48 hours. Strain and give a wineglassfull every fifteen minutes when the fit is threatening; the patient fasting. Resume it every six or eight days.

The properties and uses of the flowers are as a diaphoretic and gentle stimulant; in cold infusions they are diuretic, alterative, and cooling, and may be used in all diseases requiring such action, as in hepatic (liver) derangements of children, erysipelas and erysipelatous diseases, etc.

The expressed juice of the berries, evaporated to the consistency of a syrup is a valuable aperient and alterative; one ounce of it will purge.

The flowers and expressed juice of the berries are beneficially employed in scrofula, cutaneous diseases, syphilis, rheumatism, etc.

The inner green bark is cathartic. An infusion of it in wine or in the expressed juice will purge moderately, in doses from one half to a fluid ounce. Large doses produce vomiting; in small doses it proves an efficacious deobstruent promoting all the fluid secretion, and is very useful in dropsy, especially that following scarlet fever, and other febrile diseases as well as in many chronic diseases.

The juice of the root in half ounce doses daily acts as a hydrogogue cathartic and diuretic and will be found valuable in all dropsical affections.

1918

Herbs

Aloe, Angelica

Anise, Arnica

Ash, Asarum, Walnut, Balm Mint
Rhubard, Barbery

Green Beanpods, Mistle, Betony, Bearberry

Lavender, Birch, Black Alder,
Black Currant, Blackthorn

Blessed Thistle, Blueberry, Briar Hips, Basil

Black Thorn, Bramble, Burnet, Borage

Buckbean, Buckthorn, Broom

Burdock, Chamomile, Carline Thistle

Benedict Lust, N.D.

HERB BOOK

A COMPREHENSIVE LIST OF COMMON MEDICINAL HERBS, ROOTS, BARKS, FLOWERS AND LEAVES

Giving their popular and botanical names, together with their therapeutic properties. Alphabetically arranged under both their common and their scientific names.

This is just the book you have hunted for

Price, postpaid, 60c. (foreign 2s., 6); with the HERALD OF HEALTH one year, $2.25 (foreign 9s.) Address all orders to

B. Lust, N.D., M.D., Butler, N. J.

PHYTOTHERAPY

A new book giving the

KNEIPP NATUROPATHIC HERBS AND THEIR USES

Regeneration of the blood through herbal remedies, by Benedick Lust, N.D., M.D.

50 cents Postpaid

KNEIPP PUBL. CO.

110 E. 41st Street, New York

Benedict Lust's comprehensive herbal book promoted his Kneipp herbal sales.

Herbs

by Benedict Lust, N.D.

Herald of Health and Naturopath, XXIII (3), 253. (1918)

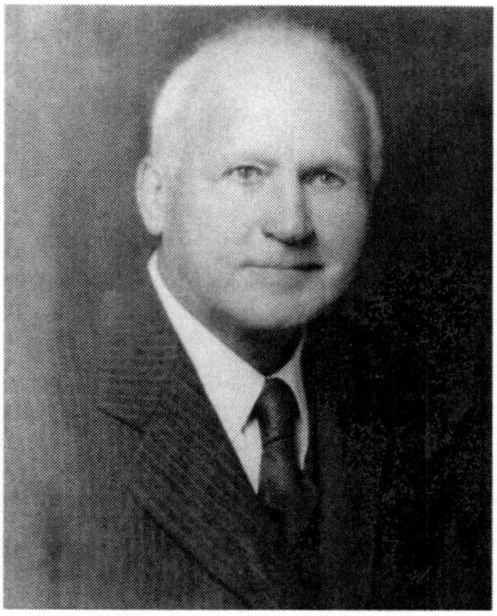

Benedict Lust (1872-1945)

Many simple herbs in their natural state or made into teas afford relief for the severest ailments. Only those which are non-poisonous and produce natural physiological action are recommended in Naturopathy.

It is the aim of *The Naturopath* to also educate the people as to make the use of even mild herbal remedies unnecessary. Part of a most ancient prayer says: "May I live my life in such a manner that herbal remedies need never pass my lips."

There are those cases, however, in which the individual's power of resistance is so low, his will-power so weak, that he will not make an effort in his own behalf. The medical profession believes in dope for such a one, and according to their new doctrine, it is not a crime to put such a one out of his misery.

Naturopathy is here to save that individual, if possible, and in most cases of such a character offers herbal remedies to assist the elimination of poisons and bring the individual to a point where he can help himself.

Preparation Of Herb Teas

To prepare tea from any of the herbs mentioned hereafter, take a tablespoonful of the dried herb, root, bark, blossom, or fruit in question, add 1 ½ cups of hot water and boil in a covered vessel for from 5 to 10 minutes, allow it to settle and decant carefully or strain through a fine sieve. One tablespoonful of honey may be added for sweetening. If not otherwise directed, a cupful of this tea should be taken three times daily.

Tea of Mountain Arnica (leopard's bane) should be used in much smaller quantities only one tablespoonful should be taken once a day.

AGAVE

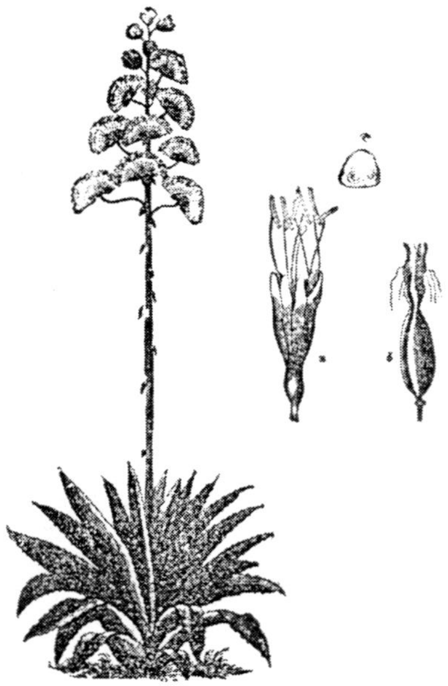

Bitter Aloe (*Agave americana*)

a. Flower, b. receptacle after the time of flowering, c. cross-section.

Latin, *Agave americana*; German, *Agaven*; French, *Agavé*; Spanish, *Pita*

This plant comes originally from Mexico, but has been successfully cultivated in southern Europe and other hot countries. In the north, it is cultivated in hot-houses.

It has long, fleshy, thorny leaves of a dark-green color.

Action: mild, laxative, diuretic, anti-syphilitic. It is also recommended in liver congestion and jaundice.

Dose: One tablespoonful boiled in one and half cupfuls of water, taken three times a day. Instead of the tea, one-half teaspoonful of the powder may be taken three times a day.

SOUR OR MORELLO CHERRY LEAVES

Latin, *Cerasus vulgaris*; German, *Weichsel*; French, *Griotte*; Spanish, *Guindo común*

The leaves of the morello cherry tree are used for coughs and sore throat as are likewise the stems of the fruit.

Dose: One tablespoonful boiled in one and half cupful of water, taken three times daily.

Selected Herbs A Review of the Most Useful Herbs as a Curative Factor for Numerous Ailments

Aloe, Angelica

by Benedict Lust, N.D.

Herald of Health and Naturopath, XXIII (4), 379. (1918)

Aloe

Latin, *Aloe vulgaris*; German, *Aloe*; French, *Alo*; Spanish, *Acibar*

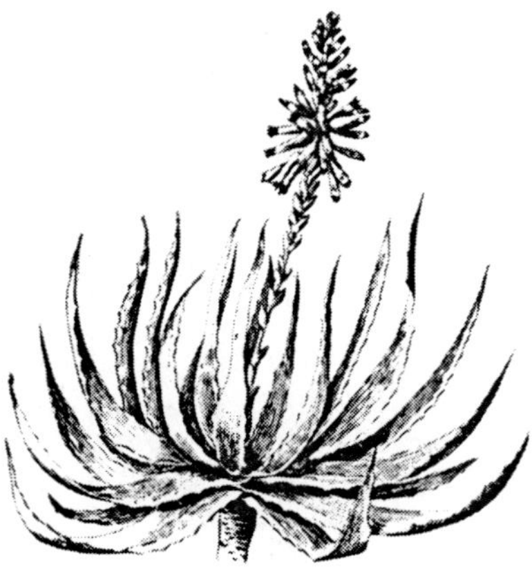

Aloe (*Aloe vulgaris*)

Aloe is the dried and powdered juice of aloe leaves. This plant grows principally in South Africa. Its taste is very bitter, and its action is that of a purgative. It is rarely used of itself, however, it is of better value when combined with other and milder herbs. The following mixture is effective in cleansing the stomach and bowels: one-half teaspoonful aloe, one tablespoonful of elder blossoms, two teaspoonful of [*Trigonella*] *foenum graecum* (Fenugreek), and one teaspoonful ground fennel seed. Make one pint of tea from above, which will provide a two days' supply. This mixture will not act violently, but will allow ample time for the digestion of food, and produce a normal stool in from 8 to 24 hours.

Aloe as tea can be used to good advantage as an eye lotion and for washing wounds of all kinds.

In inflammation of the eyes, take one-half teaspoonful of aloe and dissolve in one half pint of water. Use to bathe the eyes.

Wild Angelica

Latin, *Angelica silvestris*; German, *Angelika, Engelwurzel*; French, *Angelique*; Spanish, *Angelica*

In bloom from July to September, it is generally found near running brooks or in richly watered meadows. It has long been known for its

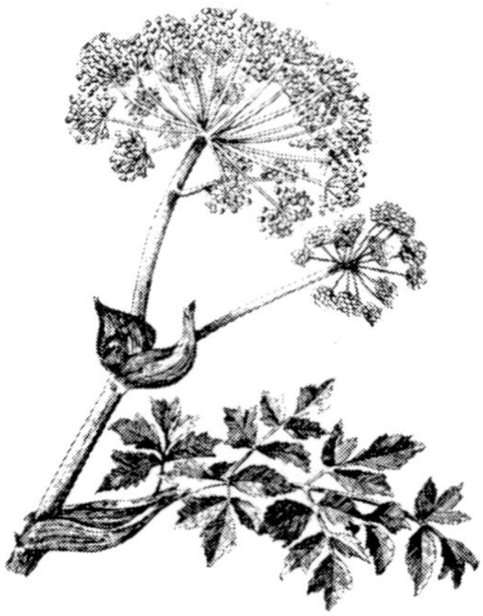

Angelica (*Angelica silvestris*)

healing properties, and is a very good remedy for colic, particularly in children, and for ordinary stomach and digestive troubles. Results from its administration are very prompt.

Angelica tea is especially recommended for gases on the stomach and pressure in the abdomen.

A cupful of angelica tea should be prepared and divided into three parts, one third being taken morning, noon and evening.

Mothers should always keep this excellent colic remedy in the house.

This mixture [of aloe, elder flower, fenugreek, and fennel seed] will not act violently, but will allow ample time for the digestion of food, and produce a normal stool in from 8 to 24 hours.

[Angelica] has long been known for its healing properties, and is a very good remedy for colic, particularly in children, and for ordinary stomach and digestive troubles. Results from its administration are very prompt.

Selected Herbs — A Review of the Most Useful Herbs as a Curative Factor for Numerous Ailments

Anise, Arnica

by Benedict Lust, N.D.

Herald of Health and Naturopath, XXIII (5), 479. (1918)

Anise

Latin, *Pimpinella anisum*; German, *Anis*; French, *Anis cultive*; Spanish, *Anis*

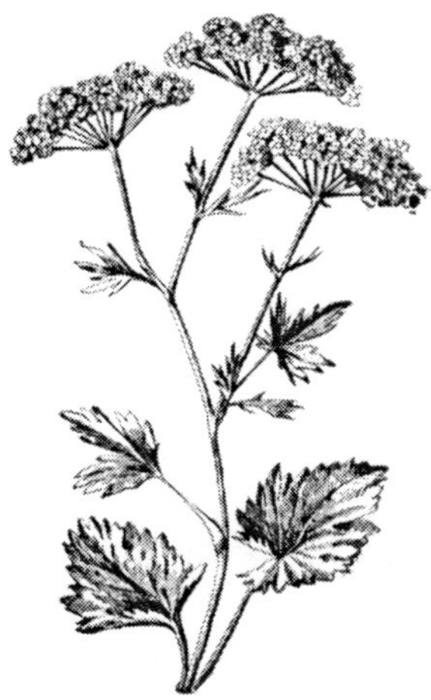

Anise (*Pimpinella anisum*)

Anise is the fruit of a plant originally cultivated in and imported from Egypt and Syria. It is now grown in colder climates. It blooms in July and August. The root and plant are edible and the seed is used for flavoring and medicinal purposes.

It is a remedy for colic and of value with other remedies in eradicating intestinal bacteria. To stop colic promptly and very effectively, take one tablespoonful of anise seed and boil in a large cupful of milk for from 5 to 10 minutes. Drink this as hot as possible. Results from this are usually very rapid; the colic disappearing in a short time.

Anise seed may be combined with equal parts of caraway and fennel seeds, and used for the same purposes. This combination is an excellent intestinal purifier.

Anise water is an excellent eye lotion; ½ teaspoonful boiled in a half of pint of water.

Arnica Flowers, Leopard's Bane

Latin, *Arnica montana*; German: *Arnika*; French: *Arnica*; Spanish: *Arnica*

This plant has been well known for its remedial properties from the olden times. It grows in mountainous districts near running waters or on well-watered meadows, at an elevation as high as 6,000 feet. It is in bloom from June to September.

To be used internally, **arnica tea must be taken very weak.** It is more

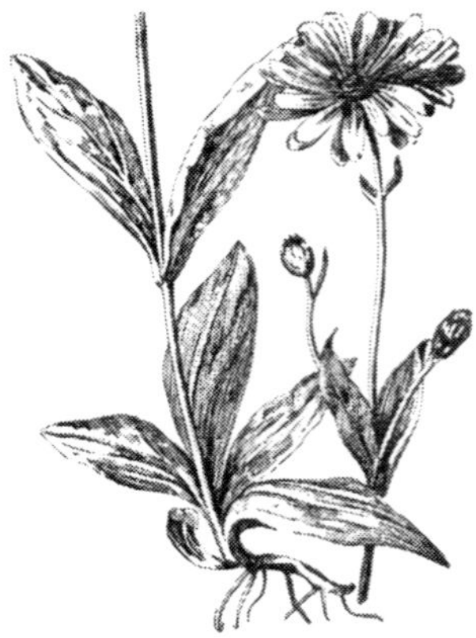

Arnica (*Arnica montana*)

to be recommended as an external application.

In cases of violent stomach and abdominal pains, apply compresses of arnica tea made by boiling the entire plant in vinegar and water. It will give quick relief.

The plant, if preserved in alcohol, makes the tincture of arnica, which is an excellent remedy to rub on stiffened, sore or painful joints and in rheumatism.

The tincture, diluted with five times the same amount of water, can be used for washing and cleansing wounds and for compresses to be applied to swellings.

[Anise] is a remedy for colic and of value with other remedies in eradicating intestinal bacteria. To stop colic promptly and very effectively, take one tablespoonful of anise seed and boil in a large cupful of milk for from 5 to 10 minutes. Drink this as hot as possible.

To be used internally, ***arnica tea must be taken very weak.*** *It is more to be recommended as an external application.*

In cases of violent stomach and abdominal pains, apply compresses of arnica tea made by boiling the entire plant in vinegar and water. It will give quick relief.

Selected Herbs — A Review of the Most Useful Herbs as a Curative Factor for Numerous Ailments

Ash, Asarum, Balm Mint, Rhubarb, Barberry*

by Benedict Lust, N.D.

Herald of Health and Naturopath, XXIII (6), 577. (1918)

Ash Tree Leaves

Latin, *Fraxinus*; German, *Eschenblätter*

This is a good remedy for gout, rheumatism and rheumatic pains. This tea should be taken steadily for some time in order to give good results.

Asarum, Wild Ginger**

Latin, *Asarum europaeum*; German, *Haselwurz*

Asarum is used practically for the same purposes as ribwort [plantain], and should be preferably mixed with the other to remove slimy mucus in respiratory passages; also for incipient consumption.

Balm Mint

Latin, *Melissa officinalis*; German, *Melisee*

This plant grows wild in mountainous districts on hilly declivities and vineyards. It is in bloom from July to September. This tea is recommended for abdominal troubles arising from nervous complaints; also for chlorosis and hysteria.

It is soothing for cramps in the stomach, gases and dyspepsia. It is also good for nervous headache and nervous tooth and earache. Tincture of balm mint will stop nausea and vomiting if taken ten to fifteen drops on a lump of sugar.

---

*To eliminate repetition, the section of walnut leaves was deleted. Walnut appears on page 318. —*Ed.*

**The following common names were cited by Lust for this plant: Asarabacca, European Snakeroot, Hazelwort, Wild Nard. —*Ed.*

RHUBARB

Latin, *Rheum palmatum*; German, *Rhabarber*; French, *Rhubarbe*; Spanish, *Ruibarbo*

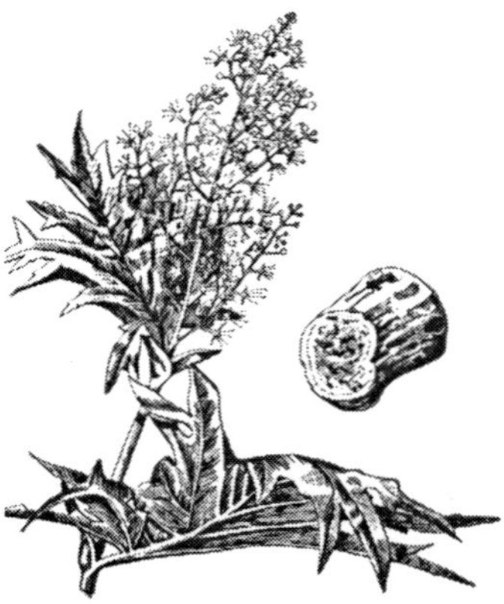

Rhubarb (*Rheum palmatum*)

The genuine rhubarb plant grows in China. And only the root of rhubarb plants growing in that country are valuable for their medicinal properties. Rhubarb is an excellent remedy for stomach and intestinal troubles. It is a very mild purgative and a good blood purifier. The world-celebrated and famous Kneipp pills partly contain some rhubarb or rhubarb tincture.

Generally, a decoction of the root is used, or some of the root pulverized half a teaspoonful in water may be taken. Some prefer to chew pieces of the root.

BARBERRY

Latin, *Berberis vulgaris*; German, *Berberitzenbeeren*; French, *Epine vinette*; Spanish, *Berbero*

A decoction of these berries, which are found nearly all over the country, is used for liver and spleen troubles. The juice of the fruit boiled with sugar, if enough water is added, makes a very toothsome cooling beverage.

Asarum is used practically for the same purposes as ribwort [plantain], and should be preferably mixed with the other to remove slimy mucus in respiratory passages; also for incipient consumption.

Tincture of balm mint will stop nausea and vomiting if taken ten to fifteen drops on a lump of sugar.

Rhubarb is an excellent remedy for stomach and intestinal troubles. It is a very mild purgative and a good blood purifier.

Selected Herbs A Review of the Most Useful Herbs as a Curative Factor for Numerous Ailments

Green Beanpods, Mistletoe, Betony, Bearberry

by Benedict Lust, N.D.

Herald of Health and Naturopath, XXIII (7), 674. (1918)

Green Beanpods, Kidney Bean

Latin, *Phaseolus vulgaris*; German, *Bohnenhülsen*; French, *Haricots blanc*

A good remedy for dropsy, kidney trouble, sciatica, gout and rheumatism.

Mistle, European Mistletoe

Latin, *Viscum album*; German, *Mistel*; French, *Gui*; Spanish, *Hierba de la liga (Muérdago)*

This plant is a parasite growing on the branches of twigs of various trees. It is in bloom in March and April and grows in winter glossy and sticky berries. As it is a parasite living on the juice extracted from others, we should despise it, if it were not for its excellent remedial properties. Its effects are not to be surpassed for stopping hemorrhages. Mistle tea is excellent also for other disturbances in the blood circulation. Mistle may be mixed to advantage with shavegrass in equal parts.

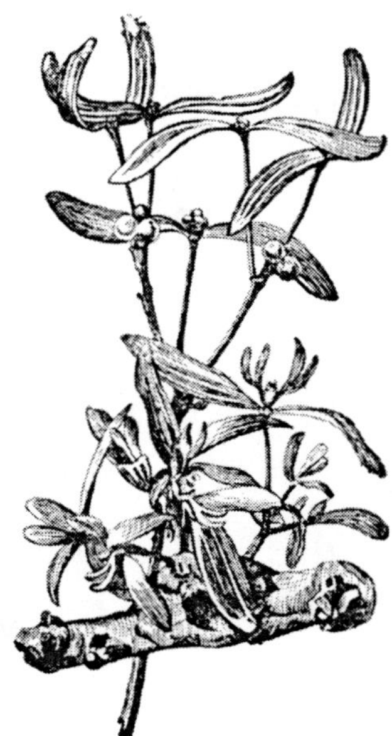

Mistletoe (*Viscum album*)

Betony

Latin, *Stachys officinalis*

This plant was formerly highly prized for its medicinal virtues. It was generally used as an emetic and also a purgative. In our present times, this plant is practically used very little only.

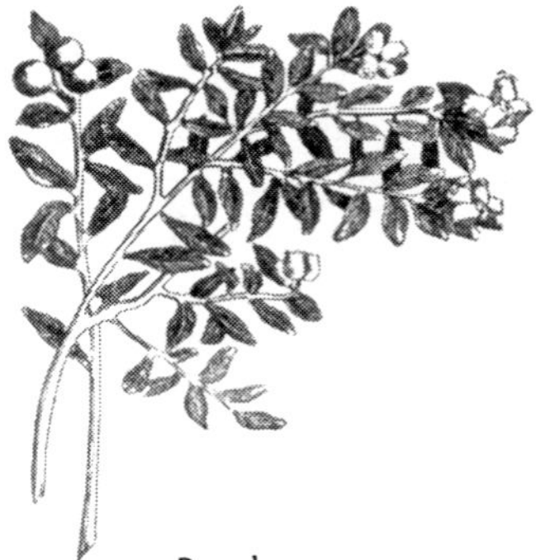

Bearberry
(*Arctostaphylos uva ursi*)

BEARBERRY

Latin, *Arctostaphylos uva ursi*; German, *Bärentraubenblätter*; French, *Bousserole*; Spanish, *Gayuba*

This shrub grows extensively in the high mountainous districts of Europe. Its leaves are recommended in kidney and bladder diseases to cause increased flow of urine.

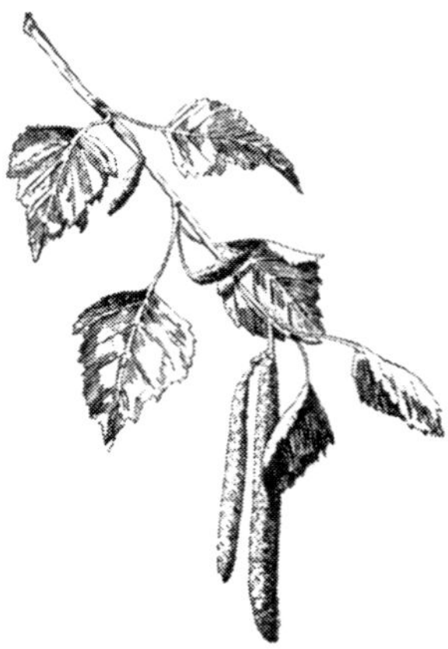

Birch leaves (*Betula alba*)

BIRCH LEAVES

(Latin, *Betula alba*; German, *Birkenblätter*; French, *Boulon blanc*; Spanish, *Abedul*

The leaves of this well-known tree are an exceptional blood purifier, and are also recommended in diseases of the kidney and bladder and also for rheumatic pains.

The bark of the tree acts similarly.

> *[Mistle's] effects are not to be surpassed for stopping hemorrhages. Mistle tea is excellent also for other disturbances in the blood circulation. Mistle may be mixed to advantage with shavegrass in equal parts.*

Selected Herbs A Review of the Most Useful Herbs as a Curative Factor for Numerous Ailments

Lavender, Birch, Black Alder, Black Current, Blackthorn

by Benedict Lust, N.D.

Herald of Health and Naturopath, XXIII (8), 740. (1918)

Lavender

Latin, *Lavandula vera*; German, *Lavendel;* French, *Lavande commuse*; Spanish, *Espliego*

This plant was originally imported from southern Europe, but is now also found in this country.

A decoction of the blossoms is used for gases in the stomach, headache, giddiness and faintness, and for congestion. Spirit of lavender is used for rubbing the sore joints in rheumatic pains.

Birch

Latin, *Betula alba*; German, *Birke;* French, *Bouleau écorce*; Spanish, *Corteza de abedul*

Tea of the leaves of the birch tree used internally is for rheumatism, gout, dropsy, urinary complaints, etc.

Externally, it is used for eruptions of the skin. The juice of the birch tree is valuable for kidney disease and is also an excellent blood purifier.

Alder Buckthorn Tree Bark

Latin, *Rhamnus frangula*; German, *Faulbaumrinde*; French, *Bourgène*; Spanish, *Arraclán*

Of this tree, which grows extensively in shrubberies and forests, the berries, but especially the bark, is used as tea as a splendid purgative.

If preferred, the bark may be preserved in wine, and may be taken a tablespoonful at a time.

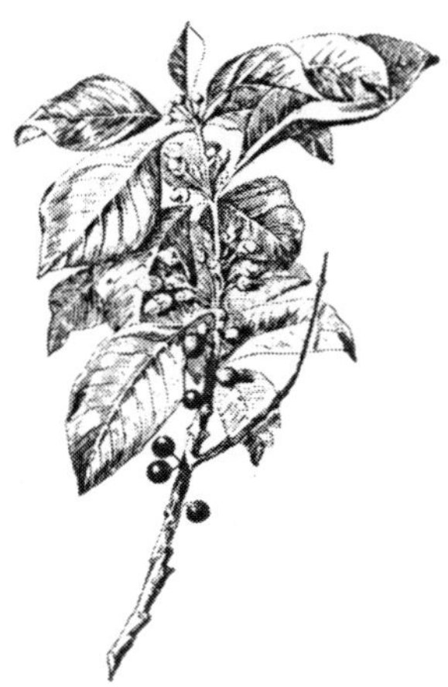

Alder Buckthorn tree (*Rhamnus frangula*)

BLACK CURRANT LEAVES

Latin, *Ribes nigrum;* German, *Schwarze Johannisbeerblätter*; French, *Grosellier noir*; Spanish, *Grosello negro*

Leaves of this shrub prepared as tea, also its extract preserved in sugar are used for whooping cough and catarrh of the chest.

BLACKTHORN BLOSSOMS

Latin, *Prunus spinosa;* German, *Dornschlehblüten;* French, *Prunier sauvage*; Spanish, *Endrino*

Tea of blackthorn blossoms are one of the mildest purgatives.

The leaves should be boiled one minute in water, and this tea should be taken three to four days one cupful at a time. It acts very gently, without griping in the least. The juice of the fruit boiled in sugar makes a good cough remedy.

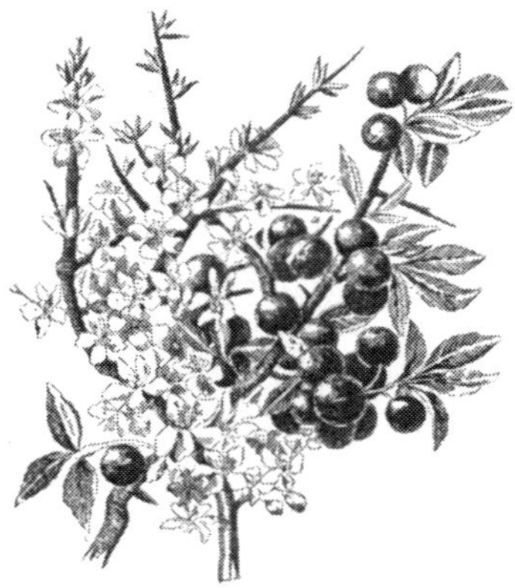

Blackthorn blossoms
(*Prunus spinosa*)

Spirit of lavender is used for rubbing the sore joints in rheumatic pains.

Leaves of [Black currant] shrub prepared as tea, also its extract preserved in sugar are used for whooping cough and catarrh of the chest.

Tea of blackthorn blossoms is one of the mildest purgatives.

Selected Herbs
A Review of the Most Useful Herbs as a Curative Factor for Numerous Ailments

Blessed Thistle, Blueberry, Briar Hips, Basil

by Benedict Lust, N.D.

Herald of Health and Naturopath, XXIII (9), 790. (1918)

Blessed Thistle

Latin, *Conicus benedictu;* German, *Kardo-Benediktenkraut*; French, *Chardon bévit*; Spanish, *Cardo santo*

The tea of this plant is used extensively in cases of nervous prostration, melancholia and hysterics and may be taken three times a day.

Blueberry (Bilberries)

Latin, *Vaccinum myrtillus;* German, *Heidelbeeren*; French, *Myrtille*; Spanish, *Arándano*

The berries, boiled and preserved, or better still, as a tincture, are one of the best specifics against diarrhea. Tea of the dried berries is also used for the same purpose.

This shrub is in common growth everywhere. The leaves of the blueberry shrub prepared as a tea are one of the best antidiabetic remedies in the world. This tea should be taken continuously for a long period.

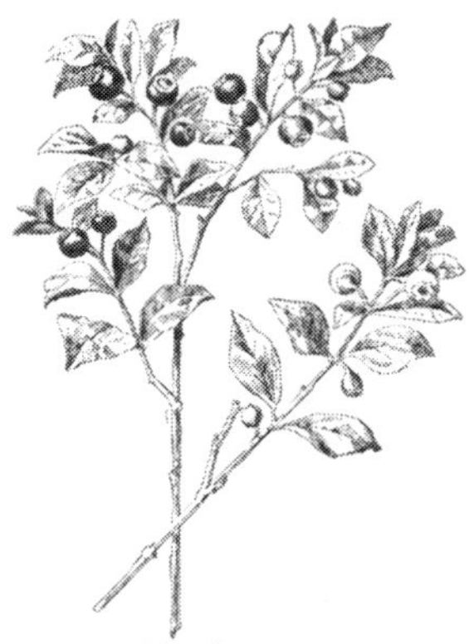

Blueberries (*Vaccinum myrtillus*)

Briar Hip

Latin, *Rosa canina;* German, *Hagebutten*; French, *Gratte cul*; Spanish, *Calumbrujo cirosbatos*

This is a plant that is as yet only little appreciated. Tea of briar hip is used to advantage in disease of the kidneys and the bladder, also against stoppages in the urinary canal, and stone in the bladder.

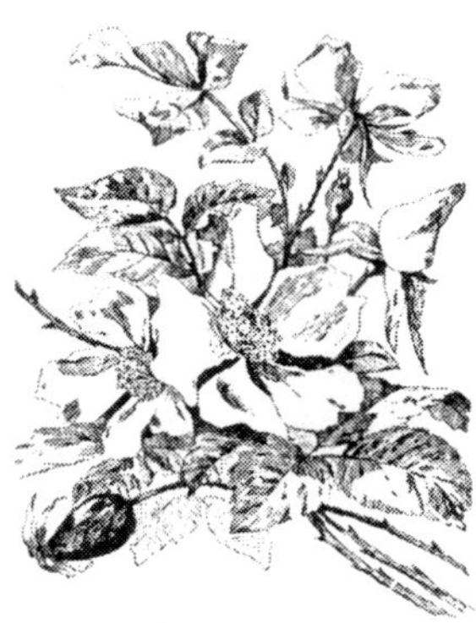

Briar hip (*Rosa canina*)

SWEET BASIL

Latin, *Ocimum basilicum;* German, *Basilicum-Kraut* or *Josephskräutlein*; French, *Grand Basilic*; Spanish, *Albahaca*

This plant is generally imported from southern Asia, and is now cultivated in some of our gardens.

A decoction of this herb, mixed with some honey, aids and increase the throwing off of the mucus and slime in catarrh of the chest and obstruction of mucus in the lungs.

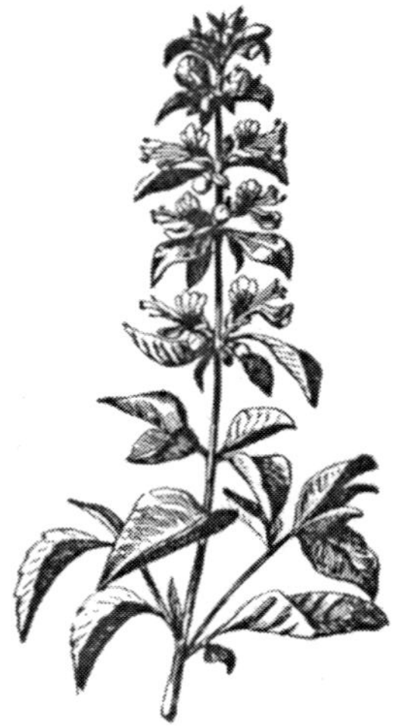

Basil
(*Ocimum basilicum*)

The tea of [blessed thistle] is used extensively in cases of nervous prostration, melancholia and hysterics and may be taken three times a day.

A decoction of [sweet basil], mixed with some honey, aids and increase the throwing off of the mucus and slime in catarrh of the chest and obstruction of mucus in the lungs.

Selected Herbs — A Review of the Most Useful Herbs as a Curative Factor for Numerous Ailments

Blackthorn, Bramble, Burnet, Borage

by Benedict Lust, N.D.

Herald of Health and Naturopath, XXIII (10), 842. (1918)

Blackthorn Blossoms

Latin, *Prunes spinosa;* German, *Dornschlehblüten;* French, *Prunier sauvage*; Spanish, *Endrino*

This plant grows in mountainous districts on hills and in forests. It is in bloom in April and May.

The tea of this plant is one of the gentlest purgatives of the entire pharmacopeia. It should be taken three to four days regularly a cupful morning, noon and night. It will not only purify the system, but also strengthen the digestive apparatus.

Bramble (Blackberry) Leaves

Latin, *Rubus fructicosus;* German, *Brombeer-Blaetter*; French, *Ronce noir*; Spanish, *Zarzamora*

The bramble leaf grows almost without exception throughout the country. Taken in tea form, it makes an excellent and desirable substitute for ordinary breakfast tea. It is a splendid blood purifier.

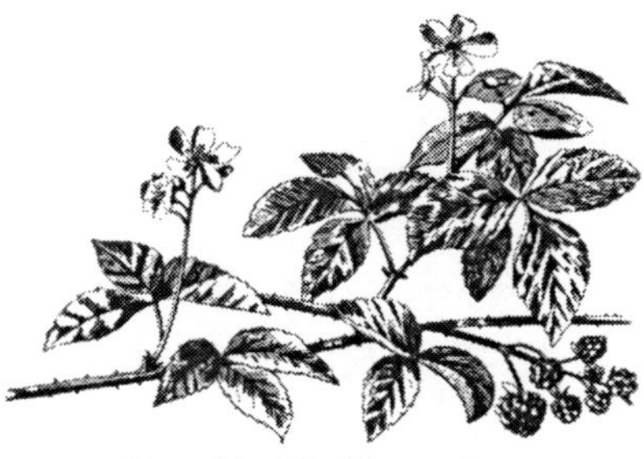

Bramble, Blackberry leaves (*Rubus fructicosus*)

Burnet Saxifraga

Latin, *Pimpinella saxifrage*; German, *Bibernelle, Pimpernelle*; French, *Pimpernelle*; Spanish, *Pimpinela*

This common weed will be found growing nearly everywhere. Its roots are used either dried and pulverized or as a tincture. It is a sudorific and diuretic, and is also used for affections of the throat, catarrh of the throat, articular rheumatism, gout, inflammation of the kidneys and stone in the bladder. For a sore throat, take twenty drops of the tincture on a lump of sugar. For other complaints, take the tea three times a day, or one-half teaspoonful of the powder in water, three times a day.

Borage

Latin, *Borago officinalis*; German, *Boretsch*

This is a blood purifier and nerve tonic. It is rich in nutritive salts, and is recommended for cases of hysteria and nervous palpitation of the heart.

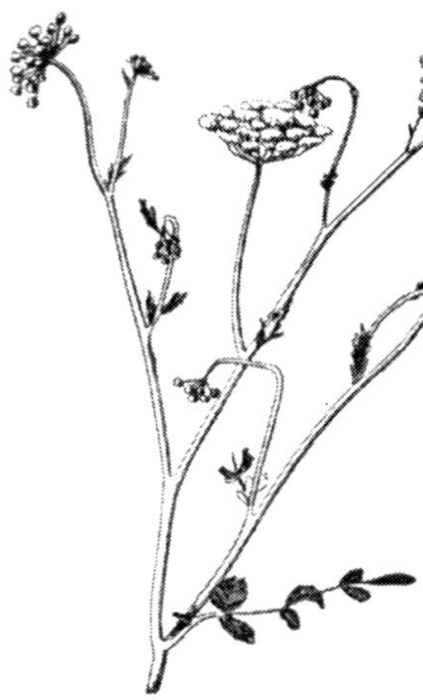

Burnet (*Pimpinella saxifrage*)

> *The tea of [Black thorn] is one of the gentlest purgatives of the entire pharmacopeia.*
>
> *[Burnet] is a sudorific and diuretic, and is also used for affections of the throat, catarrh of the throat, articular rheumatism, gout, inflammation of the kidneys and stone in the bladder.*
>
> *[Borage] is a blood purifier and nerve tonic. It is rich in nutritive salts, and is recommended for cases of hysteria and nervous palpitation of the heart.*

Selected Herbs A Review of the Most Useful Herbs as a Curative Factor for Numerous Ailments

Buckbean, Buckthorn, Broom

by Benedict Lust, N.D.

Herald of Health and Naturopath, XXIII (11), 896. (1918)

Buckbean

Latin, *Menyanthes trifoliata*; German, *Bitterklee*; French, *Trefle d'eau*; Spanish, *Trébol*

This plant grows mostly in swamps, bogs, ditches and beneath the surface of the water. It blooms from April to June, is a splendid remedy for dyspepsia, sour stomach, and similar ailments, and of great benefit in cases of torpid life. Tea of buckbean and tincture of buckthorn act as a blood purifier, restore the appetite, and may be mixed with other herbs, such as wormwood, centaury and sage.

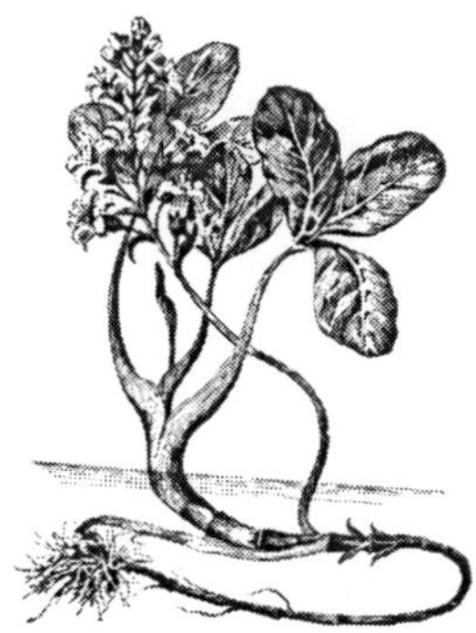

Buckbean
(*Menyanthes trifoliate*)

Common Buckthorn Bark And Berries

Latin, *Rhamnus cathartica*; German, *Kreuzdorn*; French, *Neprien,* Spanish, *Espino Cerval*

This is a very good purgative. A decoction of the dried berries may be made for tea purposes, or the juice of the crushed fresh berries, passed through a cloth and boiled with sugar, will act effectively as a strong purgative. For adults, about one or two spoonfuls is necessary while for children, about half a teaspoonful of the juice of the berry is sufficient.

The bark of buckthorn may be used as tea to good advantage, and for similar purposes as buckthorn berries.

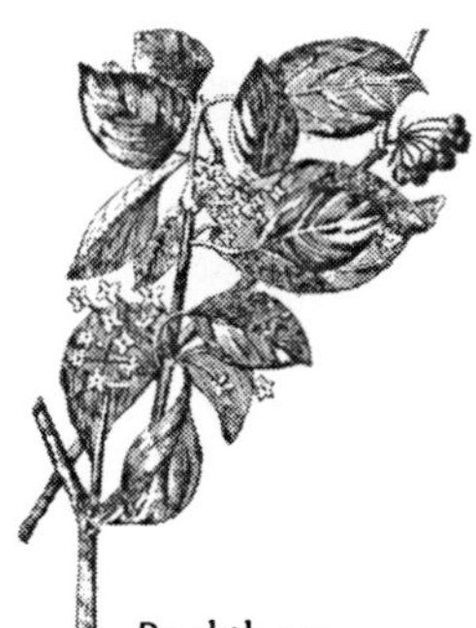

Buckthorn
(*Rhamnus cathartica*)

Broom (Geniste)

Latin, *Genista germanica*; German, *Ginster*; French, *Genête*; Spanish, *Retama*

This bush grows on sandy soil and blooms during the summer months.

It acts on the kidneys to great advantage, as well as against stone in the bladder. In cases of herpes or tetters,* it is an effective blood purifier. The tincture of this herb is used for the same purposes.

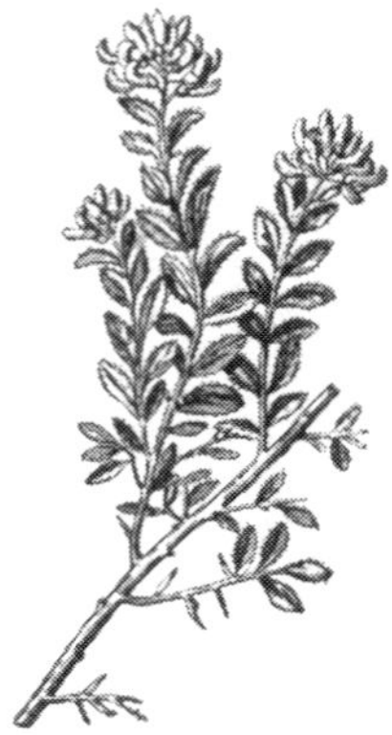

Broom
(*Genista germanica*)

Tea of buckbean and tincture of buckthorn act as blood purifiers, restore the appetite, and may be mixed with other herbs, such as wormwood, centaury and sage.

In cases of herpes or tetters, it is an effective blood purifier. The tincture of this herb is used for the same purposes.*

---

* Tetters is a skin disease with symptoms of itching and pustules patches such as eczema or ringworm. —*Ed.*

Selected Herbs A Review of the Most Useful Herbs as a Curative Factor for Numerous Ailments

Burdock, Chamomile, Carline Thistle

by Benedict Lust, N.D.

Herald of Health and Naturopath, XXIII (12), 940. (1918)

Burdock Roots

Latin, *Arctium lappa*; German, *Klettenwurzel*; French, *Bardane*; Spanish, *Lampazo*

The root of the common burdock boiled in water for from five to ten minutes, is very beneficial for the growth of the hair. Results are even better if burdock roots and blind nettle leaves*, in equal quantities, are boiled in two parts of water and one part of vinegar. Let this decoction settle for some days; then strain through a cloth sieve, and add some Cologne. Rub the roots of the hair well several times a week, but in order not to make the skin of the scalp over-sensitive, rub the scalp once a week with some good hair oil. For baldness, in which case the roots of the hair are dead, this recipe will be of no use.

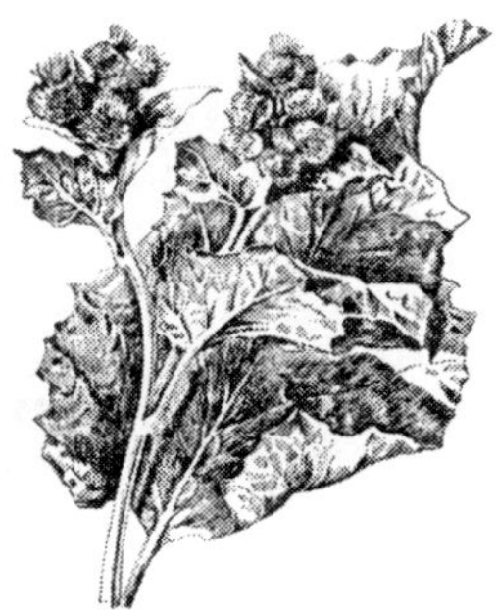

Burdock
(*Arctium lappa*)

Chamomile

Latin, *Matricaria chamomilla;* German: *Kamillen*; French: *Camomille*; Spanish: *Camomilla*

This plant has been known for centuries for its remedial properties. Even the regular physician of our present day recognizes its medical value. It grows almost everywhere, and is in bloom in May and June.

In cases of severe colds, fevers, or other similar diseases of an acute nature, chamomile tea is a very simple and effective remedy. It is also applicable in cases of griping, pains, or cramps in the stomach, strong congestions, etc. As a stomach tonic, it is a great success.

Preparation of chamomile tea is quite simple, and may be made to suit the taste.

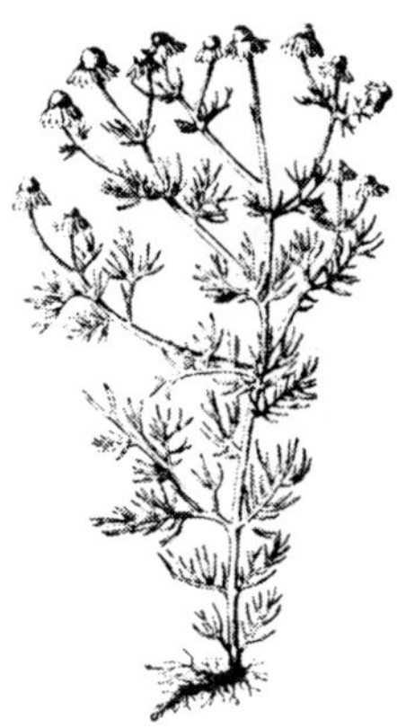

Chamomile
(*Matricaria chamomilla*)

---

*Blind nettle refers to *Lamium album*, please refer to page 306. —*Ed.*

CARLINE THISTLE (DWARF CARLINE)

Latin: *Carlina acaulis*; German: *Eberwurz*; French: *Carlin sans tige*; Spanish: *Carlina*

This plant grows in chalk-regions and on stony declivities in mountainous districts. As a decoction, its roots are used to great advantage in catarrh of the bladder and inflammation of the kidneys, as well as for a weak stomach.

The root of the common burdock boiled in water for five to ten minutes is very beneficial for the growth of the hair.

In cases of severe colds, fevers, or other similar diseases of an acute nature, chamomile tea is a very simple and effective remedy.

As a decoction, [Carline thistle] roots are used to great advantage in catarrh of the bladder and inflammation of the kidneys, as well as for a weak stomach.

1919

Caraway, Cherry, Centaury, Commack

Chicory, Coltsfoot, Chickweed

Dandelion, Dwarf Elder, Elder

Cloves, Elecampane, Eyebright, Eucalyptus, Fern

Fenugreek, Galium, Fennel

Ground Ivy, Heartsease, Hay Flowers, Heather, Iceland Moss, Juniper

Benedict Lust, N.D.

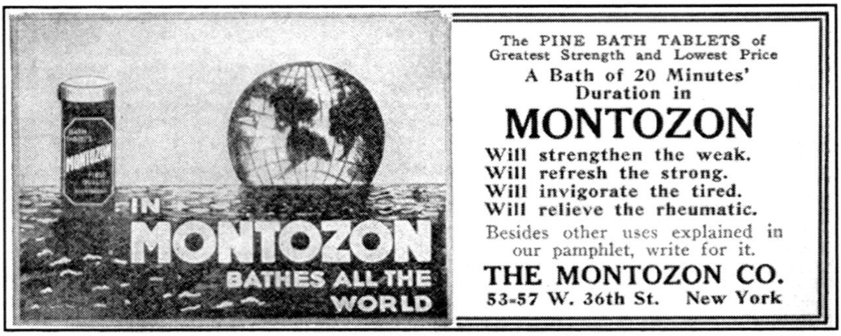

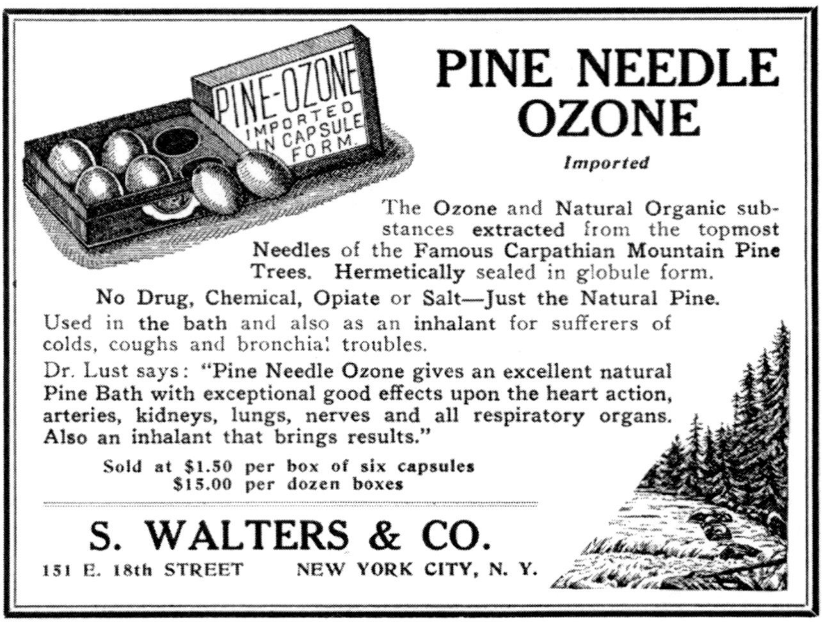

Kneipp was fond of pine needles and used them for baths to treat kidney, bladder and skin and especially strengthen the blood vessels in the elderly.

Caraway, Cherry, Centaury, Commock

by Benedict Lust, N.D.

Herald of Health and Naturopath, XXIV (1), 35. (1919)

Caraway

Latin, *Carum carvi*; German, *Kömmel*; French, *Cumide prés*; Spanish, *Alcaravea*

Caraway grows, to a large extent, in dry meadows, and is found abundantly in nearly all parts of the country. A decoction of this plant is used to cure gases, cramps in the stomach, and general stomach disorders.

Oil of caraway is used for similar purposes. Of the latter, take one drop on a piece of sugar. For infants troubled with wind in the stomach, rub one drop of the oil on the infant's abdomen, until absorbed. Relief will come as a consequence.

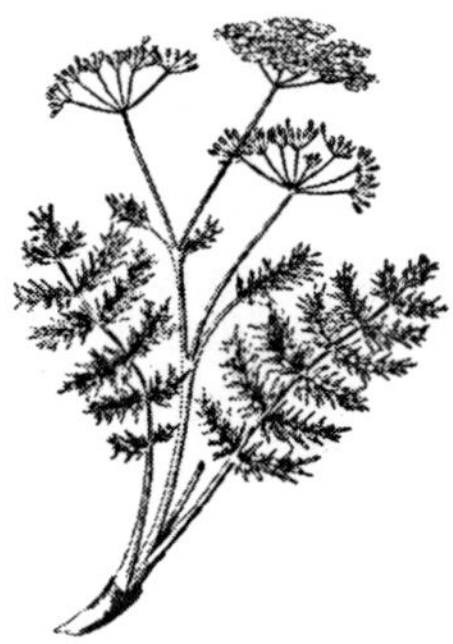

Caraway
(*Carum carvi*)

Cherry Stalks [Stems]

Latin, *Prunus serotina*; German, *Kirschenstiele*; French, *Cerise*; Spanish, *Tallo de Cereza*

Tea of cherry stalks can be used to advantage as a tonic. It is efficient in the promotion of digestion, will alleviate coughing, and is very valuable for its sedative and antispasmodic effects in cases of whooping cough, gripping and nausea, as well as spasmodic affections of the breathing organs.

Centaury

Latin, *Centaurium erythaea*; German, *Tausendguldenkraut*; French, *Centaurée*; Spanish, *Centaura menor*

This plant, which is in bloom all summer, grows mostly in forests. Like most of the bitter herbs, it is valued for its remedial properties in all kinds of ailments.

Centaury tea will dissolve all hard and effete matter which has stagnated in the bowels, and will abate any constipated condition.

People of sedentary habits, who cannot take the time for out-door exercises, will find this tea very beneficial. In cases of pains in the stomach, bowels, chest, liver or spleen, or for irregularities of the bowels, this tea is very favorably recommended.

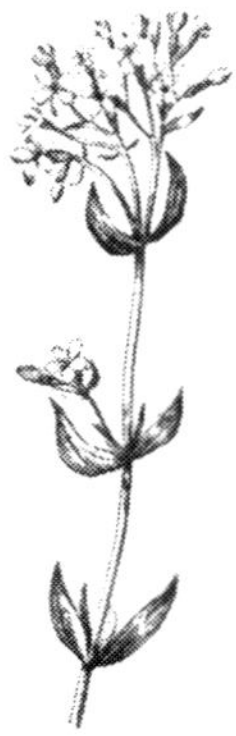

Centaury
(*Centaurium erythaea*)

Commock, Restharrow

Latin, *Ononis spinosa;* German, *Haubechel (Garnkraut)*

For rheumatism and gout, this tea is of great advantage. It is of splendid help in cases of dropsy, gravel in the bladder, and induration of the glands. It is a very mild dissolvent, diuretic, and laxative.

For infants troubled with wind in the stomach, rub one drop of [caraway] oil on the infant's abdomen, until absorbed.

[Tea of cherry stem] is efficient in the promotion of digestion, will alleviate coughing, and is very valuable for its sedative and antispasmodic effects in cases of whooping cough, gripping and nausea, as well as spasmodic affections of the breathing organs.

Centaury tea will dissolve all hard and effete matter which has stagnated in the bowels, and will abate any constipated condition

Selected Herbs A Review of the Most Useful Herbs as a Curative Factor for Numerous Ailments

Chicory, Coltsfoot, Chickweed

by Benedict Lust, N.D.

Herald of Health and Naturopath, XXIV (2), 92. (1919)

Chicory (Succory)

Latin, *Cichorium intybus*; German, *Wegwart*; French, *Chicorée*; Spanish, *Achicoria Amarga*

This weed, which blooms from early spring to the close of autumn, grows wild in various places and is also manufactured abroad as a substitute for coffee.

Although it is not considered of special importance, chicory has wonderful remedial properties. It acts with pleasing result against slime in the stomach and overflowing of the gall, and purifies the liver, kidneys and spleen. Dyspeptics would do well to take this tea.

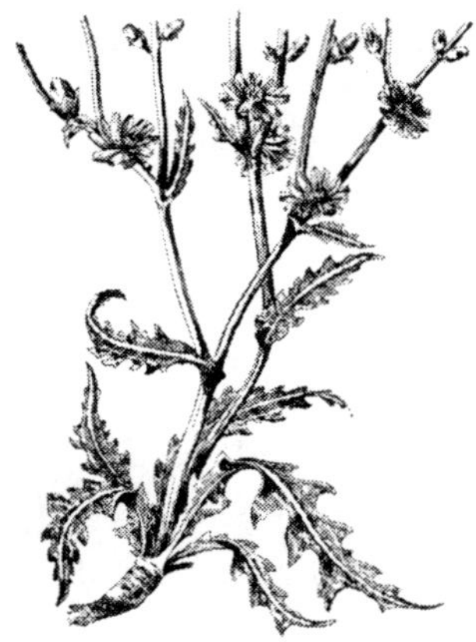

Chicory or Succory
(*Cichorium intybus*)

Coltsfoot

Latin, *Tussilago farfara*; German, *Huflattich*; French, *Pas d'âne*; Spanish, *Uña de Caballo*

This plant, although it grows quite extensively in the spring, is noticed very little. Tea of coltsfoot is very beneficial in cases of phlegm on the chest or coughing. It cleans the breast, purifies the lungs, and stops the harmful cough. For those who show an inclination to sickness of whatever nature, tea made from the leaves of this plant offers relief.

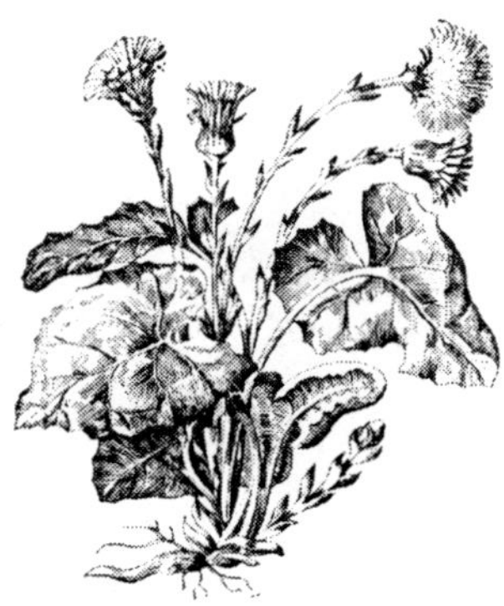

Coltsfoot
(*Tussilago farfara*)

Chickweed

Latin, *Stellaria media*; German, *Höhnerdarm*; French, *Mouron de Oiseaux*; Spanish, *Pamplinas*

This plant is generally considered a weed of no account. It grows wild almost everywhere, and in nearly all season of the year. Chickweed tea is used to great advantage in cases of catarrh of the chest.

The extract of this tea boiled in sugar is also used for the same purpose and is highly recommended.

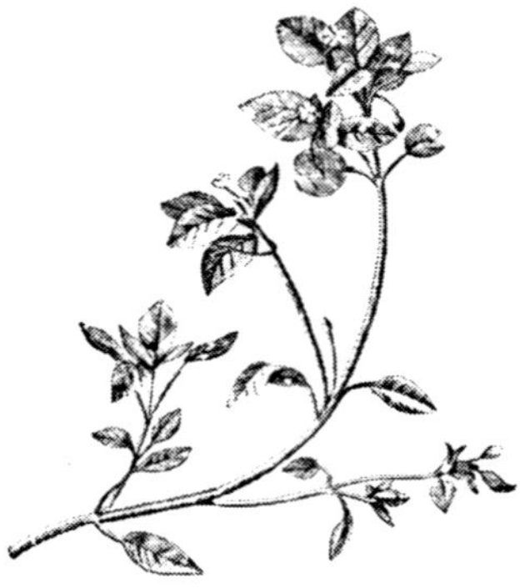

Chickweed
(*Stellaria media*)

[Chicory] acts with pleasing result against slime in the stomach and overflowing of the gall, and purifies the liver, kidneys and spleen. Dyspeptics would do well to take this tea.

Chickweed tea is used to great advantage in cases of catarrh of the chest.

Tea of coltsfoot is very beneficial in cases of phlegm on the chest or coughing.

Selected Herbs A Review of the Most Useful Herbs as a Curative Factor for Numerous Ailments

DANDELION, DWARF ELDER, ELDER

by Benedict Lust, N.D.

Herald of Health and Naturopath, XXIV (3), 144. (1919)

DANDELION

Latin, *Taraxacum officinale*; German, *Löwenzahn*; French, *Pissenlit*; Spanish, *Diente de león*

This plant grows as a weed in meadows, clover fields or pastures throughout the spring and summer. A decoction of the roots of the dandelion is a splendid blood purifier.

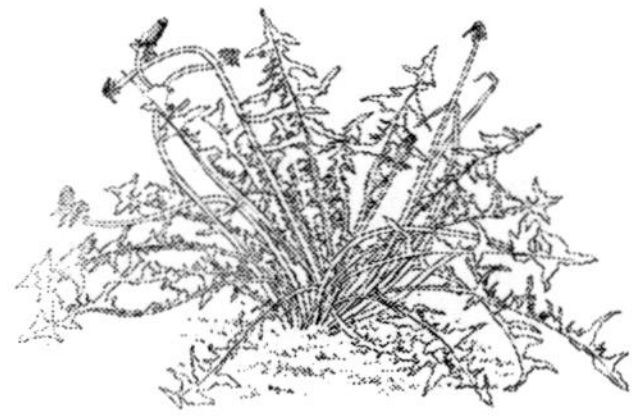

Dandelion
(*Taraxacum officinale*)

DWARF ELDER

Latin, *Sambucus ebulus*; German, *Attichwurzel*; French, *Hièble*; Spanish, *Yezgo*

Dwarf Elder tea is prepared from the dried roots of the plant, which must be either cut up fine, or ground into a powder. The effect is the same in both cases. It may also be taken as a powder, half a teaspoonful at a time.

This tea is one of the best remedies for dropsy. It compels the segregation of water in very large quantities by acting directly on the kidneys. Rev. Father Kneipp states in several of his reports that he was able to cure advanced cases of dropsy simply with this tea and proper water applications.

Whenever effete humors of the body cause abdominal disturbances, the tea of the dwarf elder will assist the segregation of these humors through the urine. Its leaves are used for similar purposes.

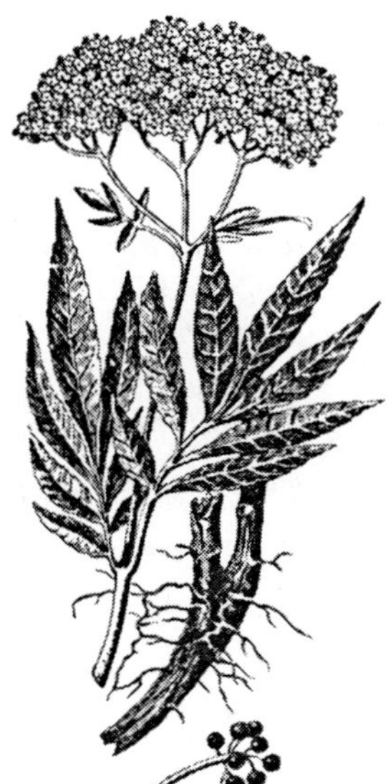

Dwarf elder
(*Sambucus ebulus*)

ELDER BERRIES

Latin, *Sambucus nigra*; German, *Hollunderbeeren*; French, *Sureau noir*; Spanish, *Sauco*

The dried berries made into a tea are an excellent remedy against colic and diarrhea.

ELDER FLOWERS

Latin, *Sambucus nigra*; German, *Hollunderblätter*

Tea made from elder flowers is a splendid spring medicine. It should be taken home for some weeks every morning before breakfast. It is an excellent blood purifier.

ELDER LEAVES

Latin, *Sambucus nigra*; German, *Hollunderblätter*

The leaves of this plant are used for practically the same purposes as the blossoms. They should be cut into long strips before boiling.

ELDER ROOTS

Latin, *Sambucus nigra*; German, *Hollunderwurzeln*

Tea made from elder roots is an excellent prevention against incipient dropsy. There is perhaps no other remedy so effective as this root in such cases.

> *[Dwarf elder root] compels the segregation of water in very large quantities by acting directly on the kidneys. Rev. Father Kneipp states in several of his reports that he was able to cure advanced cases of dropsy simply with this tea and proper water applications.*
>
> *The dried [elder] berries made into a tea are an excellent remedy against colic and diarrhea.*
>
> *Tea made from elder roots is an excellent prevention against incipient dropsy. There is perhaps no other remedy so effective as this root in such cases.*

Selected Herbs A Review of the Most Useful Herbs as a Curative Factor for Numerous Ailments

Cloves, Elecampane, Eyebright, Eucalyptus, Fern

by Benedict Lust, N.D.

Herald of Health and Naturopath, XXIV (5), 248. (1919)

Cloves

Latin, *Genum urbanum;* German, *Nelkenwurzel;* French, *Clou de l'huile;* Spanish, *Aceite de Jiroflé*

Oils (or extract) of cloves is used principally for remedial purposes. It is an aid for foul gases in the stomach, and for putrefied matter and juices in the abdominal passages. Several drops of the extract on a lump of sugar are sufficient for one time.

Elecampane

Latin, *Inula helenium;* German, *Alant;* French, *Année;* Spanish, *Ala*

The root of this plant, which grows in nearly all countries of medium climate, is an excellent remedy for throwing out phlegm and quieting pains in catarrh of the chest. It also promotes segregation of sweat and urine and is a good blood purifier.

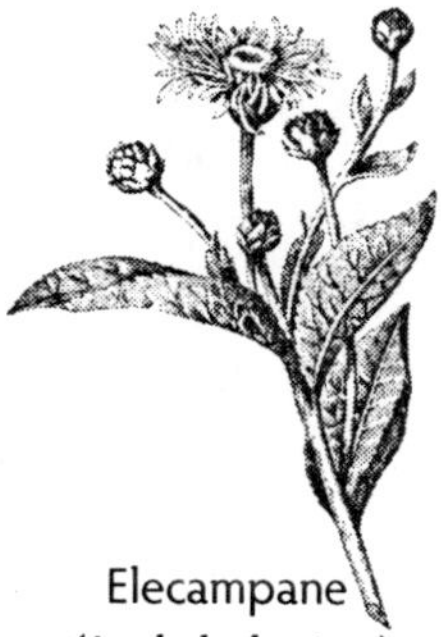

Elecampane (*Inula helenium*)

Eyebright

Latin, *Euphrasia offinalis;* German, *Augentrost;* French, *Euphrasie;* Spanish, *Eufrasia*

This plant grows in nearly every field and meadow and is in bloom from June to October.

Its leaves should be dried and boiled for tea. With this decoction wash the diseased eye several times during the day, also apply cold compresses of the same over the eye. This will clean and heal the optic and increase the power of sight. Taken internally, it is good for indigestion and gastric trouble.

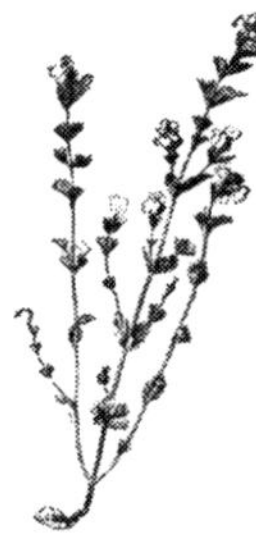

Eyebright (*Euphrasia officinalis*)

EUCALYPTUS

Latin, *Eucalyptus globulus;* German, *Eukalyptus*

This makes an aromatic bitter tea promoting digestion. It is very valuable in dyspepsia and is recommended for intermittent fevers.

FERN (POLIPOD)

Latin, *Aspidium (filix-mas);* German, *Farnkraut;* French, *Fongère (male)*

This is a specially recommended remedy for tapeworm.

Take some of the fresh root, peel it, and chew about one quarter ounce each time about five times a day. At the same time take a purgative, for example, castor oil, in doses of one tablespoon each time. This is sure to remove the entire tapeworm. Be sure that the head of the tapeworm has been passed out of your system.

Oils (or extract) of cloves is used principally for remedial purposes. It is an aid for foul gases in the stomach, and for putrefied matter and juices in the abdominal passages. Several drops of the extract on a lump of sugar are sufficient for one time.

The root of [Elecampane], which grows in nearly all countries of medium climate, is an excellent remedy for throwing out phlegm and quieting pains in catarrh of the chest.

[Fern] is a specially recommended remedy for tapeworm.

Selected Herbs A Review of the Most Useful Herbs as a Curative Factor for Numerous Ailments

Fenugreek, Galium, Fennel

by Benedict Lust, N.D.

Herald of Health and Naturopath, XXIV (6), 298. (1919)

Fœnum Graecum (Fenugreek)

Latin, *Trigonella fœnum graecum*; German, *Bockshornklee*; French, *Fenugrec*; Spanish, *Fenogreco*

This plant grows in countries with medium temperature, coming originally from Southern Europe. Rev. Kneipp recommends the seeds of this plant should be pulverized. As a tea it has remarkable cooling effects. Sore throat, with great heat in the throat, may be treated with this tea used as a gargle. One teaspoonful dissolved in a cup of water is sufficient. It may be taken either every hour, or the throat may be gargled every hour with it. This remedy is recommended especially for children, as it never fails to give relief. Dissolved in warm water to the consistency of a thick paste it may be used as a warm poultice for drawing out swellings and ulcers.

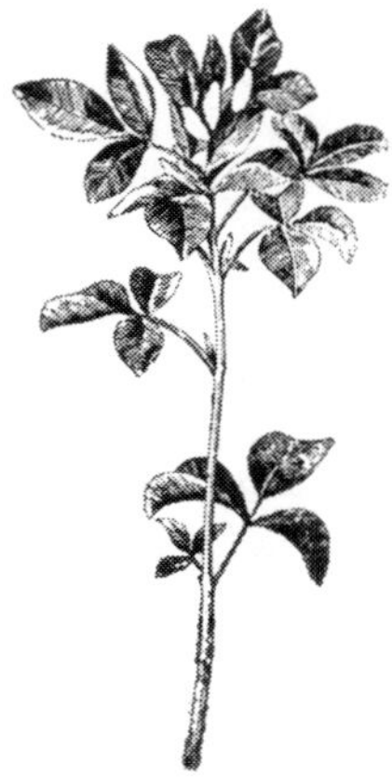

Fenugreek (*Trigonella fœnum graecum*)

Galium

Latin, *Galium aparine*; German, *Klebkraut*

A decoction of this plant is used to wash out and cleanse wounds. As a tea it is recommended as a good remedy for epilepsy, dropsy, and cutaneous eruptions.

Fennel Seed

Latin, *Foeniculum vulgare*; German, *Fenchel*; French, *Fenouille*; Spanish, *Hinojo*

This plant grows in any temperate climate and may be found almost everywhere.

Fennel tea is a most effective remedy for colic and wind. Mothers should not be without it, for delay, in the case of small babies, may result in grave consequences.

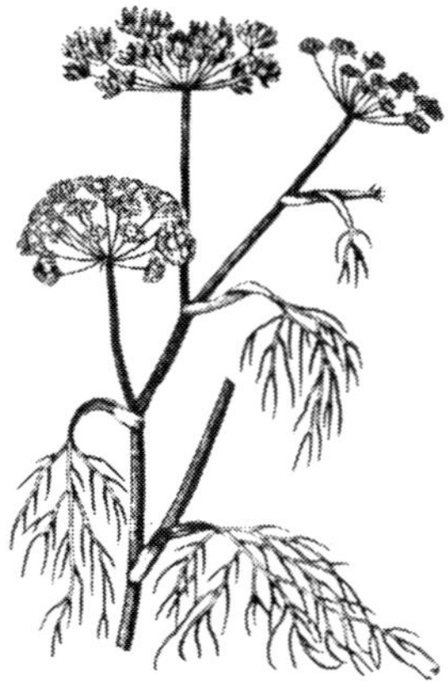

Fennel
(*Foeniculum vulgare*)

The tea is made by adding one teaspoonful to a cup of milk and boiling five to ten minutes. This beverage (after passing through a sieve) should be taken as hot as possible. It will stop colic like magic. It should also be rubbed on the abdomen of the child at the same time.

Half a teaspoonful of fennel seed boiled in water makes an excellent eye wash. Wash the eyes within three times a day.

Rev. Kneipp recommends the seeds of [fenugreek] should be pulverized. As a tea it has remarkable cooling effects. Sore throat, with great heat in the throat, may be treated with this tea used as a gargle.

Dissolved in warm water to the consistency of a thick paste [fenugreek] may be used as a warm poultice for drawing out swellings and ulcers.

As a tea [galium] is recommended as a good remedy for epilepsy, dropsy, and cutaneous eruptions.

[Fennel tea] will stop colic like magic.

Selected Herbs
A Review of the Most Useful Herbs as a Curative Factor for Numerous Ailments

Ground Ivy, Heartsease, Hay Flowers, Heather, Iceland Moss, Juniper

by Benedict Lust, N.D.

Herald of Health and Naturopath, XXIV (10), 513. (1919)

Ground Ivy (See Ivy)

Latin, *Nepeta hederacea*; German, *Gundelrebe*; French, *Lierre terrestre*; Spanish, *Hiedra*

This plant is in bloom from April till autumn. It is quite common and is found nearly all over the country. Its tea is used specifically for enhancing the elimination of phlegm in diseases of the chest and the stomach.

Heartsease (Violet)

Latin, *Viola odorata*; German, *Stiefmötterchen*; French, *Pensée sauvage*; Spanish, *Pensamiento*

The violet, or heartsease, grows almost in every garden, as well as in meadows and cultivated fields. There are many varieties of color. It is in bloom from early spring till late in the fall. The tea of this plant acts as a gentle purgative, and as such is given especially to children. Its use in the family is to be recommended.

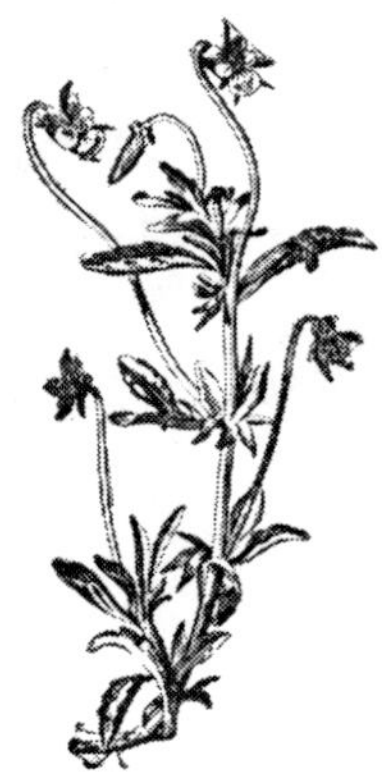

Heartsease (*Viola odorata*)

Hay Flowers

Latin, *Flores graminis*; German, *Heublumen*; French, *Fleurs de foin*; Spanish, *Flores de heno*

These are the residue of newly mown hay as they come from the hay loft, freed of dust and all coarse particles. Hay flowers stewed in water are mostly used in vapor baths and compresses, applied directly to the affected parts. Hay flower vapor baths are especially to be recommended in diseases of the generative organs for their drawing-out and soothing qualities.

HEATHER

Latin, *Calluna vulgaris*; German, *Heidekraut*; French, *Bruyère*; Spanish, *Brezo*

This plant supplies an excellent cough remedy, which serves also in catarrhal affections of the throat and nose.

ICELAND MOSS

Latin, *Certraria islandica*; German, *Isländisches Moos*

The tea of this moss is used internally for chest and lung troubles, and also for consumption and general debility.

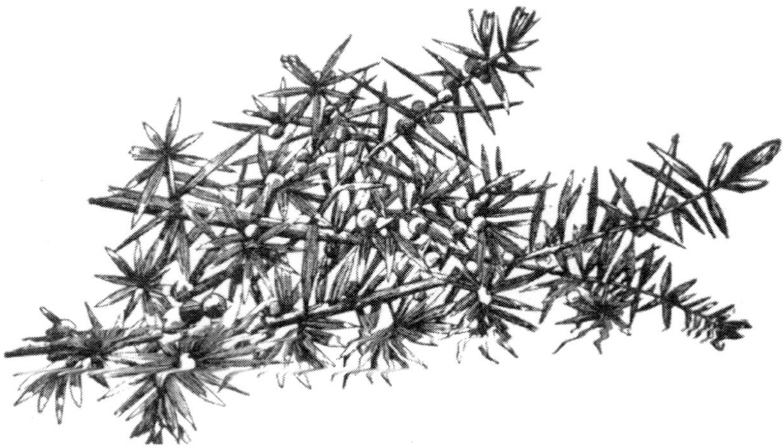

Juniper (*Juniperus communis*)

JUNIPER

Latin, *Juniperus communis*; German, *Wacholder*; French, *Geneviève*; Spanish, *Enebro*

This plant grows in Northern forests and on hillsides, and is not hard to find. Chewing its berries has proved efficacious in cases of weak stomachs, foul breath, and flatulence. Tea made of the berries as well as of the sprigs may be used for the same troubles, and also for liver and kidney complaints and stones or gravel in the bladder.

The tea [of ground ivy] is used specifically for enhancing the elimination of phlegm in diseases of the chest and the stomach.

As a gentle purgative [Violet] tea acts as a gently purgative, and as such is given especially to children.

Hay flowers stewed in water are mostly used in vapor baths and compresses, applied directly to the affected parts. Hay flower vapor baths are especially to be recommended in diseases of the generative organs for their drawing-out and soothing qualities.

[Heather] supplies an excellent cough remedy, which serves also in catarrhal affections of the throat and nose

Chewing [juniper] berries has proved efficacious in cases of weak stomachs, foul breath, and flatulence.

1920

Daisy, Hen's Feet, Hyssop, Iris, Knotgrass, Licorice, Linden Flower, Lungwort, Liverwort, Veronica, Marjoram

Mallow, Calendula, Althea, Yarrow, Milkwort, Mouse Ear, Mustard, Mullein, Nettle, Oak

Nettle, Oat, Onion, Peony, Peppermint, Pepperwort, Periwinkle, Pine, Pimpernel, Primrose, Pumpkin Seeds, Ribwort, Rosemary, Rue

St John's Wort, Sage, Sallow, Sandalwood, Sanicle, Sarsaparilla, Sassafras, Scurvy Grass, Sea Onion, Shavegrass, Silverweed, Shepherd's Purse

Soapwort, Sorrel, Strawberry, Sweet Flag, Thyme, Tormentil, Valerian, Vervaine, Violet, Wallwort, Walnut, Wormseed

Watermint, Woodruff, Watercress, Wormwood, Kneipp's Formulas

Benedict Lust, N.D.

PAGE 486 NATUROPATH—MAY, 1925

The Celebrated

FATHER SEBASTIAN

Kneipp Pills

are free from all injurious aperients, being exclusively composed of herbal ingredients, and are universally considered the best for keeping the bowels open without weakening the stomach. *The pills may be taken for years without any injury to the system and with only beneficial result.*

The best and most pleasant laxative in the world

PRICE, 50 Cents Small Size
$1.00 Large Box; Postage, 2c

DIRECTIONS FOR USE

1. To procure a regular opening of the bowels which is particularly desirable with females take 1 or 2 pills at bed time; *for the first time 3 or 4 pills are often necessary.*
2. To prevent wind and spasms, take one pill in the morning.
3. To procure a thorough cleansing of the bowels, take 2 pills at bedtime and 2 or 3 pills in the morning.

☛ Persons of *very strong constitution* require in these three cases 1 or 2 pills more. *The pills usually act after 12 hours, in some cases after 24 hours only.*

The best way of taking these pills is to swallow them as they are or wrapped up in a wafer with some water.

Manufactured and Guaranteed by

DR. BENEDICT LUST

New York, N. Y., and Butler, N. J.

Die berühmten

PFARRER SEBASTIAN

Kneipp-Pillen

sind frei von allen drastischen Abführmitteln, enthalten *nur reine pflanzliche* Stoffe, welche als Schleim abführende, windtreibende, *magenstärkende* und den *Stuhlgang befördernde* Mittel im höchsten Ansehen stehen.

Sind das angenehmste magenstärkende und blutreinigende Abführmittel, welches existiert

Weltberühmt wegen ihrer **grossartigen Wirkung** bei anhaltender (habitueller) **Verstopfung, Verdauungsstörungen, Hämorrhoidalbeschwerden** und **Blutanstauungen gegen Kopf, Brust, Leber** und **Milz.**

Pfarrer Sebastian Kneipps Pillen sind **leicht** und **bequem** zu nehmen. Sind mit Rhabarber rationell verbunden und wirken **sicher** bei schlechtem Stuhlgang und wegen ihres Rhabarbergehaltes **dabei noch günstig auf den Magen,** so dass sie sich **vornehmlich zu langandauerndem Gebrauche eignen!** Sie sind ein **blutreinigendes magenstärkendes** Abführmittel; enthalten nur reine pflanzliche Stoffe und werden deshalb benützt bei **anhaltender Verstopfung, schlechter Verdauung, Hämorrhoidal-Beschwerden** und **Blutanstauungen,** besonders geeignet für **Frauen** bei Leiden, die ihren Grund in trägem Stuhlgange und schlechter Verdauung haben.

PREIS: kleine Schachtel 50c
grosse $1.00; Porto 2c

GEBRAUCHSANWEISUNG

1. Zur Herbeiführung eines einfachen, **regelmässigen** Stuhlganges, wie es hauptsächlich bei Frauen erwünscht ist, nehme man abends vor dem Schlafengehen 1—2 Pillen; **das erste Mal sind oft 3—4 Pillen nötig.**
2. Sollen die Pillen nur **windtreibend** gegen Blähungen wirken, nehme man morgens nur 1 Pille.
3. Soll ein **reichlicher,** mehrmaliger Stuhlgang erfolgen, nehme man abends 2 und morgens 2—3 Pillen.

☛ **Nur sehr starke Naturen brauchen in diesen drei Fällen je 1—2 Pillen mehr. Die Wirkung tritt meistens in 12, manchmal erst in 24 Stunden ein.**

Am leichtesten nimmt man die Pillen in der Weise, dass man dieselben wie sie sind, oder in etwas feuchte Oblate eingewickelt, mit ein wenig Wasser verschluckt.

Hergestellt und garantiert von

DR. BENEDICT LUST

New York, N. Y., und Butler, N. J.

Benedict Lust's confidence in Sebastian Kneipp's herbal products endured and is evidenced by the advertisements that Lust placed in his magazines.

Selected Herbs A Review of the Most Useful Herbs as a Curative Factor for Numerous Ailments

Daisy, Hen's Feet, Hyssop, Iris, Knotgrass, Licorice, Linden Flower, Lungwort, Liverwort, Veronica, Marjoram*

by Benedict Lust, N.D.

Herald of Health and Naturopath, XXV (5), 249-251. (1920)

Daisy

Latin, *Bellis perennis*; German, *Gänseblümchen*; French, *Marguerite*; Spanish, *Margarita*

Tea made of the daisy is used to reduce stiffness of muscles in all parts of the body caused by exposure to draughts, and it is especially recommended for stiff neck. Taking, first, a cupful of tea, and then every hour a tablespoonful, with suitable application of compresses to the affected parts, will bring prompt relief.

Hen's Feet

Latin, *Fumaria officinalis*; German, *Erdrauch*

Tea made of this plant is recommended for jaundice, hypochondria, hysteria, and also for piles, dropsy, and eruptions of the skin.

Hyssop

Latin, *Hyssopus officinalis*; German, *Ysop*

Tea made of this plant is prescribed in cases of chronic catarrh of the respiratory and digestive organs, asthma and rheumatism. It is invigorating and anti-spasmodic, and acts as an excellent vermifuge. A decoction of hyssop may also be used advantageously as an eye-water.

Iris

Latin, *Iris germanica*; German, *Schwertlilie*; French, *Flambé*

This plant furnishes perhaps the best-known remedy for dropsy in all its stages. It should be taken regularly, as it is a powerful diuretic and will rapidly improve the condition of the patient.

---

*To eliminate repetition, I did not include Anise, Arnica and Beanpods. —*Ed.*

KNOTGRASS

Latin, *Polygonum aviculare*; German, *Wegtritt [Knöterich]*; French, *Renouée or Centinode*; Spanish, *Sanguinaria mayor or Centinodia*

This plant abounds along almost every ditch and in all meadows. It is so common and grows so rapidly that it is looked upon as a useless weed; but it has properties which make it of great value in a number of diseases, such as gravel or stone in the bladder.

People suffering from these complaints are often without the means for consulting high-priced specialist, which is fortunately not always absolutely necessary. This little weed, which is kicked away and trodden down by the heedless passerby, if taken regularly as a tea will dissolve gravel or stone in the bladder. Try it.

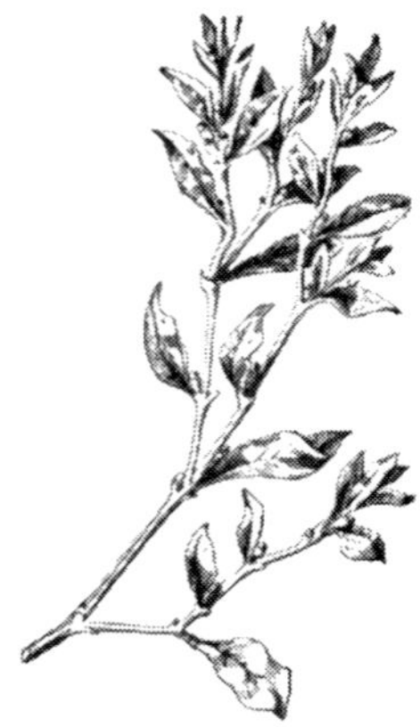

Knotgrass
(*Polygonum aviculare*)

LICORICE

Latin, *Glycyrrhiza glabra*; German, *Süssholz*; French, *Réglisse*; Spanish, *Orozuz*

Licorice furnishes an excellent expectorant. It is also much used as an excipient in pills, etc.

LINDEN FLOWERS

Latin, *Tilia europaea*; German, *Lindenblüten*; French, *Tilleul;* Spanish, *Tilo*

The linden tree is in bloom in June and July. In olden times the tea made of its flower was used to make fever patients sweat profusely. The fumes of a steam vapor bath made from linden flowers will cause profuse sweating, and where such baths are indicated they should be resorted to. Linden flower tea is especially to be recommended for people who suffer from chronic cough. It is also efficacious in removing obstructions from mucus in the lungs or trachea or in healing bronchial catarrh. Mucus in the kidneys often causes abdominal troubles which this tea will alleviate promptly.

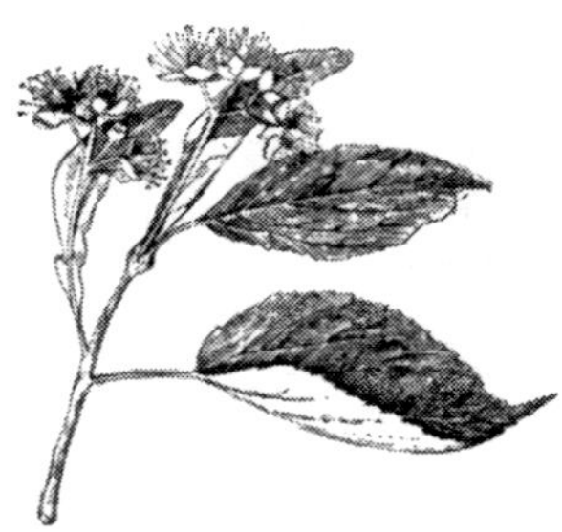

Linden flowers
(*Tilia europaea*)

Lungwort

Latin, *Pulmonaria officinalis*; German, *Lungenkraut*; French, *Grande Pulmonaire*; Spanish, *Pulmonaria*

This herb grows in shady nooks in many of our forests and is in bloom from March till May. For use as an herbal remedy it is generally mixed with ribwort, and prepared as a tea it is a specific for catarrh of the lungs. To make the beverage palatable honey may be mixed with it.

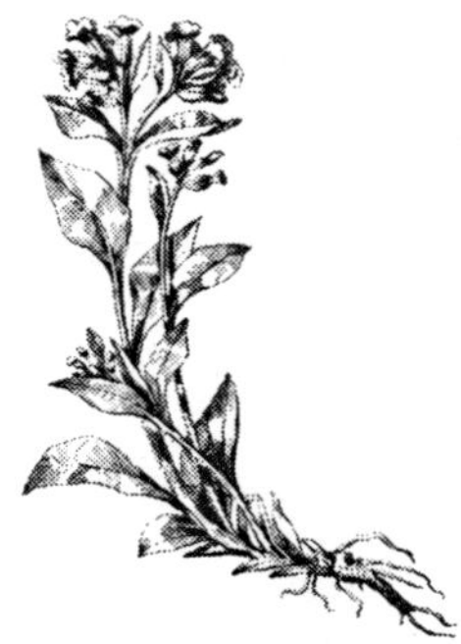

Lungwort
(*Pulmonaria officinalis*)

Liverwort

Latin, *Hepatica triloba*; German, *Leberblümchen*

Tea made of this plant may be used to advantage in cases of gastric hemorrhages, vomiting of blood, and in diseases of sexual organs.

Male Speedwell (Veronica)

Latin, *Veronica officinalis*; German, *Ehrenpreis*; French, *Véronique*; Spanish, *Verónica*

This well-known plant that grows everywhere in the United States and in Europe supplies an excellent blood purifier and renovator, which is used to great advantage especially in cases of scurvy. It should be taken as a tea as per directions given elsewhere.

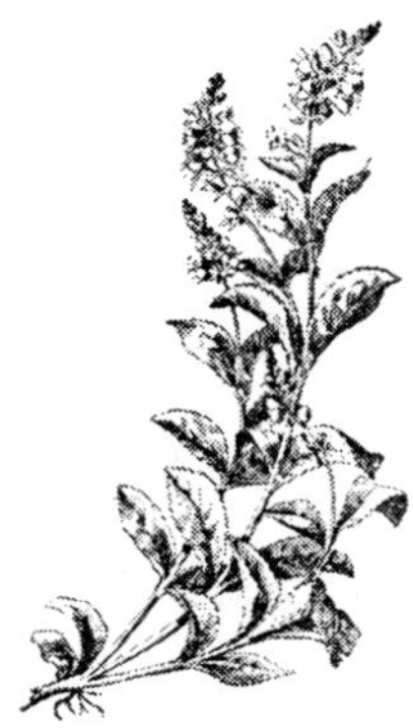

Speedwell
(*Veronica officinalis*)

Marjoram

Latin, *Origanum vulgare*; German, *Majoran*; French, *Marjolaine*; Spanish, *Mejorana*

The tea prepared from this plant is especially to be recommended to women troubled with irregular menstruation. Taken three or four days before the usual time, it will regulate the monthly periods. A tonic and a stimulant, it acts beneficially on the stomach.

Tea made of the daisy is used to reduce stiffness of muscles in all parts of the body caused by exposure to draughts, and it is especially recommended for stiff neck.

[Hyssop] is invigorating and anti-spasmodic, and acts as an excellent vermifuge.

[Iris} furnishes perhaps the best-known remedy for dropsy in all its stages

This little weed [knotweed], which is kicked away and trodden down by the heedless passerby, if taken regularly as a tea will dissolve gravel or stone in the bladder.

Licorice furnishes an excellent expectorant.

The fumes of a steam vapor bath made from linden flowers will cause profuse sweating, and where such baths are indicated they should be resorted to.

For use as an herbal remedy [lungwort] is generally mixed with ribwort, and prepared as a tea it is a specific for catarrh of the lungs.

[Veronica, a] well-known plant that grows everywhere in the United States and in Europe supplies an excellent blood purifier and renovator, which is used to great advantage especially in cases of scurvy.

The tea prepared from [marjoram] is especially to be recommended to women troubled with irregular menstruation. Taken three or four days before the usual time, it will regulate the monthly periods.

Selected Herbs A Review of the Most Useful Herbs as a Curative Factor for Numerous Ailments

Mallow, Marigold, Althea, Yarrow, Milkwort, Mouse Ear, Mustard, Mullein, Nettle, Oak

by Benedict Lust, N.D.

Herald of Health and Naturopath, XXV (6), 297-299. (1920)

Mallow Flowers (Hollyhock)

Latin, *Althea rosea*; German, *Malve*; French, *Mauve noir*; Spanish, *Malva real*

The tea prepared from the flowers of this plant is very effective in removing mucous obstructions in the chest, and it is often prescribed for many troubles of the throat and the larynx. It is advisable to mix the mallow flowers with mullein flowers. People distressed by earache will find relief by applying local vapor baths or fomentations prepared from these flowers. An excellent gargle for sore throat is obtained from a decoction of mallow flowers to which a half a teaspoonful of alum has been added.

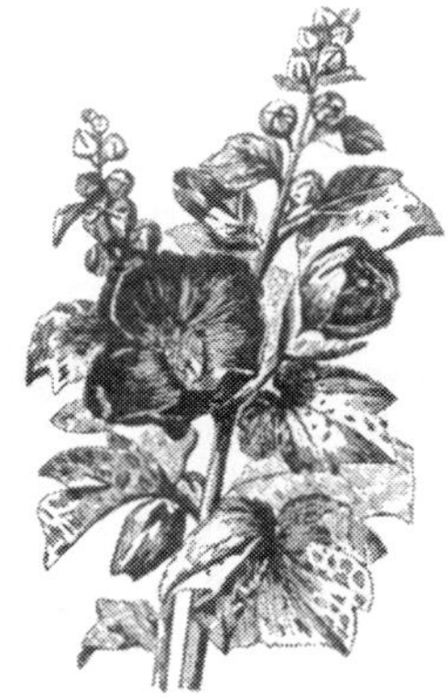

Hollyhock or Mallow
(*Althea rosea*)

Marigold (Calendula) Flowers

Latin, *Calendula officinalis*; German, *Ringelblumen*; French, *Souci*; Spanish, *Maravilla*

This is an imported plant, its native habitat being southern Europe. It now grows in our hot houses and gardens, and is in bloom from June till October. The tea made from this plant is strongly to be recommended to persons afflicted with boils, ulcers, or abscesses, especially abscesses in the stomach, and it is perhaps the best remedy for stopping recurring vomiting, but it should not be taken like other tea, a cupful at a time, but a few sips only every two hours or so.

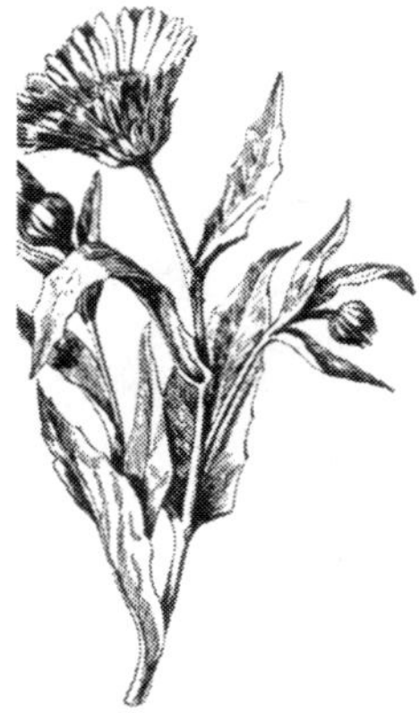

Calendula or Marigold
(*Calendula officinalis*)

MARSHMALLOW (ALTHEA)

Latin, *Althaea officinalis*; German, *Eibischwurzel*; French, *Guimauve*; Spanish, *Malavisco*

This is a cultivated plant growing in Northern latitudes. Its leaves and roots, preferable the latter, are used for a tea prescribed for all affections of the throat, especially cough and hoarseness, or for what is generally known as "frog in the throat."

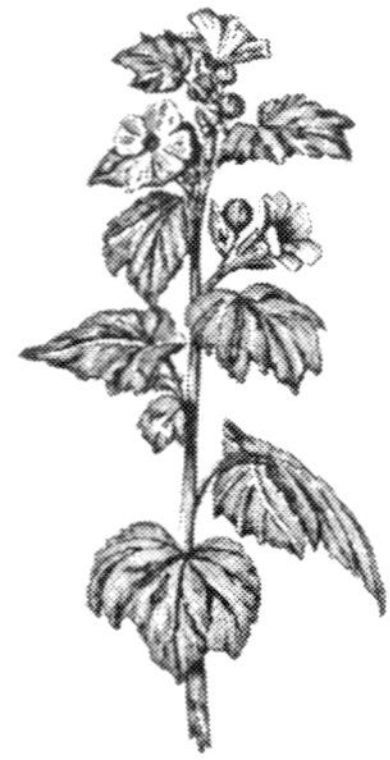

Marshmallow
(*Althaea officinalis*)

MILFOIL (YARROW)

Latin, *Achillea millefolium*; German, *Schafgarbe*; French, *Millefeuille*; Spanish, *Milefolio*

This plant, which is very common and grows in all fields, meadows, and hillsides, is in bloom from May to October. Its leaves, preferable however its blossoms mixed with St. John's wort, are used for cramps in the stomach, irregular menstruation of women, and pain in the abdomen.

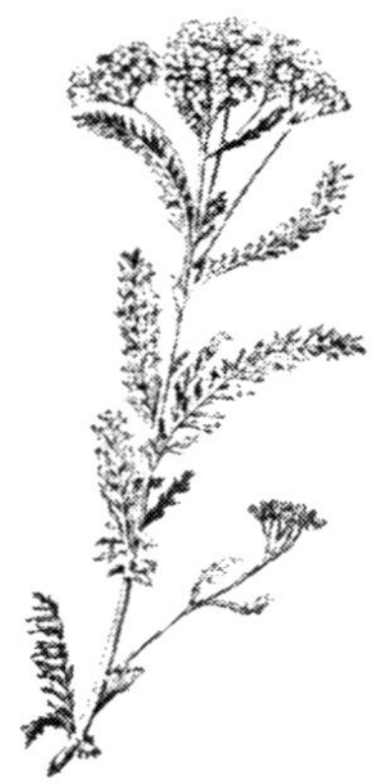

Yarrow or Milfoil
(*Achillea millefolium*)

MILKWORT

Latin, *Polygala vulgaris*; German, *Kreuzblume*; Spanish, *Polígala*

This plant does not grow in the United States, but is imported from Europe. It is used extensively for its milk giving properties. Any mother suckling her own baby and not having an abundant supply of milk is recommended to drink regularly tea made of milkwort.

Mouse Ear

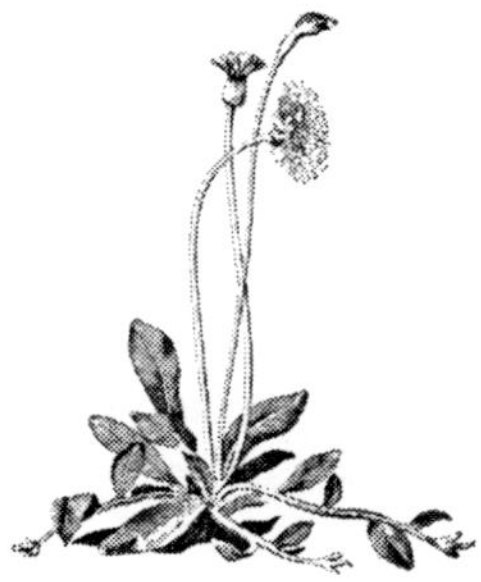

Mouse ear
(*Hieracium pilosella*)

Latin, *Hieracium pilosella*; German, *Mausöhrchen*; French, *Oreille de souris*, *Piloselle*; Spanish, *Pilosella*

This is a plant that grows in all dry meadows and fields, and it is in bloom from early spring till late fall. A decoction made of this plant is used to advantage in all diseases of the liver and spleen and in cases of dropsy and stone in the bladder. It also furnishes an excellent gargle for all affections of the throat.

Mullein Flowers

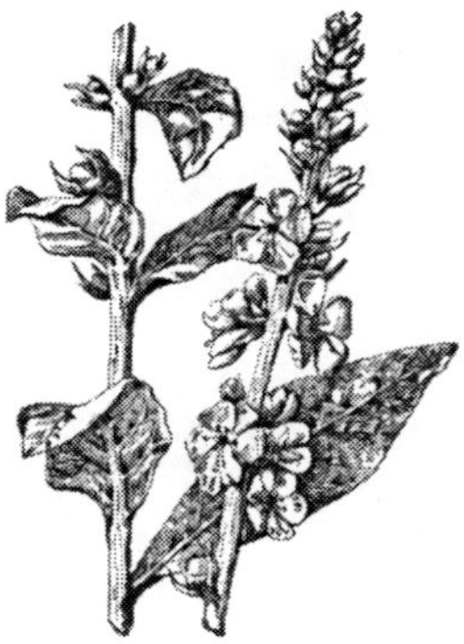

Mullein flowers
(*Verbascum thapsus*)

Latin, *Verbascum thapsus*; German, *Wollkrautblumen*; French, *Bouillon-blanc;* Spanish, *Gordolobo*

This plant grows on stony hillocks and in quarries, and it is also cultivated in many parts of the country. It is in bloom all summer. Old people and peasant immigrants from the old world hold it in great repute, and there's a reason. It will be found to furnish an excellent remedy, especially in the winter, for the affections of the throat incident to that season, and also for catarrhs, mucus on the chest, and scantiness of breath.

Mustard

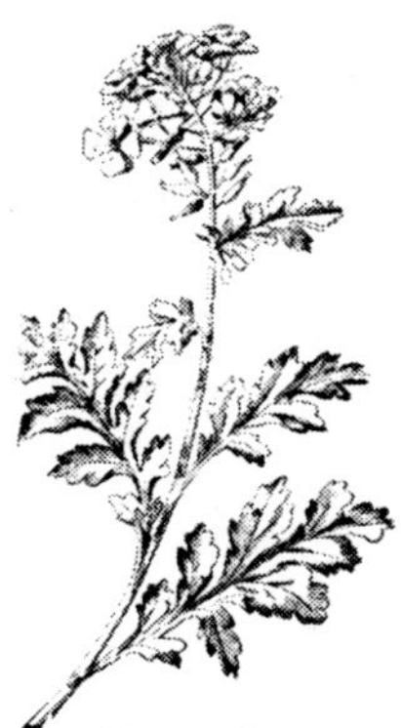

Mustard
(*Sinapis alba and nigra*)

Latin, *Sinapis alba et nigra*; German, *Senf*; French, *Moutarde*; Spanish, *Mostaza*

Sufferers from weak stomach may now and then eat some mustard seeds to advantage. The plant is principally used for poultices on the breast or back in cases of rheumatism or pains in any part of the body, and also for plasters.

NETTLE (COMMON NETTLE)

Latin, *Urtica dioica*; German, *Brennessel*; French, *Ortie*; Spanish, *Ortiga mayor*

This plant, which is generally considered as a common weed, blooms from May till July. Although people may smile at the assertion, it is nevertheless true that this little regarded plant is one of the most useful in the entire pharmacopoeia. The tea made from its fresh leaves, after these have been dried in the sun, will clear the breast and lungs of all mucus and slime and force out through the urinary canal all matter oppressive to the stomach. Tea made from the roots is an effective remedy for incipient dropsy. The entire plant, boiled in vinegar and water and preserved in Cologne, yields the world-famed Kneipp hair remedy.

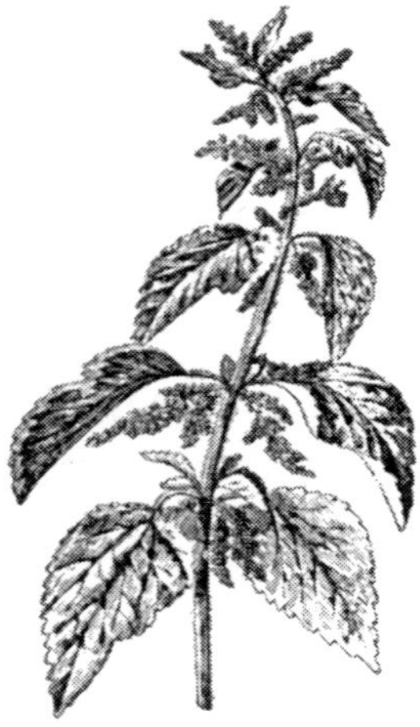

Nettle (*Urtica dioica*)

OAK BARK

Latin, *Quercus robur;* German, *Eichenrinde*; French, *Chêne*; Spanish, *Encina Roble*

Tea made from the bark of oak may be used both internally and externally, and is prescribed especially for the removal of swollen throat and goiter. For external use dip a cloth (preferably linen) into the boiled decoction and place it around the swollen part. For internal use take three tablespoonful of the tea mornings and evenings. Goitre may be successfully cured if the growth is not yet too hard. Tea of the bark of oak is also used as a tonic after overexertion of any kind. Coffee made from acorns (acorn coffee) is used either alone or together with Kneipp malt coffee for invigorating the bones of weak and rachitic young children.

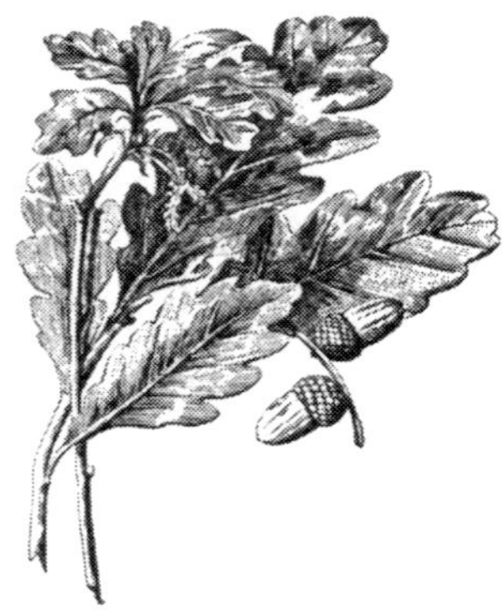

Oak (*Quercus robur*)

The tea made from calendula is strongly to be recommended to persons afflicted with boils, ulcers, or abscesses, especially abscesses in the stomach, and it is perhaps the best remedy for stopping recurring vomiting, but it should not be taken like other tea, a cupful at a time, but a few sips only every two hours or so.

[Yarrow's] leaves, preferable however its blossoms mixed with St. John's-wort, are used for cramps in the stomach, irregular menstruation of women, and pain in the abdomen.

The tea made from fresh [nettle] leaves, after these have been dried in the sun, will clear the breast and lungs of all mucus and slime and force out through the urinary canal all matter oppressive to the stomach.

Tea made from the bark of oak may be used both internally and externally, and is prescribed especially for the removal of swollen throat and goiter.

Selected Herbs A Review of the Most Useful Herbs as a Curative Factor for Numerous Ailments

BLIND NETTLE, OATS, ONION, PEONY, PEPPERMINT, PEPPERWORT, PERIWINKLE, PINE, PIMPERNEL, PRIMROSE, PUMPKIN SEEDS, RIBWORT, ROSEMARY, RUE

by Benedict Lust, N.D.

Herald of Health and Naturopath, XXV (7), 353-355. (1920)

BLIND NETTLE (OR WHITE OR DEAD NETTLE)

Latin, *Lamium album*; German, *Taubnessel*; French, *Ortie blanche*; Spanish, *Ortiga muerta*

A decoction made of the flowers of this plant is used as an excellent blood purifier in cases of rash, eczema, etc.

OATS AND OATSTRAW

Latin, *Avena sativa*; German, *Haferstroh*; French, *Avoine*; Spanish, *Avena*

Oatstraw cut into small strips boiled one hour, with a little honey added, makes an excellent tea for diseases of the chest. A decoction of oatstraw is also frequently used as an addition to the warm bath or for packs and compresses. Oat gruel with honey is a fine food or beverage for convalescents. Oatmeal makes a splendid porridge for everybody, being very invigorating.

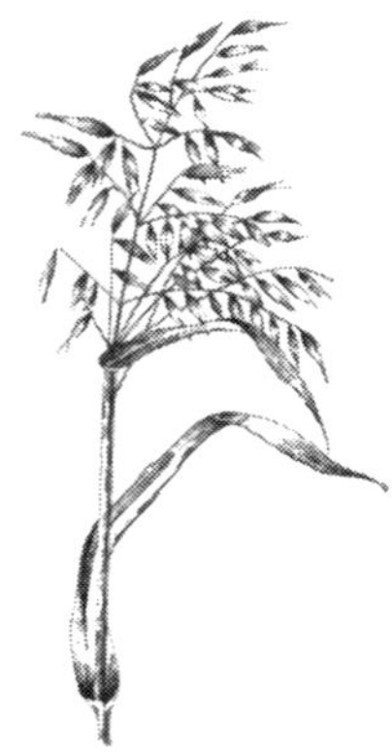

Oat and Oatstraw (*Avena sativa*)

ONION

Latin, *Allium cepa*; German, *Zwiebel*; French, *Ognon*; Spanish, *Cebolla*

Onion syrup and onion poultices are much used for domestic purposes. The juice of the plant is stimulating, aids expectoration, and is a powerful diuretic.

Peony

Latin, *Paeonia officinalis*; German, *Pfingstrose*; French, *Pivoine*; Spanish, *Peonia*

This flower yields a remedy which is very beneficial in cases of epilepsy, cramps, gout, and asthma. It is antispasmodic and a sedative.

Peppermint, Watermint*

Latin, *Mentha piperita*; German, *Pfeffermünz*; French, *Menthe poivrée*; Spanish, *Menta piperita*

These two plants are recognized by the regular medical faculty as possessing high remedial qualities. The pleasant aromatic smell of the mint is a sure sign that it has special merit. Among all the remedies recommended for strengthening the stomach and improving digestion the mint should occupy first place. Tea made of these two plants is prescribed for those who suffer from palpitation of the heart or from nausea. For abdominal pains boil some peppermint in milk and drink hot.

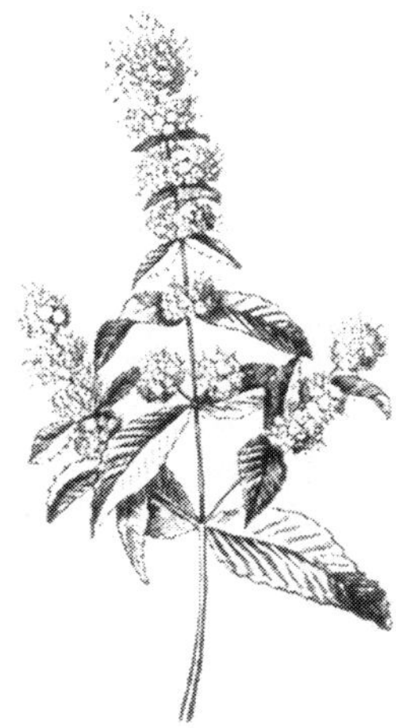

Peppermint
(*Mentha piperita*)

Pepperwort

Latin, *Satureja hortensis*; German, *Pfefferkraut*

The tea made of this plant is recommended for colic, griping pain, and vomiting. It is a dissolvent remedy and also an excellent stomach tonic.

Periwinkle

Latin, *Vinca minor*; German, *Immergrün*; French, *Pervenche*; Spanish, *Vincapervinca*

The tea made of this plant furnishes an excellent remedy for diarrhoea, obstructions of mucus in the intestines and lungs, congestions and hemorrhages, etc., and it is also to be recommended as a gargle in cases of scurvy.

---

*Lust elaborates upon the watermint on page 320. —Ed.

Pine Sprigs

Latin, *Pinus*; German, *Fichtenspros-sen*; French, *Pin*; Spanish, *Pino*

The sprigs of the pine made into an extract furnish an excellent cough remedy. Pine sprig honey is especially recommended for small children in severe attacks of cough; also in cases of bronchitis and catarrhal affections of the chest. Pine needle baths are used by convalescents, weak persons, and other for their bracing and stimulating qualities.

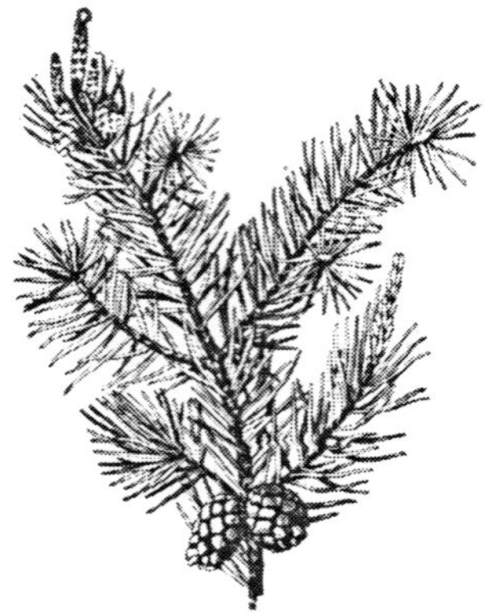

Pine Sprigs (*Pinus*)

Red Pimpernel

Latin, *Anagallis arvensis*; German, *Gauchheil*; French, *Mouron rouge*; Spanish, *Anagálida*

This plant is generally considered as a useless weed, growing nearly all over the country and blossoming (commonly red) from June to October. As a tea it is used to excellent purpose in cases of dyspepsia, liver complaint, and jaundice. It is also a powerful diuretic and sudorific.

Primrose, Odorous Cowslip

Latin, *Primula officinalis*; German, *Schlüsselblume*; French, *Primevère*; Spanish, *Primavera*

This plant grows freely on every meadow. The tea made from it is an excellent remedy for articular rheumatism, which is one of the most painful of diseases. Whoever is liable to be afflicted with it should not delay, on the appearance of the preliminary symptoms, taking primrose tea regularly three times a day, with the assurance that he will soon feel the beneficial effects. This tea will also alleviate, and even completely cure, chronic headache. Finally, people are cautioned against confounding this plant with its odorless namesake.

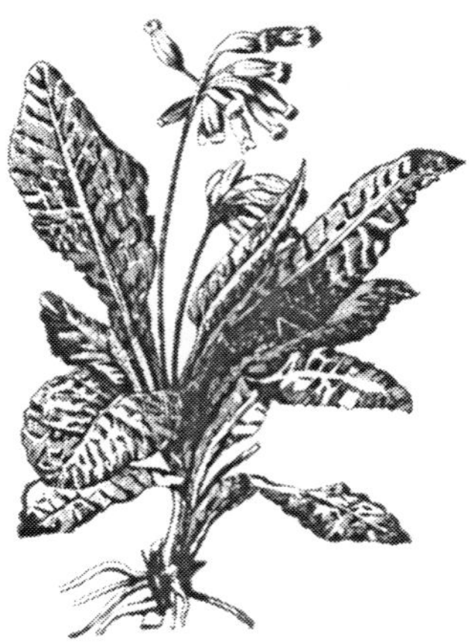

Primrose
(*Primula officinalis*)

Pumpkin Seeds

Latin, *Cucurbita pepo*; German, *Kürbiskerne*; French, *Citrouille*; Spanish, *Calabaza*

Pumpkin seeds are a specific remedy for tapeworm. A large quantity, about 100, of the inner seeds of this well-known fruit should be thoroughly chewed and eaten. It may be also had in extract form, which is a better way to give it to small children.

Ribwort

Latin, *Plantago lanceolata*; German, *Spitzwegerich*; French, *Plantain lanceolé*; Spanish, *Llantén*

Like so many others, this plant also is considered by many people as a useless weed, though they should really know better. The tea made of ribwort loosens mucus and slime in the inner organs. In conjunction with lungwort it is often used for pulmonary complaints and as an infallible cough remedy.

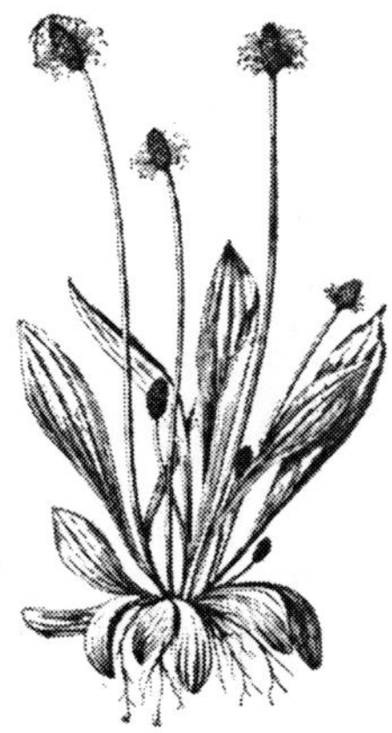

Ribwort or Plantain
(*Plantago lanceolata*)

Rosemary

Latin, *Rosmarinus officinalis*; German, *Rosmarin*; French, *Rosmarin*; Spanish, *Romero*

This plant was originally imported from Italy, but may now be found in many of our gardens. It is in bloom in April and May. On account of its exceeding bitterness the tea made of rosemary is an excellent stomach remedy. Especially people with a bad or torpid liver should not forget rosemary tea. It expels all morbid matter from the system, and it is also a preventive of the much dreaded dropsy which it cures entirely in its incipient stages.

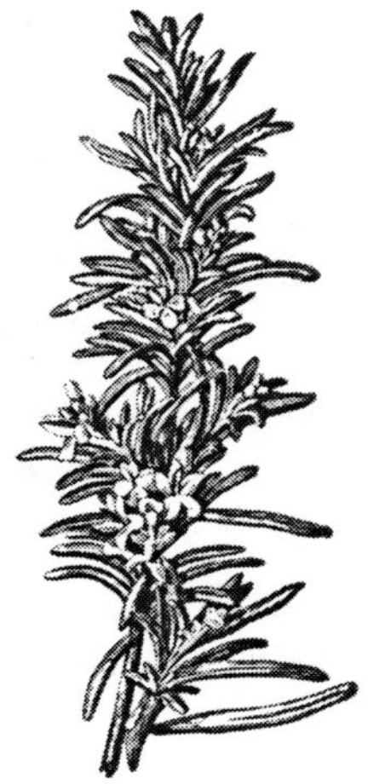

Rosemary
(*Rosmarinus officinalis*)

RUE

Latin, *Ruta graveolens*; German, *Raute*; French, *Rue*; Spanish, *Ruda*

This plant was originally imported from southern Europe, and is in bloom during June and July. It has excellent qualities which are, however, scarcely appreciated in this country. Tea made from rue is highly to be recommended for congestions or acute pains in the head, also for nausea, fainting spells, difficult breathing, abdominal troubles, and cramps in the stomach.

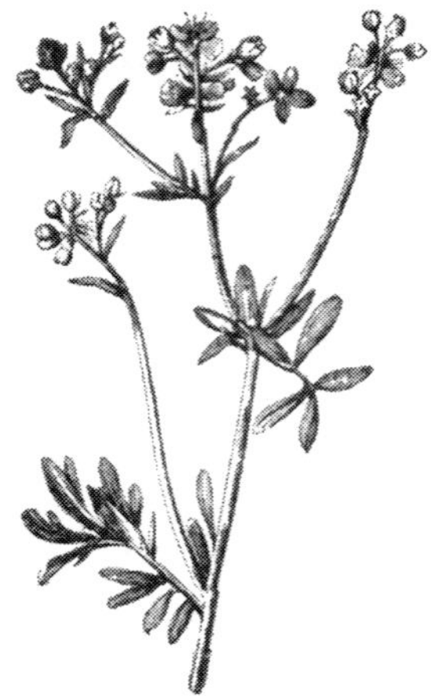

Rue (*Ruta graveolens*)

The juice of the [onion] is stimulating, aids expectoration, and is a powerful diuretic.

Peony yields a remedy which is very beneficial in cases of epilepsy, cramps, gout, and asthma. It is antispasmodic and a sedative.

Among all the remedies recommended for strengthening the stomach and improving digestion [peppermint] should occupy first place.

The tea made of [periwinkle] furnishes an excellent remedy for diarrhoea, obstructions of mucus in the intestines and lungs, congestions and hemorrhages, etc., and it is also to be recommended as a gargle in cases of scurvy.

Pine sprig honey is especially recommended for small children in severe attacks of cough; also in cases of bronchitis and catarrhal affections of the chest.

The tea made from [Primrose] is an excellent remedy for articular rheumatism, which is one of the most painful of diseases.

Selected Herbs — A Review of the Most Useful Herbs as a Curative Factor for Numerous Ailments

St. John's Wort, Sage, Sallow, Sandalwood, Sanicle, Sarsaparilla, Sassafras, Scurvy Grass, Sea Onion, Shave grass, Silverweed, Shepherd's Purse

by Benedict Lust, N.D.

Herald of Health and Naturopath, XXV (8), 406-408. (1920)

St. John's Wort

Latin, *Hypericum perforatum*; German, *Johanniskraut*; French, *Millepertuis*; Spanish, *Corazoncillo*

In the dark ages witches were supposed to banish disease by means of this plant, but in the present time it is but little known. It furnishes however, a splendid remedy for diseases affecting the liver, and if mixed with bitter aloe powders its healing properties are considerably increased. It is also recommended in cases of constipation and mucous obstructions in the chest and lungs. To mothers who have trouble in breaking their children of the bed-wetting habit, tea made from St. John's wort, if taken regularly for some time, will prove a real blessing.

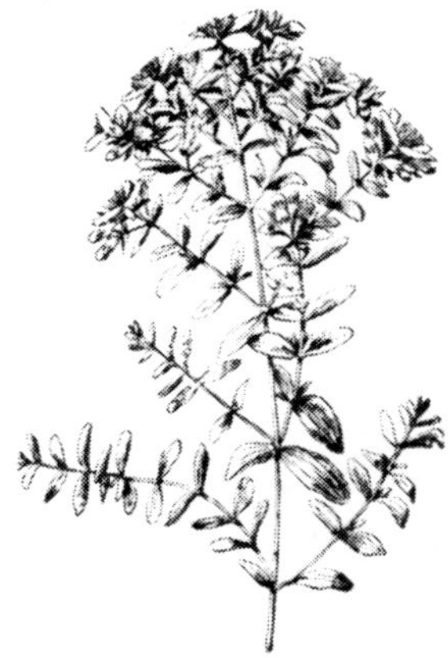

St. John's Wort
(*Hypericum perforatum*)

Sage

Latin, *Salvia officinalis*; German, *Salbei*; French, *Sauge*; Spanish, *Salvia*

Sage grows wild on many hills and stony declivities near the sea coast. It is in bloom June and July. This plant furnishes one of the old remedies that have been used for centuries by country folk. A tea made from it is recommended for all diseases of the liver and kidneys, also for mucous obstructions in the palate, throat, and stomach. A decoction of sage to which is added a teaspoonful of alum makes an excellent gargle.

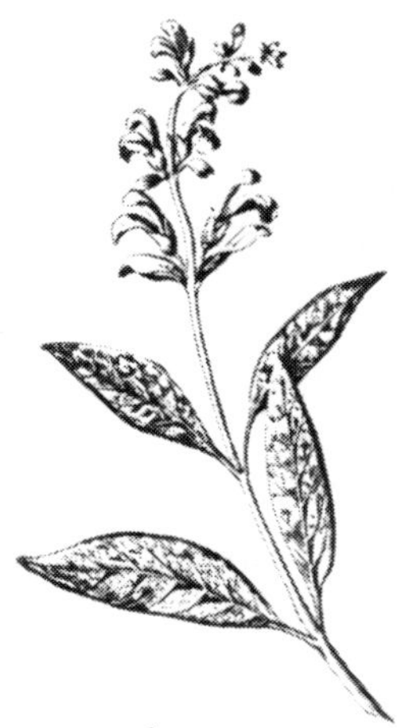

Sage
(*Salvia officinalis*)

SALLOW

Latin, *Salix caprea*; German, *Salweide*; French, *Saule*

A tea made from the bark of this plant will prove highly beneficial in cases of catarrh, whooping cough, and also of acute and chronic rheumatism, dyspepsia, etc. An extract made from it, used externally, promotes the growth of the hair. It is also used for disinfecting bandages.

SANDALWOOD

Latin, *Pterocarpus santalinus*; German, *Sandelholz*; French, *Santal rouge*; Spanish, *Sándalo*

The red wood of the red saunders tree is pulverized into a fine powder and two teaspoonfuls of this tea, added to tea of mistletoe, may be used for stopping the flow of blood in all kinds of hemorrhages.

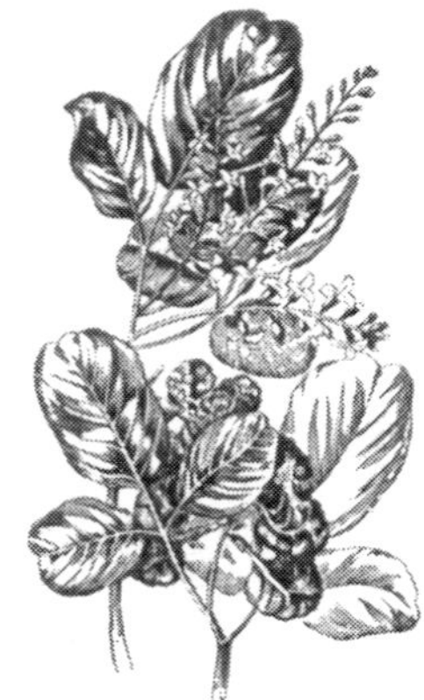

Sandalwood
(*Pterocarpus santalinus*)

SANICLE

Latin, *Sanicula europaea*; German, *Sanicle [Heildolde]*; French, *Sanicle*; Spanish, *Sanícula*

This plant grows in moist, shady nooks in mountainous forests and is in bloom from May to July. A tea is made from it for violent attacks of catarrh of the chest, and a pure decoction of it is used for washing out wounds of all sorts.

SARSAPARILLA, REEDGRASS

Latin, *Smilax officinalis;* German, *Sarsaparille*; French, *Salsepareille*; Spanish, *Zarzaparrilla*

This plant grows very extensively in Mexico. A decoction made of its roots provides a most effective blood purifier. It is also an excellent remedy in cases of rheumatism and syphilis. If taken regularly for an extended period of time it will remove all impurities from the blood.

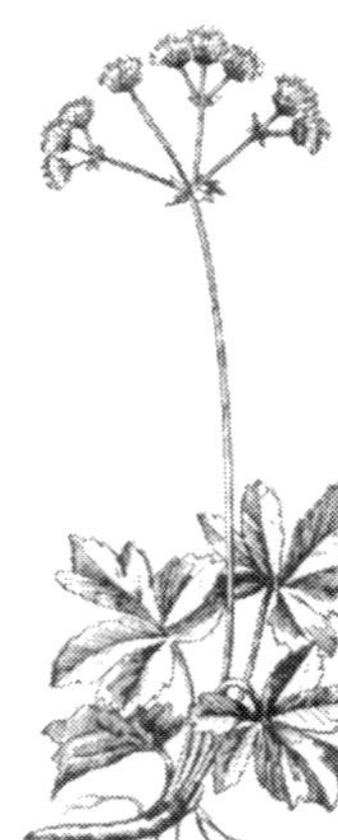

Sanicle
(*Sanicula europaea*)

Sassafras

Latin, *Sassafras officinalis*; German, *Sassafras*; French, *Sassafras*; Spanish, *Sasafrás*

Sassafras yields a diaphoretic stimulant used to advantage in cases of asthma and catarrh of the lungs.

Scurvy Grass, Spoonwort

Latin, *Cochlearia officinalis*; German, *Löffelkraut*

Tea made from this herb is used for rheumatism in any form; also in cases of dropsy, scurvy, and sexual diseases of both sexes.

Sea Onion

Latin, *Urginea maritime*; German, *Meerzwiebel*

This plant is recommended for its expectorant and diuretic qualities. It is also used in large doses as a purgative.

Shavegrass, Common Horsetail Or Pewter Grass

Latin, *Equisetum arvense*; German, *Zinnkraut*; French, *Prîbe des champs*; Spanish, *Cola de caballo*

This plant, which grows on potato fields and marshy ground, is not generally known to possess other qualities than such as make it available in preparations for cleaning metal and pewterware; but a decoction made of shavegrass serves excellently for compresses in sores of all kinds containing evil-smelling pus. A steam bath of shavegrass is beneficial in all cases of bladder and kidney troubles, especially stone in the bladder. Tea of shavegrass cleans the stomach and alleviates the pain of suffers from stone in the bladder. It may also be used to advantage by those who are suffering from painful urinating. In cases of hemorrhage and vomiting of blood it is most effective. Bleeding of the nose is promptly stopped by it.

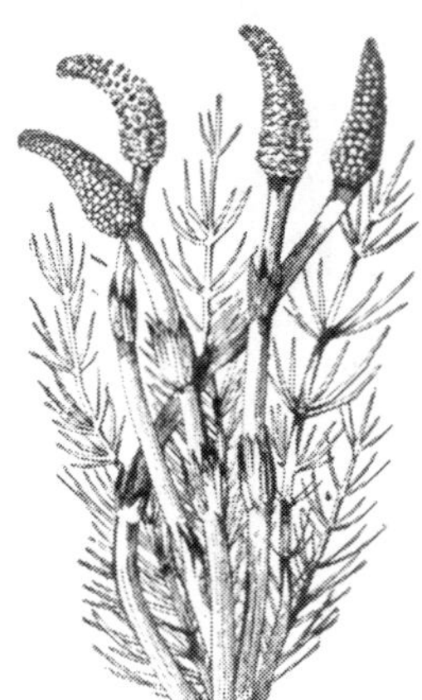

Shavegrass or Horsetail (*Equisetum arvense*)

Silverweed

Latin, *Potentilla anserina*; German, *Anserine, Gänsefingerkraut*; French, *Anserine vulgaire*; Spanish, *Argentina*

This plant grows nearly everywhere in the vicinity of water. It is in bloom from early spring till late fall, and has beautiful yellow flowers.

A tablespoonful added to a cup of boiled milk and the mixture boiled a few minutes longer provides an effective remedy in the case of one of the most dreaded of diseases: tetanus or lockjaw. The tea should be drunk as hot as possible. Continue taking the tea, with the assurance that the disease will finally be routed. In cases where the patient dislikes milk, boiling water may be used. It is also an excellent remedy for cramps of the stomach, heart, and abdomen. In addition to the tea taken internally, it is advisable to apply to the affected parts compresses dipped into it.

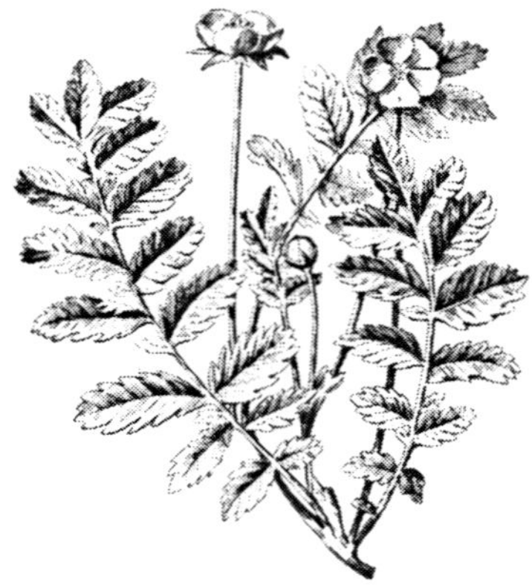

Silverweed (*Potentilla anserine*)

SHEPHERD'S PURSE

Latin, *Capsella bursa pastoris*; German, *Hirtentäschchen*; French, *Bourse á Pasteur*; Spanish, *Bolso de pastor*

This plant is generally considered to be one of the many useless weeds growing wild on all cultivated land, but it yields a tea which is one of the best specifics for stopping hemorrhages of all kinds, such as hemorrhage of the stomach, of the lungs, and of the uterus.

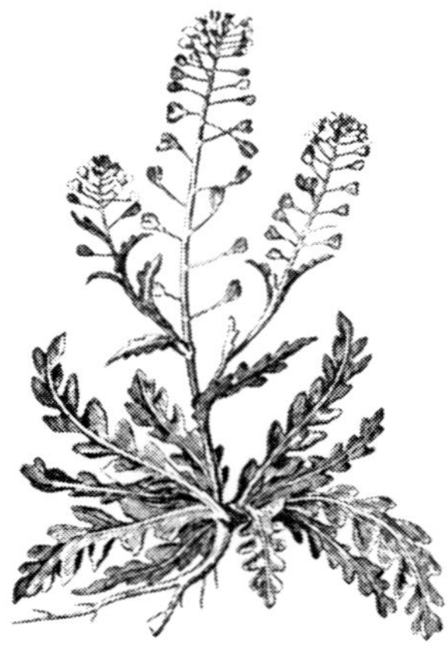

Shepherd's purse
(*Capsella bursa pastoris*)

> *A tablespoonful [of silverweed] added to a cup of boiled milk and the mixture boiled a few minutes longer provides an effective remedy in the case of one of the most dreaded of diseases: tetanus or lockjaw.*

Selected Herbs A Review of the Most Useful Herbs as a Curative Factor for Numerous Ailments

Soapwort, Sorrel, Strawberry, Sweet Flag, Thyme, Tormentil, Valerian, Vervaine, Violet, Wallwort, Walnut, Wormseed

by Benedict Lust, N.D.

Herald of Health and Naturopath, XXV (9), 450-452. (1920)

Soapwort

Latin, *Saponaria officinalis*; German, *Seifenkraut*

The tea made of this herb is used internally for catarrh, while the tea made of its roots is used in cases of gout, syphilis, eruptions of the skin, and hard cancerous tumors.

Sorrel

Latin, *Rumex acetosa*; German, *Sauerampfer*; French, *Oseille*; Spanish, *Acedera*

Persons suffering from ulcers in the mouth or throat should take tea (mixed with a little honey) made from sorrel. Boiled in wine, this herb yields an excellent remedy for abdominal pains, which it will positively cure. It will also promote secretion of the urine.

Strawberry Leaves

Latin, *Fragaria vesca*; German, *Erdbeere*; French, *Fraisier*; Spanish, *Fresera*

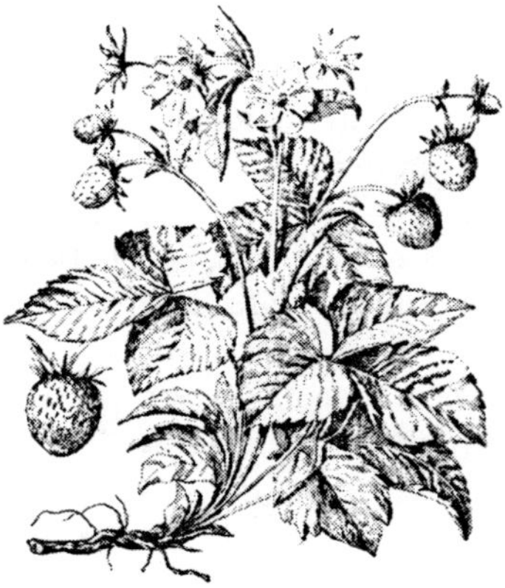
Strawberry leaves (*Fragaria vesca*)

The strawberry plant gives us not only its tasty berries, but also leaves which possess great remedial properties. For the invigoration of convalescents, and also as a blood purifier, make a tea by boiling a quantity of strawberry leaves in a pint of water for fifteen minutes. Strained through a sieve, with hot milk and some sugar added, the tea is ready for use. Those also suffering from liver complaint and eczema should not fail to provide themselves with this simple, cheap, and effective remedy.

Sweet Flag, Calamus

Latin, *Acorus calamus*; German, *Kalmus*; French, *Acorus odorant*; Spanish, *Cálamo aromático*

This plant is imported from Asia and grows near rivers, ponds, and swamps. The tea made of it is an effective remedy for gases in the stomach, also scrofula in children. Candied sweet flag root may be eaten in small pieces at a time. Sweet flag furnishes the principal condiment of many stomach bitters advertised in the papers.

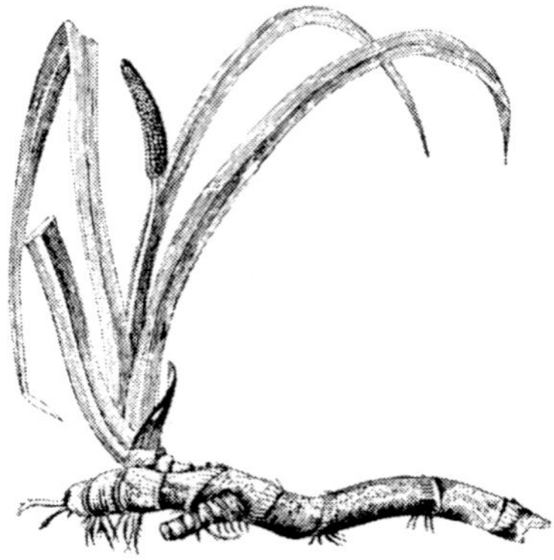

Sweet flag or Calamus (*Acorus calamus*)

Thyme

Latin, *Thymus vulgaris*; German, *Thymian [Quendel*]; French, *Thym commun*; Spanish, *Tomillo*

This plant comes from southern Europe and is not cultivated in this country. A decoction made of thyme is beneficial in cases of cramps in the stomach and diarrhoea.

Tormentil

Latin, *Potentilla tormentilla*; German, *Tormentil [Fünffinger-kraut]*; French, *Tormentille*; Spanish, *Tormentila*

This plant grows on meadows, fields, etc., and is in bloom in June and July. In the form of a tincture its root is used for stopping hemorrhages, and it is also prescribed for chronic diarrhoea, gonorrhea, fluor albus*. For internal use one teaspoonful three times a day and a decoction of the root as an injection. For sore and tender gums and inflammations of the throat and larynx a gargle and mouthwash is prepared from the decoction and diluted tincture.

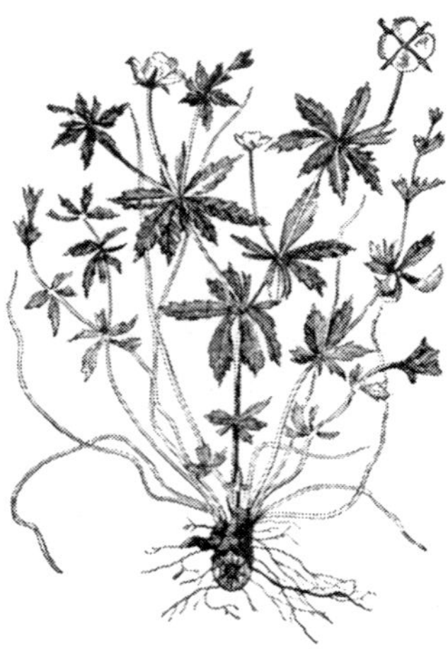

Tormentil (*Potentilla tormentilla*)

---

*Ed. Note: Fluor albus refers to leucorrhea.

Valerian Root

Latin, *Valeriana officinalis*; German, *Baldrian*; French, *Valérian*; Spanish, *Valeriana*

This plant grows in marshy forests and it is also cultivated in gardens. Its root is the only part adapted for remedial purposes. Out of the root, a tea is made which should be taken only in small quantities at a time. This tea is an excellent remedy for congestion in the head, attacks of giddiness, and fainting fits. It is highly prized also in cases of nervous stomach troubles, sleeplessness, and hysteria. Cramp-like conditions, abdominal troubles, and palpitation of the heart, too, are readily reduced by tea of valerian root. In the form of a powder it may be taken one-half a teaspoonful at a time.

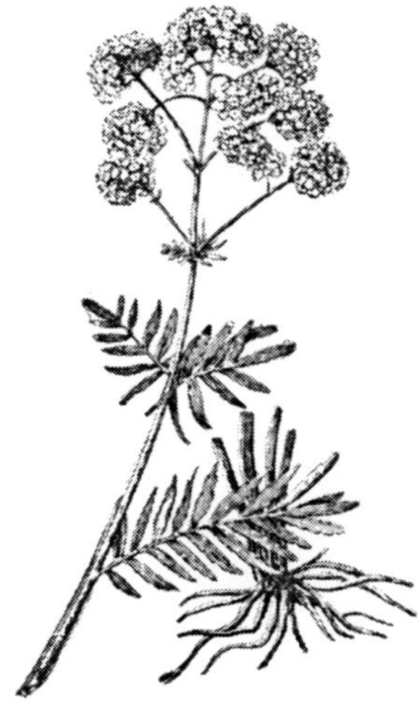

Valerian
(*Valeriana officinalis*)

Violet (Sweet)

Latin, *Viola odorata*; German, *Veilchen*; French, *Violette*; Spanish, *Violeta*

The leaves of this beautiful and fragrant flower, which is known to everyone, supply a healing remedy of great value. Tea made of violet leaves is effective in alleviating severe cough, even the dreaded whooping cough in children. To consumptives it is recommended for dissolving mucus, and it is also used to advantage in cases of severe headache and congestion in the head. It makes a splendid gargle for swollen throat, a procedure which should be supplemented by applying compresses dipped into warm tea. Violet tea will furnish relief to those suffering from shortness of breath. Of the root of the violet a remedy is made for dissolving mucus in cases of severe cough.

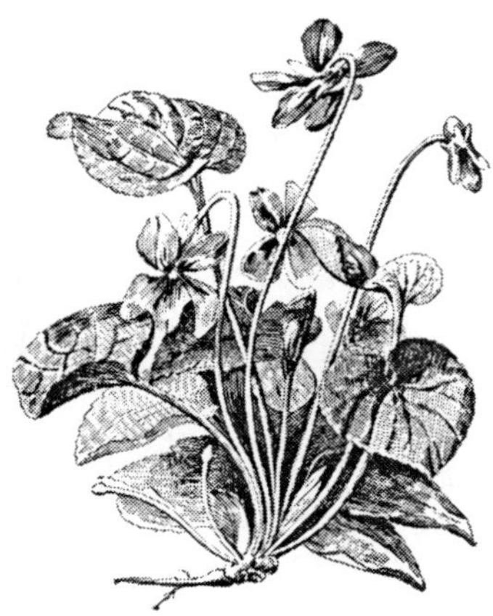

Violet (*Viola odorata*)

VERVAINE

Latin, *Verbena officinalis*; German, *Eisenkraut*; French, *Verveine*; Spanish, *Verbena*

This plant grows everywhere. Made into a tea and in powder form it is used to great advantage in whooping cough, kidney trouble, dropsy, liver complaint, and jaundice. The root is the part of the plant mostly used.

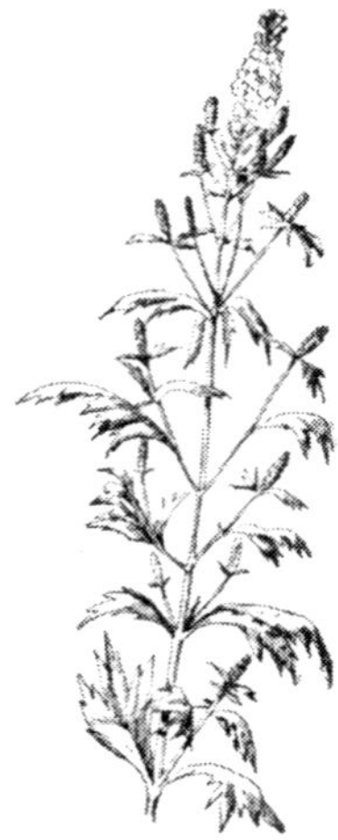

Vervaine
(*Verbena officinalis*)

WALLWORT (GREATER CONSOUND) [COMFREY]

Latin, *Symphytum officinalis*; German, *Wallwurz*; French, *Grand Consoude*; Spanish, *Consuelda mayor*

This plant grows on watery meadows and on the banks of rivers and rivulets and is in bloom from May till July. A decoction made of the roots is used for washing out wounds, and it may be used internally for spitting blood and intestinal troubles.

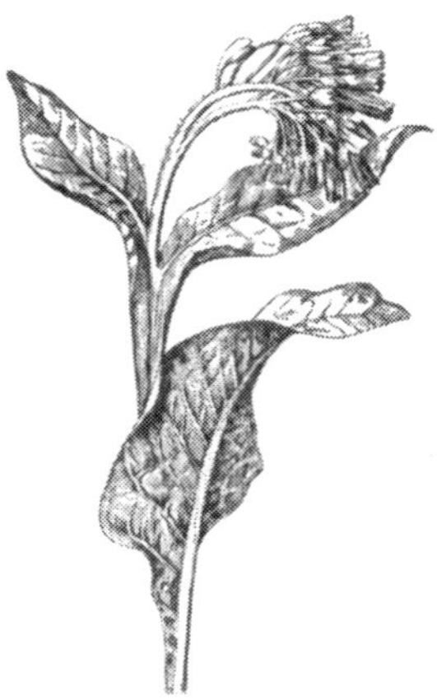

Wallwort or Comfrey
(*Symphytum officinalis*)

WALNUT

Latin, *Juglans regia*; German, *Walnuss*; French, *Noyer commun*; Spanish, *Nogal*

For purifying the blood a decoction made of the leaves of the walnut tree is used, while from the shells of the green walnut a splendid hair dye is prepared.

The tea made of the leaves of the tree as well as of the green peels of the ripe nut is very salutary in internal use for removing obstructions with phlegm in the stomach or intestines, eruptions of the skin, gout, scrofula, syphilis, poisoning by mercury, etc., etc.; used externally for scrofulous, syphilitic, etc., etc., cancers, as well as scrofulous inflammations of the eyes.

Wormseed

Latin, *Chenopodium ambrosioides var. anthelminticum*; German, *Wurmsamen*

This plant, indigenous to the United States, yields a mild cardiac stimulant, which also promotes the secretions of the skin and kidneys. To people afflicted with round worm it is moreover to be recommended as a most effective anthelmintic.

Boiled in wine, sorrel yields an excellent remedy for abdominal pains, which it will positively cure. It will also promote secretion of the urine.

For the invigoration of convalescents, and also as a blood purifier, make a tea by boiling a quantity of strawberry leaves in a pint of water for fifteen minutes.

In the form of a tincture, [Tormentil] is used for stopping hemorrhages, and it is also prescribed for chronic diarrhoea, gonorrhea, fluor albus [leucorrhea].

[Valerian root] tea is an excellent remedy for congestion in the head, attacks of giddiness, and fainting fits.

[Vervaine] grows everywhere. Made into a tea and in powder form it is used to great advantage in whooping cough, kidney trouble, dropsy, liver complaint, and jaundice.

A decoction made of the roots of wallwort [mullein] is used for washing out wounds, and it may be used internally for spitting blood and intestinal troubles.

[Wormwood], indigenous to the United States, yields a mild cardiac stimulant, which also promotes the secretions of the skin and kidneys.

Selected Herbs A Review of the Most Useful Herbs as a Curative Factor for Numerous Ailments

WATERMINT, WOODRUFF, WATERCRESS, WORMWOOD, KNEIPP'S FORMULAS

by Benedict Lust, N.D.

Herald of Health and Naturopath, XXV (10), 509-511. (1920)

WATERMINT

Latin, *Mentha aquatica*; German, *Wassermünze*; French, *Menthe aquatique*

The tea made of this plant is an excellent remedy for various complaints of the stomach and bowels. A decoction of watermint prepared with vinegar stops blood vomiting.

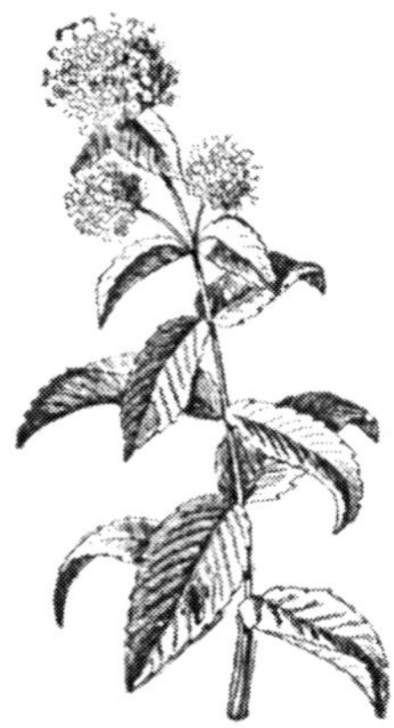

Watermint
(*Mentha aquatica*)

WOODRUFF

Latin, *Asperule odorata*; German, *Waldmeister*; French, *Aspérule*; Spanish, *Enebro*

This plant grows in shady forests and is in bloom in the spring and early summer. It is generally mixed with strawberry leaf tea, to give it a better flavor and to increase its blood-purifying and invigorating qualities. These two herbs combined constitute an excellent spring cleaning medicine, and they not only clean, but also strengthen the system.

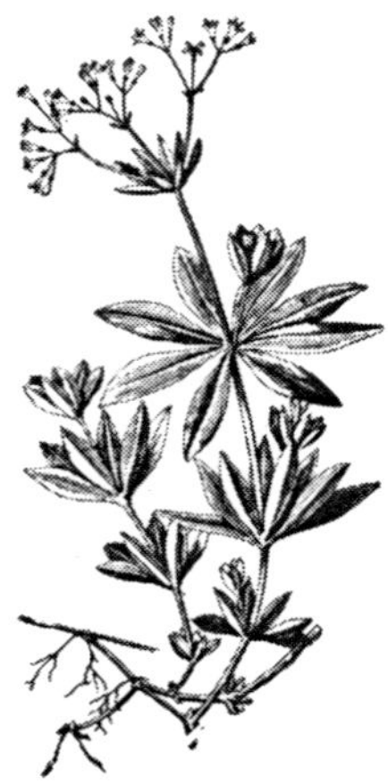

Woodruff
(*Asperule odorata*)

Watercress (Common)

Latin, *Nasturtium officinale*; German, *Brunnenkresse*; French, *Cresson de fontaine*; Spanish, *Berro*

This plant grows along fresh-water courses and is in bloom in June and July. It should be eaten as a salad for purifying the blood. Also if dried and prepared as a tea it serves as an excellent blood purifying beverage, provided it is taken regularly for some time.

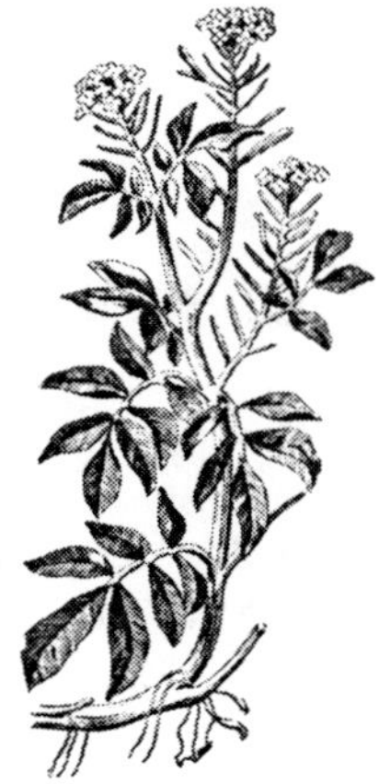

Watercress
(*Nasturtium officinale*)

Wood Ashes

Latin, *Tilia parviflora, grandiflora;* German, *Holzasche*

Ashes of the linden tree especially are recommended to people suffering from a weak stomach. These ashes should be taken in milk three or more times a day, to regulate the bowels and at the same time strengthen the digestive organs. This cheap remedy, although very effective, is too little known. It is to be recommended to convalescents who generally suffer from a weak stomach.

Wormwood

Latin, *Artemisia absinthium*; German, *Wermut*; French, *Absinthe*; Spanish, *Ajenjo*

This plant grows wild in the central parts of Europe and in the Tyrol. The tea made of wormwood is an excellent stomach remedy, promptly correcting loss of appetite and impaired digestion. If you have a feeling of something heavy lying on your stomach, wormwood tea will afford instant relief. There is no better remedy to be recommended for incipient dropsy and jaundice than this tea. Children troubled with worms should be given wormwood tea on arising, on their empty stomach. The tea is rarely taken pure, but mostly mixed with St. John's wort and centaury.

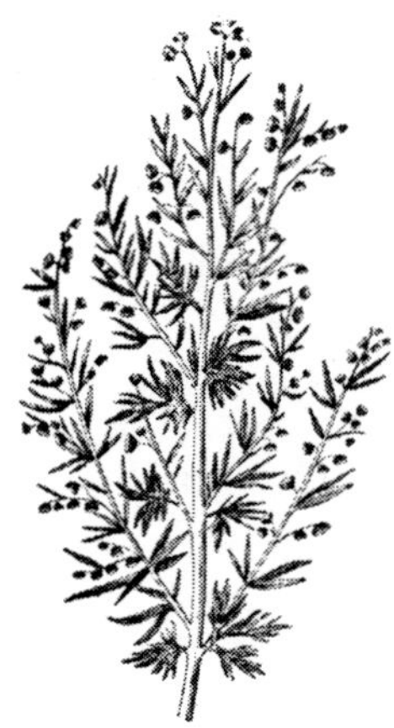

Wormwood
(*Artemisia absinthium)*

Kneipp's Aromatic Nourishing Tea

This is a combination of dietary nourishment and strength-giving tea. This very valuable nourishing and strength-giving tea was used by Father Kneipp to a great extent and with constant success for weak patients, convalescents, anaemic persons, for improving the appetite and physical strength. The best substitute for any breakfast tea.

Kneipp's Bone Powder

Nourishes the blood and the bones, strengthens the nerves. There is no powder used in the same ailments which is as easy to digest as this one, so that even little children and adults with the weakest stomachs can take it without disturbance. To this property may be attributed the marvelous cures often produced in anaemic persons, scrofulous and rachitic children, and in cases of nervousness, headache, and vertigo.

Kneipp has three kinds of Bone Powder:

The White Powder is the best remedy for nervousness, nervous headache, anaemia, and vertigo.

The Gray Powder is the best remedy for lung, kidney, and bladder diseases.

The Black Powder is the best remedy for scrofulous and rachitic children.

Children take a small pinch of powder; adults a quarter of a teaspoonful three times a day during meals.

Kneipp's Cough Tea

This is an excellent remedy for all cases of catarrh of the respiratory organs; it cannot be too highly recommended to those who suffer in the chest, throat, or lungs. We have seen the most obstinate cases of catarrh disappear in a few days, especially when the appropriate applications of water were made at the same time. Full directions enclosed in each package.

Cramp Drops And Cramp Tea

The best remedy for cramps of all kinds, especially of the womb, and a good anti-hysteric remedy. Three times a day one teaspoonful of the drops in a cup of cramp tea.

Kneipp's Depurative Tea

It is the best depurative; it rids the blood of morbid matter and acts slightly upon the bowels. For a radical depuration of the system in cases of eruptions, itch, lupus, and cancerous affection, this tea must be used for quite a long while and suitable applications of water be made at the same time to insure a radical cure. Each package contains directions for use.

Kneipp's Diuretic Tea

A highly pronounced diuretic hydragogue. Its virtues have often been proven in cases of dropsy, diseases of the kidneys (Bright's disease), and diseases of the bladder (stone, gravel). Each package contains directions for use.

Pfarrer Sebastian Kneipp's Liver Regulator # 1, Tonic Laxative I, Wühlhuber # I

This is a strong purgative which cleanses the stomach and bowels of all morbid matter. It must be rarely used, that is, only in cases of necessity. Put one-half to one teaspoonful in a cup of boiling water, let it draw during a quarter of an hour. This tea is taken either hot or cold at bed time.

Pfarrer Sebastian Kneipp's Liver Regulator # 2, Tonic Laxative II., Wühlhuber # 2

This tea has less purgative properties than No. 1, but acts especially upon the kidneys and the bladder. It is employed with great success in the beginning of dropsy and in affections of the urinary canal, also in acute pains of the bladder and kidneys. It is prepared and taken in the same manner as No. 1.

A decoction of watermint prepared with vinegar stops blood vomiting

[Woodruff] is generally mixed with strawberry leaf tea, to give it a better flavor and to increase its blood purifying and invigorating qualities. These two teas combined constitute an excellent spring cleaning medicine, and they not only clean, but also strengthen the system.

{Wood ashes} should be taken in milk three or more times a day, to regulate the bowels and at the same time strengthen the digestive organs.

If you have a feeling of something heavy lying on your stomach, wormwood tea will afford instant relief. There is no better remedy to be recommended for incipient dropsy and jaundice than this tea.

1921

Are Drugs Herbs? An Answer

Benedict Lust, N.D.

Tonic Of The Pines Bottled For You in Bing's Pine-Needle Baths

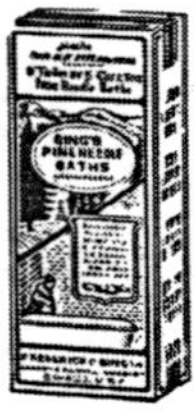

Is a new process **"Pine-Needle Extract"** which embodies the magic curative qualities with which Nature has endowed the Pine. Used in the Bath it exhales the wonderful aromatic odors of countless pine tree forests. It relaxes and soothes, acting as a strengthening nerve tonic.

Just as as sojourn among the pines helps restore the ailing to health, so do the **Pine-Needle Baths** benefit both sick and well. Tired people, nervous people, fagged mental workers—all who suffer from stress and strain, are wonderfully refreshed and strengthened. Even the robust should indulge in the Luxury of

Bing's Pine-Needle Baths

They cost but 8 cents and less per bath. Use it in hot, warm or cold bath, the one you most enjoy. After you have experienced the feeling of ease and well being—the relaxing of nerve strain—the general rest of a **Pine-Needle Bath,** you will retain it as an indispensable toilet article. Any physician will testify to the value of **Pine-Needle Baths** and their great aid to those seeking better health or greather efficiency.

Bing's Pine-Needle Baths come in 3 size pkgs. No. 1: Individual, holds 10 baths, $1.00. Size 2: Family pkg., holds 75 baths, $5.00. Size 3: Hospital or Sanitarium pkg. holds 160 baths, $10. Sent Exp. Prepaid on receipt of price. Personal checks accepted.

Live Agents wanted.

Fred. K. Bing, Jr.
906 Great Lakes Building
Chicago

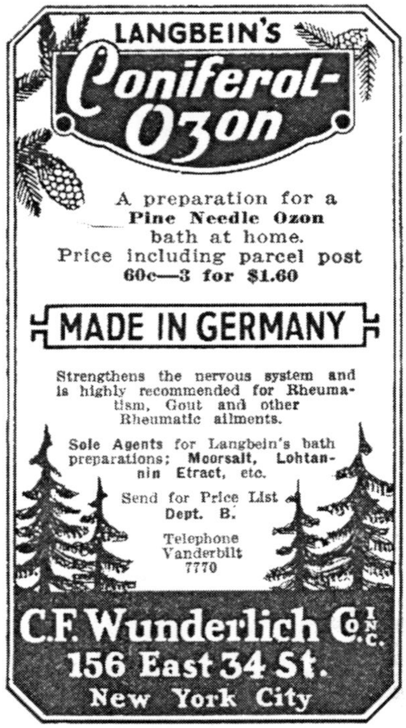

Pine needle baths were used to alleviate rheumatism. Kneipp would pick the pine needles to be used fresh in the therapeutic bath.

Are Herbs Drugs? An Answer

by Benedict Lust, N.D.

Herald of Health and Naturopath, XXVI (6), 291. (1921)

A new health publication in a recent issue refers to us as a hypocrite for carrying herb advertisements when we profess to be drugless. Sebastian Kneipp, one of the greatest natural physicians of recent times, used herbs but condemned drugs. The practice of herbalism in England is outside of the practice of medicine. Non-poisonous herbs vary little from our common garden vegetables such as celery, parsley, onions, etc., and can be used to good advantage on occasion to supply certain needs of the body. The principle behind the use of these simple remedies is quite different from the administration of poisonous and metallic drugs which contain no vital principle and cannot be metabolized by the animal body. But as Omar the poet expressed it, "Perhaps a hair divides the false from the true," and for one who is educated to the use of powerful drugs it would be a hard matter to find this hair line. It does not worry us to be called a hypocrite by one who does not understand how Nature cures. It is not therapeutic substances or treatments that cure but the forces of the body through its natural power of reaction. Cure is brought about through the elimination of encumbrance and the raising of vitality. Anything which operates to the contrary lowering vitality, or increasing encumbrance is detrimental and acts to prevent the cure. Fruits, vegetables and herbs supply the different glands of the body with vital, organic material to chemicalize the accumulated wastes that they are readily eliminated. Many of our garden vegetables were crude *herbs* before they were put under cultivation. Over-cultivation has robbed many of their choicest properties and it is sometimes necessary to go back to the cruder forms when we require eliminators. Herbs are vegetables. If *medicine* has extracted their active principles and concocted therefrom poisonous, life-destroying drugs, shall we condemn the herbs? Reason is all that is required in this matter.

But we notice all hypocrites have the tendency to quibble over words and terms. The hypercritical gentleman who questions our honesty is starting out to do a very laudable thing: teach Rational Living, but he has a fault-finding tendency that does not mix well with constructive effort. Through reading his magazine, we have found out a good deal of what he dislikes and of what he doesn't believe but very little in the five issues of it that gives us a clue to what he considers a rational life.

1922

Kneipp Herbs Advertisement

French Botanist Angers Doctors By Competition

Naturopathic News

Benedict Lust, N.D.

"INNER-CLEAN"

A scientifically prepared, Effective, Blood Purifier and System Cleaner

A Drugless Herb Compound perfected By PROF. ARNOLD EHRET

The special efficiency of this wonderful discovery is not through any laxative qualities, but rather through its ability to effectively remov : from the intestines hardened feces and other age-old, uneliminated, imperfectly digested fatty substances produced through the wrong eating of various foods of modern civilization and consequent lack of natural efficiency.

Inner-clean remedies this condition and rejuvenates the bowel's action. Severe cases of chronic constipation of long standing have been **permanently** cured.

Postpaid to any part of the U. S., 60 cents package.

HEALTH STORE

110 E. 41st ST., NEW YORK, N. Y.

"INNER-CLEAN" A Scientifically Prepared, Effective Blood Purifier and System Cleaner

A Drugless Herb Compound Perfected By Prof. Arnold Ehret

The special efficiency of this wonderful discovery is not through any laxative qualities, but rather through its ability to effectively remove from the intestines hardened feces and other age-old, uneliminated, imperfectly digested fatty substances produced through the wrong eating of various foods of modern civilization and consequent lack of natural efficiency.

Inner-Clean remedies this condition and rejuvenates the bowel's action. Severe cases of chronic constipation of long standing have been **permanently** cured.

Postpaid to any part of the United States, 60 cents a package; 6 for $3.00.

HEALTH STORE, 110 EAST 41st ST., NEW YORK

Arnold Ehret's book, *Mucusless Diet Healing System* would have a deep and lasting impact upon health seekers long after his untimely death. Ehret developed a herbal product to "clean" the bowels.

Kneipp Herbs

by Benedict Lust, N.D.

The Naturopath and Herald of Health, XXVII (9), 463. (1922)

Commonly Prescribed With Water Cure And Naturopathy. Selected Qualities

Directions how to use herbs in different ailments are given in Kneipp's books and in the booklet, *Kneipp's Naturopathic Herbs and Their Use.* Price, 50 cents

For postage add 20 cents per pound or 5 cents per package.

Item	Per lb.	Per pkg.
Aloe (Agave), Powder 55c.	1.75	0.55
Althea, Marsh Mallow (Eibischwurzel)	1.60	0.75
Angelica Root (Engelwurzel), Powder 40c.	1.60	0.75
Alum (Alaun) Powder		0.50
Anise Seed (Anissamen), Powder 55c.	1.50	0.50
Arnica Flowers, Leopard's Bane (Arnika-blüten, Wohlverleih)	1.60	0.50
Aromatic Nourishing Tea (Diätetuscger Nähr and Krafttee, Wörishofener Kräutertee), small pkg. large pkg.		1.00 2.00
Ash Leaves (Silbereschenblätter)	1.75	0.50
Balm Mint (Melisse)	1.75	0.50
Bark of Oak (Eichenrinde)	1.00	0.50
Bark of Black Alder Tree (Faulbaum)	1.75	0.50
Barberries (Berberitzenbeeren)	1.75	0.50
Basil (Josephskräutlein)	1.80	0.50

Item	Per lb.	Per pkg.
Bear Berry Leaves (Bärentraubenblätter)	1.50	0.60
Berries of Buckthorn (Kreuzdornbeeren)	1.50	0.50
Bilberry Leaves (Heidelbeerblätter)	1.75	0.50
Blessed Thistle (Kardobenediktenkraut)	1.65	0.50
Blind (or Dead) Nettle Flowers (Taubnesselblütne)	3.00	1.00
Birch Leaves (Birkenblätter)	1.75	0.50
Black Current Leaves (Johannisbeerblätter)	1.75	0.55
Breakfast tea (Fühstücktee), small pkg. large pkg.		1.00 2.00
Briar Hip (Hagebutten)	2.50	0.85
Briar Hip Seeds (Hagebuttenkerne)	2.50	0.85
Broomherb, Geniste (Ginster)	1.50	0.50
Bogbean (Bitterklee)	1.50	0.50
Buckthorn Bark (Kreuzdornrinde)	1.50	0.50
Burdock Roots (Klettenwurzel)	1.50	0.60
Calamus, Sweet Flag (Kalmuswurzel)	1.50	0.50
Chamomile (Kamille)	2.00	0.75
Caraway (Krümmel)	1.50	0.40
Carline Thistle (Eberwurz)	1.60	0.50
Centaury (Tausendguldenkraut)	1.75	0.50
Chalk Powder (Kreidemehl)		1.00

Item	Per lb.	Per pkg.
Charcoal Powder (Lindenholzkohle)		1.00
Chestnut Powder (Kastanienpulver)		0.40
Chicory, Succory (Wegwart)	1.50	0.50
Chickweed (Hühnerdarm, Sternmiere)	1.60	0.50
Coltsfoot (Huflattich), Powder 55c.	1.50	0.50
Common Nettle (Brennessel)	1.50	0.50
Common Nettle Roots (Brennesselwurzel)	1.60	0.50
Cough Tea (Hustentee), small pkg. large pkg.		1.00 2.00
Cramp Tea (Krampftee), small pkg. large pkg.		1.00 2.00
Depurative Tea (Blutreinigungstee), small pkg. large pkg.		1.00 2.00
Diabetic Tea (Zuckerharnruhrtee), small pkg. large pkg.		1.00 2.00
Dwarf Elder (Attichwurzel), Powder 60c.	2.00	0.80
Elder Berries (Hollunderbeeren)	1.50	0.50
Elder Flowers (Hollunderblüten)	1.75	0.75
Elder Leaves (Hollunderblätter)	1.50	0.50
Elder Roots (Hollunderwurzel)	1.75	0.50
Elecampane (Alantwurzel)	1.80	0.50
Eucalyptus (Eukalyptus)	1.50	0.50

Item	Per lb.	Per pkg.
Eyebright (Augentrost), Powder 40c.	1.50	0.50
Family Tea (Familiengesundheitstee), small pkg. large pkg.		1.00 2.00
Fenugreek, Foenum Graecum (Bockshornklee), Powder 50c.	1.60	0.50
Fennel Seed (Fenchel), Powder 55c.	1.30	0.40
Gallstone Tea (Gallensteintee), large pkg.	2.00	1.00
Gentian (Enzian)	1.40	0.50
Grains of Incense (Harzkörner)	2.00	1.00
Ground Ivy (Gundelrebe)	1.50	0.50
Hay Flowers (importierte Heubleumen)		0.75
Holy Herb (Heiliges Kraut)	2.00	0.75
Horehound (Andorn)		0.30
Iceland Moss (Isländisches Moos)	1.60	0.50
Iris (Schwertlilie)	1.50	0.50
Juniper Berries (Wachholderbeeren)	1.40	0.40
Juniper Sprigs (Wachholderspitzen)	1.50	0.50
Juniper Berries, Powder		0.50
Knotgrass (Wegtritt, Knöterich)	1.50	0.40
Laxative Tea (Stuhlgangstee)		1.00
Linden Flowers (Lindenblüten)	1.60	0.75
Liverwort (Leberblümchen)	1.80	0.50

Item	Per lb.	Per pkg.
Lungworth (Lungenkraut)	1.50	0.50
Mallow Flowers, Hollyoke (Malve)	1.75	0.80
Marigold Flowers (Ringelblumen)	1.50	0.50
Maté, small pkg. large pkg.		1.00 2.00
Mistletoe (Mistel)	1.50	0.50
Mouse Ear (Mausöhrchen)	1.50	0.50
Mullein Flower (Wollblume)	3.00	1.00
Mullein Herb (Wollblumenkraut)	1.50	0.50
Nerve Tea (Nerentee), small pkg. large pkg.		1.00 2.00
Oat Straw (importiertes Haferstroh)	1.50	0.75
Obesity Tea (Entfettungstee)	2.00	1.00
Peppermint (Pfefferminze)	2.75	0.50
Pimpernelle, Small Burnet (Gauchheil)	1.75	0.50
Pine Sprigs (Fichtensprossen)	2.00	0.50
Pine Tannin (Fichetenlohe, Tannin)	1.50	0.50
Primrose, Cowslips (Schlüsselblume)	3.00	0.80
Rheumatism Tea (Rheumatismustee), small pkg. large pkg.		1.00 2.00
Rhubarb Powder or Pills	1.50	0.50
Ribworth (Spitzwegerich)	1.50	0.50
Rosemary (Rosmarin)	1.30	0.50

Item	Per lb.	Per pkg.
Rue (Raute)	1.50	0.50
Sage (Salbei), Powder 55c.	1.50	0.40
Sandalwood, Red Saunders (Sandelholz), Powder 75c.		0.70
Sanicle (Sanikel, Heildolde), Powder 75c.		0.75
Sarsaparilla Root (Riedgras)	2.50	0.75
Sassafras (Sassafras)	2.50	0.50
Scurvy Grass, Spoonwort (Löffellkraut)	2.00	0.50
Sea Onion (Meerzweibel)	2.00	0.50
Shavegrass, Common Horse Tail, Pewtergrass (Zinnkraut)	1.50	0.40
Shepherd's Purse (Hirtentäschchen)	1.50	0.50
Silverweed (Anserine, Gänsefingerkraut)	1.50	0.50
Soapwort (Seifenkraut)	1.50	0.50
Sorrel (Sauerampfer)	2.00	0.50
St. John's Wort (Johanniskraut)	1.50	0.50
St. John's Wort, Powder		0.75
Stomach Tea (Magentee), small pkg. large pkg.		1.00 2.00
Strawberry Leaves (Erdbeerblätter)	1.50	0.50
Thyme (Thymian, Quendel)	0.75	0.50
Tonic Laxative II (Wühlhuber II), Powder		1.00
Tormentil (Tormentille, Blutwurz, Fünffingerkraut), Powder $1.00	3.00	0.75

Item	Per lb.	Per pkg.
Valerian Root (Baldrianworzel, powder 60c.	1.50	0.50
Veronica, Male Speedwell (Ehrenpreis)	1.50	0.50
Vervain (Eisenkraut)	1.50	0.50
Violet Leaves (Veilchenblätter)	1.50	0.50
Violet Root	3.00	1.00
Wallworth (Beinwell, Wallwurz)	1.50	0.50
Walnut Leaves (Wallnussblätter)	1.50	0.50
Watermint (Wasserminze)	1.50	0.50
Watercress (Brunnenkresse)	1.50	0.50
White Beanpods (Bohnenhülsen)	1.50	0.50
Woodroof (Waldmeister)	1.50	0.50
Wood Ashes (Holzasche), small box large box		1.00 2.00
Wormwood (Wermut), Powder 60c.	1.40	0.40
Wormseed (Wurmsamen)		0.50
Wormseed Chocolate		0.50
Yarrow, Milfoil (Schafgarbe)	1.50	0.50

FRENCH BOTANIST ANGERS DOCTORS BY COMPETITION

by Benedict Lust, N.D.

Herald of Health and Naturopath, XXVII (10), 498. (1922)

EFFECTS MARVELOUS CURES BY SUGGESTION SUPPLEMENTED BY HERB PREPARATIONS, PATIENTS BY THEIR TESTIMONY SAVING HIM FROM PRISON SENTENCE

Medicos of the Department of the Haute Garonne are up in arms against the constant successes of Jean Bizet, a local botanist with highly developed powers of suggestion, which are said to be cutting down the death rate simultaneously with the doctors' income. As a result, they are asking the incarceration of Bizet and damages of $4,000, alleging that his preparations infringe upon the realm of medicine.

The local court which has just heard the evidence would have granted the doctors' plea, but at the last moment the defendant's lawyers introduced a score of new witnesses, each of whom swore that he had been cured by Bizet's methods when others failed to bring any relief.

Bizet, himself, says that the suggestion consists merely in applying Nature's reasoning power, adding that botany is Nature's own method, and he has defied the court to imprison him for bringing back suffering humanity into touch with Nature herself. For the time being, the judges have decided to agree and have suspended judgment until they have further studied therapy as practiced by Bizet.

Naturopathic News

by Benedict Lust

Herald of Health and Naturopath, XXVII (11), 557. (1922)

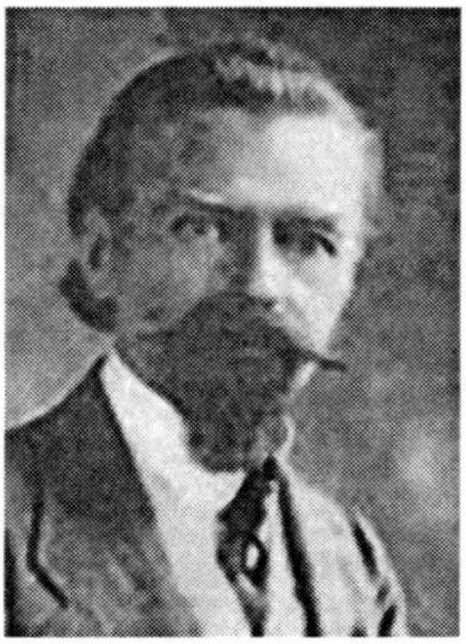

Arnold Ehret (1866-1922)

Just received the sad news that our old personal friend and pioneer of Dietetics, and well known authority in the Nature Cure line, Professor Arnold Ehret, of Los Angeles, California, lost his life by an accident on October 9th. He was delivering a lecture at Hotel Angelus, and leaving close to twelve o'clock at night and crossing the street with a number of friends who left the hotel with him, he slipped on the sidewalk and hit his head on the curbstone and never recovered consciousness. He died on the spot.

Dr. Ehret is the author of a number of famous books on dietetics in German and English, French and Portuguese. His principal work is his famous course of twenty-four lessons which he has made up for practitioners. However, of late he opened some up also for the public at large. These lessons consist of a scientific course on dietetics and are the last word on this question. The Ehret Mucousless Diet is a diet for more efficiency, more strength and more endurance and longevity. This course is also a real therapeutic system for the cure of all disease by diet. Cures have been made by Professor Ehret all over the world, and his diet seems to be far superior to any other diet so far known in the world. His lesson five on the Secret of Vitality, Lessons 23 and 24 on the Magic Mirror and Lessons 15 and 16 on the Transitional Diet, explaining also the so-called Internal Uncleanliness of Man, are absolutely new ideas in Dietetics. These lessons have been published in special little booklets. Anyone who is in harmony with Ehret's teachings should get these little booklets as long as they can be had. Dr. Ehret has also discovered an Herbal Food called Inner Clean which is a specific cure for the removal of mucous from the digestive tract and is not a medicine. With this discovery alone Ehret has rendered a great service to natural therapeutics. In the near future, we will bring a biography of Professor Ehret, also his picture. We are awaiting more news from Los Angeles in regard to his sudden death. We are all shocked and sustain a great loss, as Dr. Ehret is one of the pillars on which the drugless movement stands today in America. He was a leader, and there were many who copied him, many who used his methods, but none of them came up to him. His name will never die in the history of the drugless movement and Natural Dietetics.

R.I.P.

1923

Herbs Combined With Nature Cure

Louisa Lust, N.D.

HERBS COMBINED WITH NATURE CURE

by Louisa Lust, N.D.

Naturopath, XXVIII (8), 370-371. (1923)

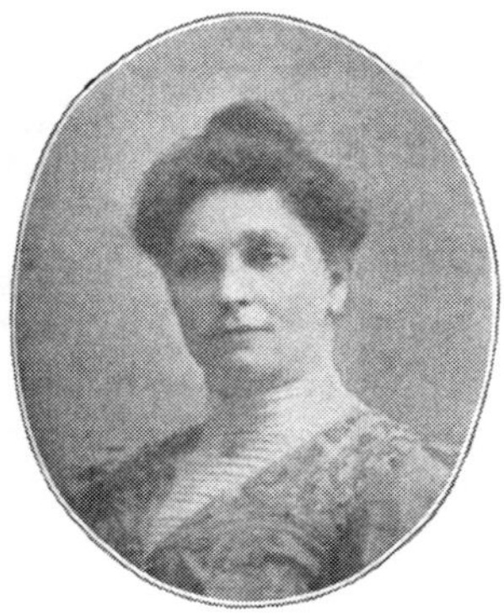

Louisa Lust (1864 –1925)

Every person desires to live as long as they can; therefore it becomes a necessity to conserve or preserve the life force. We see men and women, both young and old, with stiff joints, perhaps paralyzed, blind, hard of hearing, teeth all gone, and yet, with all these infirmities they hate to die. Perhaps with all these symptoms they are not more than 30, 40 or 50 years old. We see people with rheumatism, shortness of breath, palpitation of the heart, swollen feet and various more unpleasant diseases of no use mentioning here; and we ask: "Why should they be afflicted in this manner?" We say they should not! Neither would they be afflicted in such a manner, if they had conserved the vital force. They might have the vital force to a certain extent, but the organism is clogged with waste matter. Such conditions can be obviated by a natural regime of diet and treatment, and the results will be that a man can really renew his youth. For just such conditions the Nature Cure with the use of herbs will be of great benefit. Necessarily, we must take care of the body, remove the obstructions and have a long and useful life.

The use of herbs has a threefold aim: to dissolve morbid matters, to eliminate them, and then, to strengthen the organism. Certain herbs contain actual food value beneficial to the blood and nerves, and for upbuilding. Sage is a good eradicator for all kinds of impurities, stomach and intestinal. Tormentil, thistle and shavegrass are excellent herbs for hemorrhages; to stop bleeding of any kind, whether internal or external. Ribwort is an herb that loosens up mucus in the throat and lungs. Rosemary can be used for dropsy, kidney and liver troubles. Fenugreek surpasses any remedy for diphtheria, sore throat and nose, and it is also used in case of fever.

For kidney and bladder troubles, juniper and wormwood are most beneficial in stimulating these organs. For chronic constipation, a tea of dandelion blossoms will regulate stool; but by a proper diet of fruits and nuts and green vegetables, avoiding all bread and cereals or any mucus building food, constipation can be cured.

For diarrhea, tea of raspberry leaves used for injection. Also drink a cup of the tea morning and night, which will eliminate morbid matter. Diarrhea comes as a result of the effort of the vital force to clean the body of old material in the intestines; therefore, do not suppress it, but assist it.

There are numerous teas that a Naturopath can use for the different ailments. Anyone can see how foolish it is to use poisonous drugs and patent medicines, when Nature supplies all we need. Using these herbs will not do harm, like Calomel and doses of salts alternated by opiates, as an allopathic doctor is almost sure to give you.

Necessary for good health is a daily bath, alone for motives of cleanliness, as well as conserving the vital force. Cleanliness within as well as without will give evidence of a healthy skin and bright eyes. Not alone for the cleanliness of body, but the increased mental development and purity of mind. Every pure thought comes out on your face and leads you closer to a better and higher life. If we know and have these truths, we are happy, and we may know that we are among the wise who will understand; or need we worry because everyone will not take hold of these laws and become well?

Herbal Formulas

Aesthetic Spring Synede, *p. 196*

Around the inside edge of an oatmeal dish arrange four salad ingredients in such order as to produce the best color effect, leaving room, for the fifth ingredient which must always be flaked nuts. For example

1 ½ oz. banana cubed,
1 oz. beet shredded,
1 oz. spinach chopped,
2 oz. peanuts, flaked.

Now spin or drip over the beet and spinach ½ oz. honey (teaspoonful) and let it stand 5 or 10 minutes for the honey to mix by sinking. A combination of honey, oil and lemon juice may be used another time. Heavy opaque dressings are not used on this salad as that would obliterate its aesthetic effect. This salad admits of an endless variety by substituting an ingredient of similar color effect but the proportions should not be changed.

When you start to eat this salad, mix a little of each of the ingredients in the center and eat the mixed portion and then you mix more until finally your mix all the remainders at once and finish.

Appetite And Blood, *p. 275*

Tea of buckbean and tincture of buckthorn act as a blood purifier, restore the appetite, and may be mixed with other herbs, such as wormwood, centaury and sage.

Astringent Formula, *p. 71*

Mistletoe mixed with santala makes an astringent tea.

Refreshing Beverage, *p. 153*

If you will parch the common field peas, as you would coffee, and cut up fine, these dry roots of dandelion and parch them also, then grind each separately, then take a teaspoonful of the ground dandelion, and a sufficient quantity of the ground peas to make a pea coffee. You will have one of the best substitutes for Mocha and Java coffee you ever used.

Burn Ointment, *p. 254*

Beaten up with lard, cream, or Vaseline, the inner green bark of elder forms an excellent discutient ointment which is of much value in burns, scalds, and some cutaneous diseases.

Chest Cold, *p. 211*

Boil a quart of water, stir in 2oz. honey, and ¼ oz. of chamomile flowers, quickly remove the vessel to a table, cover the patient's head and the vessel with a rain-proof or similar cloth, let the patient inhale the vapor till cold, stirring occasionally. If the desired results are not brought about by the first treatment, repeat once or more.

Chest Obstructions, *p. 301*

The tea prepared from the [mallow] flowers of this plant is very effective in removing mucous obstructions in the chest, and it is often prescribed for many troubles of the throat and the larynx. It is advisable to mix the mallow flowers with mullein flowers.

Chronic Abscesses, Swelling, *p. 228*

Sassafras when mixed with ground mullein and boiling water poured upon it, it is a superior application for swollen face, chronic abscesses or any condition where the flesh is swollen and congested. In such cases it relieves the pain and reduces the swelling quickly, and may be used in local dropsies.

Chronic Stomach Catarrh, *p. 141*

Chronic stomach catarrh may be cured by a tea composed of wormwood, gentian and shavegrass.

Consumption, Early Stage, *p. 62*

Tea of lungwort and ribwort mixed in equal parts will remove all slimy obstructions in the lungs and chest and will cure consumption in its first stages.

Convalescence Tea, *p. 50*

For a strengthening tea for convalescents, mix strawberry leaves with woodruff and thyme

Cough, *p. 161*

Herbs as ribwort, common nettle, violets, and sage are cut to pieces, dried in the shade in the open air, mixed, pestled and strained. This powder will cure any irritating cough, if taken three times a day: a knifepoint full in water or in a wafer.

Cough, Colds, Sore Throat, *p. 211*

For coughs, colds, and sore throats, honey and lemon juice mixed together in equal quantities will be found a remedy as useful as it is old.

Coughs, *p. 311*

The tea made of ribwort loosens mucus and slime in the inner organs. In conjunction with lungwort it is often used for pulmonary complaints and as an infallible cough remedy.

Dandelion Synede, *p. 196*

Take a cup loosely filled with chopped dandelion leaves and put them in one side of an oatmeal dish. Now spin a teaspoonful of honey over the chopped leaves and then drip over them a teaspoonful of lemon juice and one of olive oil. In the vacant side of the dish put four heaping table spoonsful of ground (or flaked) almonds or flaked unroasted Spanish peanuts. Now the synede is ready to be served and the one who eats it is to mix the ground nuts with the greens, with his fork, little by little as he eats it. For those who are not acquainted with the apyrotropher diet it is best to mix the synede completely before serving it.

Detoxifying, *p. 141*

Shavegrass can be used in the most various ways. First of all, it may be added to any tea, as wormwood and gentian, thereby contributing to their strengthening and cleansing effect.

Diaphoretic, *p. 246*

To use [dandelion] for sweating and general benefit to the whole body at the same time, add to 2 parts of the dandelion, 1 part each of pleurisy root (*Asclepias tuberosa*), and 1 part boneset (sometimes called through wort; Latin, *Eupatorium perfoliatum*), boil this 15 minutes, strain and keep warm, give to patient a cupful every 15 to 20 minutes give it hot. This will be found very sure and certain cure for colds, when accompanied by biliousness. Try it.

Digestion, *p. 142*

If it is desired to strengthen the digestive organs, a pinch of agave should be added to the dwarf elder.

Digestive Tonic, *p. 140*

The gentian root is very bitter; mixed with wormwood and shavegrass, we have an excellent tea for strengthening the digestive organs.

Diuretic, *p. 142*

A composition of dwarf elder, rosemary and shavegrass is of great efficacy in dropsy.

Edema, *p. 246*

In a case of dropsy, by adding common garden parsley to the dandelion roots and tops, say 2 parts of dandelion to 1 part parsley, and boil them 20 minutes, strain the tea and drink a wine glassful or more every 2 hours, you will be greatly relieved. Be sure to use plenty of the herbs so as to have it good and strong.

ERYSIPELAS, *p. 253*

The properties and uses of the [elder] flowers are diaphoretic, and gentle stimulant; in cold infusions they are diuretic, alterative, and cooling, and may be used in all diseases requiring such action, as in hepatic (liver) derangements of children, erysipelas and erysipelatous diseases, etc. In infusion with maiden hair [*Adiantum capillusveneris L.*] and beech drops [*Orobanche virginiana*], they will be found very valuable in all erysipelatous diseases. The expressed juice of the berries, evaporated to the consistency of a syrup is a valuable aperient and alterative; one ounce of it will purge.

EVACUATING, *p. 47*

The powder of the Barbados aloe plant will cure quite a number of ailments. A little aloe powder boiled with a teaspoonful of honey thoroughly cleanses the stomach. Mixed with other herbs aloe has a very beneficial effect, not a very purging but a more evacuating effect. One mixture which cannot be recommended too highly consists of one pinch of aloe, sufficient elder flowers, a small teaspoonful *Foenum graecum* (Fenugreek) and one teaspoonful of fennel. Of this mixture two cups of tea are prepared and taken within two days.

EYE WASH AND VAPOR BATH, *p. 133*

A good eye wash, healing in its effects, is made by taking a half tablespoonful of fennel powder and boiling in water. The eyes may be washed with this three times a day. Another effective method is to use the steam of this concoction by throwing a towel over the head. A similar effect is obtained by using ground anise or caraway. Frequently these three kinds of seeds are mixed and are used together for the vapor bath.

FRECKLES, *p. 211*

Equal parts of honey and cream mixed together, rubbed on the affected parts, it is said to be a good thing for freckles.

GOUT, *p. 85*

Especially to be recommended are ground juniper berries, further dwarf elder, parsley, common nettle root; and there should be added from four to six tablespoonful of a mixture of the above remedies to a quart of water, and the lot be boiled until only ¾ of a quart remain. This "tea" should be taken two or three times a week for some length of time. The secretion of uric acid from the blood, which is most essential, is also greatly favored by drinking for some length of time daily one to two cups of tea made from a decoction of ground juniper berries, shavegrass and knotgrass, to which finally, some wormwood should be added. This tea must be taken on an empty stomach in the morning, and warm; and also in the evening, several cups at bed time.

Hair Growth, *p. 277*

The root of the common burdock boiled in water for from five to ten minutes, is very beneficial for the growth of the hair. Results are even better if burdock roots and blind nettle leaves [*Lamium album*], in equal quantities, are boiled in two parts of water and one part of vinegar. Let this decoction settle for some days; then strain through a cloth sieve, and add some Cologne. Rub the roots of the hair well several times a week, but in order not to make the skin of the scalp over-sensitive, rub the scalp once a week with some good hair oil.

Hemostatic, *p. 267*

Mistletoe's effects are not to be surpassed for stopping hemorrhages. Mistletoe tea is excellent also for other disturbances in the blood circulation. Mistletoe may be mixed to advantage with shavegrass in equal parts.

Hemostatic, *p. 312*

The red wood of the red saunders tree [sandlewood] is pulverized into a fine powder and two teaspoonfuls of this tea, added to tea of mistletoe, may be used for stopping the flow of blood in all kinds of hemorrhages.

Incipient Tuberculosis, *p. 265*

Asarum is used practically for the same purposes as ribwort [plantain], and should be preferably mixed with the other to remove slimy mucus in respiratory passages; also for incipient consumption.

Intestinal Purifier, *p. 263*

Anise seed may be combined with equal parts of caraway and fennel seeds, and used for the same purposes. This combination is an excellent intestinal purifier.

Kidney And Bladder, *p. 343*

For kidney and bladder troubles juniper and wormwood are most beneficial in stimulating these organs.

Kneipp Stomach Formula, *p. 52*

Take two tablespoonful of pounded fennel, two tablespoons of crushed juniper berries, one tablespoonful of *Foenum graceum* and one tablespoonful of aloe powder. Mix them all well together, put the mixture in a box and keep it in a dry place. The remedy operates after twelve to thirty hours. The tea is taken generally at night before bed; a small cupful is a dose. One teaspoonful of the mixture is sufficient for a cupful. It is boiled for a quarter of an hour, then poured off and drunk either cold or warm with or without sugar. Kneipp recommends to strong people to drink a cup of the tea on two succeeding days; to weak people to divide the cupful for two or three days so that they take four or six tablespoonful like medicine every evening. There will be no uncomfortable feelings, but the beneficial effect will be felt at once.

Kneipp Kidney And Bladder Formula, *p. 53*

Two tablespoonful of pounded fennel, three tablespoonful of crushed juniper berries, three tablespoonful of powder from dwarf elder roots, one tablespoonful of *Foenum graceum* and one tablespoonful of aloe powder are mixed well together.

Liver And Constipation, *p. 246*

There is perhaps no single agent of greater value to the constipated patient, whose trouble generally arises from a torpid liver, than this same dandelion. To make it more effective, add 1 part blue flag root and 1 part culvers root to 2 parts whole herb and root of dandelion. Boil 30 minutes; take a cupful 2 to 3 times daily, if you find it necessary.

Liver And Kidney, *pp. 162-163*

St. John's wort has a particular influence on the liver; its tea is an excellent remedy for it. A small admixture of aloe powder increases the effect, which can be observed chiefly in the urine; whole flakes of morbid matters are sometimes washed away with it.

Liver Cleanse Formula, *p. 243*

We will need a bitter principle to aid in the cleansing of the liver. Select dandelion root, culver's root, or yellow parilla. Either of the above. Then we want a decided stimulant select, cayenne pepper, prickly ash bark, ginger, either of these. Then we want a laxative for the bowels: mandrake root, cascaria bark, licorice root, senna leaves; either of these. Then we want a remedy to aid the blood to cleanse the mucous membranes: blue flag root, sassafras bark, stillingia, tag alder bark, sarsaparilla; either of the last named may also be used in combination with the others. Then add if obtainable a good handful of hemlock boughs, using of the other about two ounces of each. Boil this quantity in three quarts of water down to three pints, strain and add two pounds of cut loaf sugar; when this is dissolved, add about six ounces of alcohol to prevent it from souring. Dose, one-half a wine glass before each meal.

Liver Diseases, *p. 311*

St. John's wort furnishes however, a splendid remedy for diseases affecting the liver, and if mixed with bitter aloe powders its healing properties are considerably increased.

Liver, Stomach And Nervous System, *p. 236*

When cascara is aged, it may then be made into infusion or syrup with an equal quantity of Oregon grape root, licorice root, dandelion root, burdock root, and lady slipper root. This may be boiled to a moderately strong tea. This formula is a desirable medicine for the bowels because of its aid to the liver, stomach, and nervous system.

Lung Catarrh, *p. 299*

For use as an herbal remedy, [lungwort] is generally mixed with ribwort, and prepared as a tea it is a specific for catarrh of the lungs.

Menses (Irregular), Stomach Cramps, *p. 302*

Yarrows leaves, preferable however its blossoms mixed with St. John's wort, are used for cramps in the stomach, irregular menstruation of women, and pain in the abdomen.

Plantain Synede, *p. 214*

Such a plantain synede may be composed of chopped plantain leaves and ground raw peanuts (or other nuts) dressed with honey if desired sweet; though some people prefer the plantain leaves as an admixture to other synede herbs for that particular flavor they impart. Those who wish to prepare a larger variety of plantain synedes may be referred to George J. Drew's book, *Unfired Food.*

Rosemary Wine, *p. 141*

This wine is prepared in the following way. Into a bottle of common white wine put a rosemary twig; let it draw for a short time, according to the strength desired. During this process the wine must remain in a warm rom. After five or six days the twig is taken out and the wine is ready for use.

ROSEMARY WINE, *p. 173*

This wine is prepared in the following way: Young, fresh branches of the rosemary-shrub are cut into finger lengths, washed in cold water and a handful of it put into a bottle of genuine, old white wine; kept at a place of medium temperature, and then within a fortnight it is ready for use. According to the degree of the ailment, three spoonfuls of this wine, taken twice a day, will be of beneficial use.

SCIATICA AND RHEUMATIC PAIN, *p. 157*

Take the fresh plant of mayweed and smart weed, equal parts, and bruise them together and moisten them with a small quantity of spirits of turpentine. This will be found an excellent application where severe skin irritation is suffered from.

SKIN OINTMENT, *p. 218*

A very desirable ointment can be made from the green flowers and leaves of yarrow with equal parts of ground ivy and red raspberry leaves, also green, and the green bark of dogwood (sometimes called green ozier). Bruise them well, place in kettle and add sufficient Vaseline to cover the herbs. Let it simmer over a slow fire so as not to make the Vaseline too hot (and thus burn the herbs) for two or three hours. Then strain through a piece of cloth and box for use. You have now one of the best ointments for scurvy, old sores and cracked hands. If you wish it still more active, which is sometimes necessary in sores of long standing, add to each pound of Vaseline two teaspoonful of best cayenne pepper.

SPRING DETOX FORMULA, *p. 320*

Woodruff is generally mixed with strawberry leaf tea, to give it a better flavor and to increase its blood purifying and invigorating qualities. These two teas combined constitute an excellent spring cleaning medicine, and they not only clean, but also strengthen the system.

STOMACH, *p. 161*

Stomach troubles will be alleviated by a composition of wormwood, mint and gentian, prepared and taken in the same way as the just mentioned herbs. The herbs are cut in pieces, dried in the shade in the open air, mixed, pestled and strained. The powder is taken three times a day; a knife-point full in water or in a wafer.

STOMACH AND BOWEL, *p. 261*

The following mixture is effective in cleansing the stomach and bowels: one-half teaspoonful aloe, one tablespoonful of elder blossoms, two teaspoonful of [*Trigonella*] *foenum graecum* (Fenugreek), and one teaspoonful ground fennel seed. Make one pint of tea from above, which will provide a two days' supply. This mixture will not act violently, but will allow ample time for the digestion of food, and produce a normal stool in from 8 to 24 hours.

Stomach Bleeding, *p. 161*

Hemorrhages from the stomach are cured by: shavegrass, shepherd's purse and mistletoe every hour a knife-point full.

Strengthen Stomach, *p. 135*

Water trefoil can also be mixed with other herbs. Two or three leaves of water trefoil, one leaf of wormwood and a centaury flower will produce an excellent combination that will strengthen and improve the stomach.

Tape Worms, *p. 211*

The eating of honey while otherwise fasting, is said not only to provide a remedy, but also a cure for tape worms.

Teeth Powder, *p. 77*

During the cold season, when fresh sage leaves are not to be obtained, you may take sage leaf powder and finely ground linden wood coal in equal parts, mix them well together and clean the teeth therewith. This powder does not hurt the enamel and purifies the mouth very nicely.

Throat Gargle, *p. 301*

An excellent gargle for sore throat is obtained from a decoction of mallow flowers to which a half a teaspoonful of alum has been added.

Throat Tickling, *p. 211*

Old people, who suffer with a tickling sensation at the bottom of the throat will find great relief in the following: Simmer together for several hours, 8oz. of honey, 2oz. chopped onion, and strain; take a teaspoonful at a time as desired.

Tonic Laxative I, *p. 165*

Mix two tablespoonful of pounded fennel, two tablespoonful of crushed juniper berries, one tablespoonful of *Foenum graecum* and one tablespoonful of aloe powder. Mix them all well together, put the mixture in a box, and keep it in a dry place. The remedy operates after twelve to thirty hours. The tea is taken generally at night before going to bed; a small cupful is a dose. One teaspoonful of the mixture is sufficient for a cupful;

it is boiled for a quarter of an hour, then poured off and drunk either cold or warm, with or without sugar.

TONIC LAXATIVE II, *p. 165*

Mix two tablespoonful of pounded fennel, three tablespoonful of crushed juniper berries, three tablespoonful of powder from dwarf elder roots, one tablespoonful of Foenum graecum, and one tablespoonful of aloe-powder. This tea does not exclude purging effects; still its districts are (instead of the stomach and bowels) more the kidneys and bladder; it drives the morbid matters out through the urine.

VERMIFUGE FOR TAPEWORMS, *p. 321*

Children troubled with worms should be given wormwood tea on arising, on their empty stomach. The tea is rarely taken pure, but mostly mixed with St. John's wort and centaury.

WHOOPING COUGH, COUGH CANDIES, *p. 211*

A splendid candy for colds, whooping coughs, etc., can be made as follows: boil a strong solution of horehound leaves in soft water, strain through muslin, add as much honey as desired, boil until all the water evaporates, pour into shallow vessel and allow to set.

References

Bailey, L. H. (1906). *Cyclopeia of American Horticulture, (*6 volumes), Doubleday, Page & Company, New York.

Baumgarten, A. (1908). Herbs for stomach troubles. *The Naturopath and Herald of Health*, IX (2), 40-41.

Carqué, O. (1912). St. Jame's oil. *The Naturopath and Herald of Health*, XVII (2), 114-115.

Drews, G. J. (1913). Curled leaf mallow or hygeia plant. *The Naturopath and Herald of Health*, XVIII (1), 56.

Drews, G. J. (1913). Curled dock. *The Naturopath and Herald of Health*, XVIII (4), 266.

Drews, G. J. (1913). Dandelions. *The Naturopath and Herald of Health*, XVIII (4), 267-268.

Drews, G. J. (1914). Licorice. *The Naturopath and Herald of Health*, XVIX (12), 830-831.

Drews, G. J. (1915). Plantain. *The Naturopath and Herald of Health*, XX (9), 580-581.

Fritz, W. W. (1916). Comparative therapeutics.. *Herald of Health and Naturopath*, XXI (5), 314-316.

Gerard, J. (1633). The Herbal or Generall historie of plantes, of plantes, Adam Islip Joice Norton and Richard Whitakers, 1633, London.

Heinrichs, P. (1911). Our most medicinal herbs, knotgrass. *The Naturopath and Herald of Health*, XVI (12), 786-787.

Kahut, K. (1908). Phyto-therapy (plant cure). *The Naturopath and Herald of Health*, IX (8), 233-235.

Kneipp, S. (1896). *My Water Cure*, Jos. Kœsel Publisher, Kempten, Bavaria, 4th edition, pp. 395.

Kneipp, S. (1900). My medicinal herbs. *The Kneipp Water Cure Monthly*, I (8), 143-144.

Kneipp, S. (1902). Kneipp's apotheca. *The Naturopath and Herald of Health*, III (2), 384-386.

Lust, B. (1900). Herbs and their healing power. *The Kneipp Water Cure Monthly*, I (1), 11-12.

Lust, B. (1900). Strawberry and purgative remedies. *The Kneipp Water Cure Monthly*, I (2), 29-30.

Lust, B. (1900). Ribwort, Plantago lanceolata. *The Kneipp Water Cure Monthly*, I (3), 44.

Lust, B. (1900). Cowslips and violets. *The Kneipp Water Cure Monthly*, I (5), 81-82.

Lust, B. (1900). The Kneipp apotheca. *The Kneipp Water Cure Monthly*, I (7), 116-118.

Lust, B. (1901). Care of the teeth. *The Kneipp Water Cure Monthly*, II (9), 224.

Lust, B. (1901). How to heal wounds quickly by natural means. *The Kneipp Water Cure Monthly*, II (11), 300.

Lust, B. (1902). Kneipp's popular healing remedies and their application. *The Naturopath and Herald of Health,* III (8), 348-349.

Lust, B. (1903). Falling out of the hair. *The Naturopath and Herald of Health,* IV (10), 301.

Lust, B. (1904). Knotgrass. *The Naturopath and Herald of Health,* V (6), 137.

Lust, B. (1905). Birch leaf tea. *The Naturopath and Herald of Health,* VI (1), 7.

Lust, B. (1905). Allopathic thinking and naturopathic thinking. *The Naturopath and Herald of Health,* VI (2), 36.

Lust, B. (1905). Kneipp's medicinal herbs. *The Naturopath and Herald of Health,* VI (4), 108-109.

Lust, B. (1905). Father Kneipp's curative herbs, angelica. *The Naturopath and Herald of Health,* VI (6), 164-165.

Lust, B. (1906). Kneipp's medical herbs, Arnica montana. *The Naturopath and Herald of Health,* VII (1), 9-10.

Lust, B. (1906). The effect of hay flowers, heublumen. *The Naturopath and Herald of Health,* VII (1), 40-41.

Lust, B. (1907). Medicinal virtues of the oak tree. *The Naturopath and Herald of Health,* VIII (3), 67.

Lust, B. (1907). Timely talks. *The Naturopath and Herald of Health,* VIII (4), 101-103.

Lust, B. (1907). Medicinal virtues of shavegrass. *The Naturopath and Herald of Health,* VIII (5), 135.

Lust, B. (1907). Medicinal virtues of the common elder. *The Naturopath and Herald of Health,* VIII (7), 199.

Lust, B. (1907). Medicinal virtues of the mint plant. *The Naturopath and Herald of Health,* VIII (8), 231.

Lust, B. (1907). Medicinal virtues of fennel. *The Naturopath and Herald of Health,* IV (9), 263.

Lust, B. (1907). Bogbean, Menyanthus trifoliate. *The Naturopath and Herald of Health,* VIII (10), 295.

Lust, B. (1908). The science of herbotherapy. *The Naturopath and Herald of Health,* IX (6), 167-173.

Lust, B. (1909). Aromatic powders. *The Naturopath and Herald of Health,* XIV (1), 33.

Lust, B. (1909). Kneipp's herbs and their uses. *The Naturopath and Herald of Health,* XIV (8), 482-486.

Lust, B. (1909). Contents of a little Kneipp home dispensary. *The Naturopath and Herald of Health,* XIV (8), 486.

Lust, B. (1910). Rosemary wine. *The Naturopath and Herald of Health,* XV (5), 291.

Lust, B. (1911). Naturopath advocate offers elder blossoms as blood purifier. *The Naturopath and Herald of Health,* XVI (7), 443.

Lust, B. (1913). Autumn's peace, autumn's bliss. *The Naturopath and Herald of Health,* XVIII (10), 645-646.

Lust, B. (1915). Honey. *The Naturopath and Herald of Health,* XX (1), 120-121.

Lust, B. (1916). Garlic juice and medicine. *Herald of Health and Naturopath,* XXI (1), 11.

Lust, B. (1918). Herbs. *Herald of Health and Naturopath,* XXIII (3), 253.

Lust, B. (1918). Aloe, angelica. *Herald of Health and Naturopath,* XXIII (4), 379.

Lust, B. (1918). Anise seed, arnica. *Herald of Health and Naturopath,* XXIII (5), 479.

Lust, B. (1918). Ash, asarum, balm mint, rhubarb, barberries. *Herald of Health and Naturopath,* XXIII (6), 577.

Lust, B. (1918). Green beanpods, mistletoe, betony, bearberry. *Herald of Health and Naturopath,* XXIII (7), 674.

Lust, B. (1918). Lavender, birch, black alder, black current, buckthorn. *Herald of Health and Naturopath,* XXIII (8), 740.

Lust, B. (1918). Blessed thistle, blueberries, briar hips, basil. *Herald of Health and Naturopath,* XXIII (9), 790.

Lust, B. (1918). Black thorn, bramble, burnet, borage. *Herald of Health and Naturopath,* XXIII (10), 842.

Lust, B. (1918). Buckbean, buckthorn, broom. *Herald of Health and Naturopath,* XXIII (11), 896.

Lust, B. (1918). Burdock, chamomile, carline thistle. *Herald of Health and Naturopath,* XXIII (12), 940.

Lust, B. (1919). Caraway, cherry, centaury, commock. *Herald of Health and Naturopath,* XXIV(1), 35.

Lust, B. (1919). Chicory, coltsfoot, chickweed. *Herald of Health and Naturopath,* XXIV (2), 92.

Lust, B. (1919). Dandelion, dwarf elder, elder. *Herald of Health and Naturopath,* XXIV (3), 144.

Lust, B. (1919). Cloves, elecampane, eyebright, eucalyptus, fern. *Herald of Health and Naturopath,* XXIV (5), 248.

Lust, B. (1919). Fenugreek, galium, fennel. *Herald of Health and Naturopath,* XXIV (6), 298.

Lust, B. (1919). Ground ivy, hearts ease, hay flowers, heather, Iceland moss, juniper. *Herald of Health and Naturopath,* XXIV (10), 513.

Lust, B. (1920). Daisy, hen's feet, hyssop, iris, knotgrass, licorice, linden flower, lungwort, liverwort, veronica, marjoram. *Herald of Health and Naturopath,* XXV (5), 249-251.

Lust, B. (1920). Mallow, marigold, althea, yarrow, milkwort, mouse ear, mustard, mullein, nettle, oak. *Herald of Health and Naturopath,* XXV (6), 297-299.

Lust, B. (1920). Nettle, oats, onion, peony, peppermint, pepperwort, periwinkle, pine, pimpernel, primrose, pumpkin seeds, ribwort, rosemary, rue. *Herald of Health and Naturopath,* XXV (7), 353-355.

Lust, B. (1920). St. John's wort, sage, sallow, sandalwood, sanicle, sarsaparilla, sassafras, scurvy grass, sea onion, shavegrass, silverweed, shepherd's purse. *Herald of Health and Naturopath,* XXV (8), 406-408.

Lust, B. (1920). Soapwort, sorrel, strawberry, sweet flag, thyme, tormentil, valerian, vervaine, violet, wallwort, walnut, wormseed. *Herald of Health and Naturopath,* XXV (9), 450-452.

Lust, B. (1920). Watermint, woodruff, watercress, wormwood, Kneipp's formulas. *Herald of Health and Naturopath*, XXV (10), 509-511.

Lust, B. (1921). Are herbs drugs? An answer. *Herald of Health and Naturopath*, XXVI (6), 291.

Lust, B. (1922). Kneipp herbs. *Herald of Health and Naturopath*, XXVII (9), 463.

Lust, B. (1922). French botanist angers doctors by competition. *Herald of Health and Naturopath*, XXVII (10), 498.

Lust, L. (1923). Herbs combined with nature cure. *Naturopath*, XXVIII (8), 370-371.

Staden, L. (1900). How nature cures. *The Kneipp Water Cure Monthly*, I (7), 126.

Waugh, W. (1910). Drugs and drugs. *The Naturopath and Herald of Health*, XV (8), 469-471.

Young, M. G. (1915). Yarrow. *The Naturopath and Herald of Health*, XX (12), 775-776.

Young, M. G. (1916). Sage. *Herald of Health and Naturopath*, XXI (1), 50.

Young, M. G. (1916). Sassafras, Laurus sassafras. *Herald of Health and Naturopath*, XXI (4), 261.

Young, M. G. (1916). Cascara sagrada. *Herald of Health and Naturopath*, XXI (5), 335-336.

Young, M. G. (1916). Impure blood. *Herald of Health and Naturopath*, XXI (6), 398-402.

Young, M. G. (1916). Dandelion. *Herald of Health and Naturopath*, XXI (7), 461-462.

Young, M. G. (1917). Mayweed. *Herald of Health and Naturopath*, XXII (2), 97.

Young, M. G. (1917). Elder. *Herald of Health and Naturopath*, XXII (3), 169-170.

General Index

Underlined herbs were considered exceptional. —Ed.

A

B

C

E

F

G

H

I

R

T

Herb Index

A

B

C

R

S

T

V

W

Y

About the Editor, NUNM, NUNM Press

Sussanna Czeranko, ND, BBE, is a 1994 graduate of CCNM (Toronto). She is a licensed ND in Oregon. In the last twenty-two years, she has developed an extensive armamentarium of traditional naturopathic therapies for her patients. Especially interested in balneotherapy, botanical medicine, breathing and nutrition, she is a frequent international presenter and workshop leader. She is a monthly Contributing Editor (Nature Cure—Past Pearls) for NDNR and a Contributing Writer for the Foundations of Naturopathic Medicine Project. Dr. Czeranko founded *The Breathing Academy* and along with Dr. Karis Tressel *The Nature-Cure Academy*, both of which provide training and practicums for Naturopathic doctors, the former in the scientific model of Buteyko breathing therapy, and the latter in traditional Naturopathic modalities. Dr. Czeranko also founded *Manitou Waters Clinic, Spa and Health Education Centre* in Saskatchewan, Canada, on the shores of a pristine, highly mineralized northern lake.

NUNM (National University of Natural Medicine, Portland, Oregon) was founded in 1956 as National College of Naturopathic Medicine (NCNM). It transitioned to university status in June 2016. NUNM is home to the longest serving, accredited clinical doctorate naturopathic program in North America and to numerous accredited graduate research programs and undergraduate programs. NUNM's program mix also includes one of the country's most unique clinical doctorates in Classical Chinese Medicine.

NUNM Press publishes distinctive titles that enrich the history, clinical practice, and contemporary significance of natural medicine traditions. The rare book collection on natural medicine at NUNM is the largest and most complete of its kind in North America and is the primary source for this landmark series—*In Their Own Words*—which brings to life and timely relevance the very best of early naturopathic literature.

The Hevert Collection: *In Their Own Words*
A Twelve-book Series

Origins of Naturopathic Medicine

Philosophy of Naturopathic Medicine

Dietetics of Naturopathic Medicine

Principles of Naturopathic Medicine

Practice of Naturopathic Medicine

Vaccination and Naturopathic Medicine

Physical Culture in Naturopathic Medicine

Herbs in Naturopathic Medicine

Mental Culture in Naturopathic Medicine

Water Cure in Naturopathic Medicine

Clinical Pearls of Naturopathic Medicine, Vol. I

Clinical Pearls of Naturopathic Medicine, Vol. II

From the NUNM Rare Book Collection On Natural Medicine.
Published By NUNM Press, Portland, Oregon.

nunm PRESS

CPSIA information can be obtained
at www.ICGtesting.com
Printed in the USA
FFOW02n0923140517
35444FF

9 781945 785078